QUANTITATIVE METHODS IN HEALTH CARE MANAGEMENT

QUANTITATIVE METHODS IN HEALTH CARE MANAGEMENT

Techniques and Applications

Second Edition

YASAR A. OZCAN

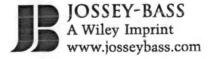

JOSSEY-BASS
A Wiley Imprint
www.josseybass.com

Published by Jossey-Bass
A Wiley Imprint
989 Market Street, San Francisco, CA 94103–1741—www.josseybass.com

Jossey-Bass books and products are available through most bookstores. To contact Jossey-Bass directly call our Customer Care Department within the U.S. at 800–956–7739, outside the U.S. at 317–572–3986, or fax 317–572–4002.

Jossey-Bass also publishes its books in a variety of electronic formats. Some content that appears in print may not be available in electronic books.

Library of Congress Cataloging-in-Publication Data

Ozcan, Yasar A.
    Quantitative methods in health care management : techniques and applications / Yasar A. Ozcan.—2nd ed.
      p. ; cm.
    Includes bibliographical references and index.
    ISBN-13: 978-0-470-43462-8

      1. Health services administration—Statistical methods. 2. Health services administration—Decision making. 3 Health services administration—Methodology. I. Title.
      [DNLM: 1. Health Services Administration. 2. Statistics as Topic. 3. Decision Making, Organizational. 4. Decision Support Techniques. 5. Models, Theoretical.
WA 950 O99q 2009]
RA394.O98 2009
362.1072'7—dc22

                                              2009001457

PB Printing   10 9 8 7 6 5 4 3 2

CONTENTS

TABLES, FIGURES, & EXHIBITS

TABLES

FIGURES

EXHIBITS

To my wife, Gulperi, and my daughters, Gunes and Nilufer

FOREWORD

I would like to congratulate Professor Yasar Ozcan on producing this excellent, comprehensive textbook, *Quantitative Methods in Health Care Management*. The field has needed such a textbook for a very long time, and Professor Ozcan is eminently qualified in bringing it to us.

The last textbook in this area was written over twenty years ago. To all of us in health services research and management, we know that health care delivery today bears little resemblance to that era. So too, the use, types, and depth of quantitative methods and techniques have progressed greatly in this time period. Professor Ozcan brings us not only the latest and best methods and techniques, but also illustrates their uses through current cases and examples.

And what I like best about this textbook is that it has been written by one of the leading and most knowledgeable health care management professors in the world. Professor Ozcan has been at the forefront in developing and applying many of the methods in the book, and as founding editor of the journal *Health Care Management Science,* he draws on the latest knowledge available from other areas.

For those of us who teach quantitative methods in health care management courses, this book will make our task far easier. More importantly, it will provide our students with a comprehensive text that they can draw on in their health care management careers. In addition, this text is a welcome, comprehensive, and up-to-date addition to the work of current managers and to all those who say, "There must be a better way to deliver health care."

Indeed there is, and the application of the methods and ideas in this book will provide many, many answers.

William P. Pierskalla, Ph.D.
Distinguished Professor and Dean Emeritus,
The Anderson School, UCLA,
and Ronald Rosenfeld Professor Emeritus,
The Wharton School, University of Pennsylvania

ACKNOWLEDGMENTS

Writing this book could not have been achieved without the help and encouragement of many individuals. I take this opportunity to thank them; if I miss anyone, it is through authorial oversight only, as all the help received was deeply appreciated. First of all, I thank my colleague Ramesh K. Shukla, who provided valuable insights and material for the productivity chapter. Many thanks go to my graduate students from the MSHA Class of 2007 and MSHA Class of 2006 who received the first draft of the manuscript and pointed out many corrections. Similarly, graduate students from the MSHA Class of 2005 lent their real-life experiences with quantitative techniques and associated materials and data, which are used in the examples and exercises throughout the text. In that vein, more specifically, I thank Adrian Amedia, Joani Brough, Mark Cotter, Sandy Chung, Suzanne Coyner, Alan Dow, and Paulomi Sanyal for their resourcefulness.

I would like to acknowledge Dorothy Silvers for her diligent editing of the manuscript from cover to cover. I extend my sincere thanks as well to Jossey-Bass/Wiley staff members Andrew Pasternack and Seth Schwartz, for their cooperativeness and help in the production of this manuscript.

No book can be written on time without the support and encouragement of loved ones. I am indebted to my wife, Gulperi Ozcan, who became my sounding board for every example in this book. Moreover, she extended her support throughout the development of the manuscript even as I deprived her of my time in favor of my desktop. I thank her for the sustained support she has given me throughout my academic career and our personal life.

Yasar A. Ozcan, Ph.D.
May 15, 2008
Richmond, Virginia

THE AUTHOR

Yasar A. Ozcan, Ph.D. is a professor in the Department of Health Administration, Virginia Commonwealth University (VCU), where he has served as a faculty member for over thirty years. Dr. Ozcan teaches quantitative health care management courses in graduate professional programs in health administration, and methodology courses at the doctoral level. He has served twice as president of the Health Applications Section in the Institute of Operations Research and Management Science. Professor Ozcan is the founding Editor in Chief of a highly regarded journal, *Health Care Management Science,* and coeditor of the *Journal of Central Asian Health Services Research.*

Dr. Ozcan has been principal and co-principal investigator on various federal and state grants and contracts. He has also provided management consultancy services to health care facilities and managed care organizations.

Dr. Ozcan's scholarly work is in the areas of systems productivity, technical efficiency, financial efficiency, and effectiveness. Specifically, he has applied data envelopment analysis to measure efficiency across the range of health care facilities and practices, including hospitals, nursing homes, health maintenance organizations, mental health care organizations, physician practices, and other facilities. He has presented numerous papers in professional meetings and published extensively in these areas.

Dr. Ozcan has long been active in distance education, having taught quantitative techniques, the content of this book, both in the traditional and on-line graduate programs at VCU since 1988.

INTRODUCTION

This book is written to meet the need for a quantitative methods curriculum in health administration or health care management programs. It is designed so that it can be used for one-semester courses in graduate programs as well as for advanced undergraduate programs in health administration. Practical and contemporary examples from the field make it a useful reference book for health care managers, as well.

The quantitative techniques offered in this book are those more amenable to the health care management environment and those most frequently used. The second edition employs the use of Excel. Although the simpler examples are demonstrated in the text, their Excel solutions are also provided. As techniques increase in sophistication, as for example in queuing models, Excel template solutions are preferred to lengthy formulas and look-up tables. The second edition also incorporates *learning objectives* at the beginning of each chapter and *key terms* at the end of each chapter to facilitate the appropriate pedagogy for learning. Because the intent of the book is to make students into able users of quantitative methods for decision making, the interpretation of the results from hand-calculated or Excel solutions to guide for informed decision making is the foremost goal. Thus, students who have had basic algebra and introductory statistics courses should be able to follow the contents of this book.

The book has fifteen chapters including the introductory chapter. The presentation of quantitative techniques starts with forecasting, which provides the data for many of the other techniques discussed, as well as for planning in health care facilities. The chapter on decision making provides the decision techniques not only for single attribute decision theory, but also for the multi-attribute methods often used in health care management decisions, especially in evaluating new contracts or in requests for proposals.

Chapters Four and Five provide techniques for facility location and layout. The techniques discussed for layout also can be used to improve flows in facilities. Hence, in Chapter Six, reengineering is introduced as the means to identify bottlenecks in operational processes and to correct them. Chapters Seven and Eight cover staffing and resource scheduling management in health care facilities; surgical suite resource management is highlighted. These two chapters can be assigned and covered together in one session. Chapter Nine, on productivity, not only presents the traditional productivity concepts and their measurements in both inpatient and outpatient settings, but also discusses more contemporary methods of productivity measurements as conducted through data envelopment analysis.

Chapter Ten explains linear programming and its use in resource allocation. Furthermore, integer programming, an extension of linear programming, is discussed and illustrated for staff scheduling. Supply chain management in health care has become popular in recent decades, and the first part of Chapter Eleven discusses that; the second part of the chapter is devoted to traditional techniques for inventory management. Quality control, essential above all in health care, is discussed in Chapter Twelve. Types of control charts and their developments are illustrated. Several approaches to quality control, including total quality management, continuous quality improvement, and six-sigma, are discussed. The tools for quality improvement are presented.

Project management is the subject of Chapter Thirteen, where program evaluation and review technique/critical path method (PERT/CPM) techniques are discussed in detail, with examples of project compression. The last two chapters cover queuing and simulation techniques with emphasis on capacity decisions using those tools. Simple queuing methods are shown with detailed examples. More sophisticated ones are illustrated by Excel solutions.

The sequence of chapters has a certain logic. For example, in Chapter Four, the location of a new facility is identified; and in Chapter Five, layout of that facility can be explored. On the other hand, Chapter Five can be also used in an independent layout analysis for existing facilities to improve flow and productivity. Similarly, Chapters Six, Seven, Eight and Nine are built to feed the knowledge onward. Chapters Fourteen and Fifteen address capacity issues using different techniques. Regardless of this sequence, however, the chapters can be selected in any order and presented to students based on the professor's preferences.

Developing exercises for the techniques explained in each chapter has been a consuming task. Any errors and oversights in that process are solely mine. I will appreciate reader comments to improve or correct the exercises, as well as suggestions for incorporating additional material in future editions.

There are on-line resources to accompany this book. On-line resources (password protected) are available to professors who adopt the book and to the students. Professors' resources include PowerPoint lectures, solutions to exercises, prototype course syllabus, Excel templates, and additional exercises with solutions. Student resources include solutions to selected exercises, Excel templates, a subset of additional exercises with solutions, and other study guide materials. These resources can be accessed via www.josseybass.com/go/ozcan2e.

CHAPTER

1

INTRODUCTION TO QUANTITATIVE DECISION-MAKING METHODS IN HEALTH CARE MANAGEMENT

LEARNING OBJECTIVES

- Recognize the quantitative techniques for decisions about delivering health care of high quality.
- Describe the historical background and the development of decision techniques.
- Describe the health care manager's role and responsibilities in decision making.
- Review the scope of health services and follow recent trends in health care.
- Describe health services management and distinct characteristics of health services.

In today's highly complicated, technological, and competitive health care arena, the public's outcry is for administrators, physicians, and other health care professionals to provide high quality care at a lower cost. Health care managers must therefore find ways to get excellent results from more limited resources. The goal of this book is to introduce aspiring health care managers to operations research models that allow decision makers to sort out complex issues and to make the best possible use of available resources. Such models are used, for example, to forecast patient demand, and to guide capital acquisition and capacity decisions, facility planning, personnel and patient scheduling, supply chain, and quality control. They use mathematical and statistical techniques: multivariate statistical analysis, decision analysis, linear programming, project evaluation and review technique (PERT), queuing analysis, and simulation, to name a few.

This book presents all these techniques from the perspective of health care organizations' delivery of care, rather than their traditional manufacturing applications. This chapter covers a brief historical background and the development of decision techniques and explains the importance of health care managers using these techniques. Finally, the scope, distinctive characteristics, and current trends of health services are emphasized. After reading this chapter, you should have a fair understanding of how important quantitative techniques are for decisions about delivering health care of high quality.

HISTORICAL BACKGROUND AND THE DEVELOPMENT OF DECISION TECHNIQUES

Beginning in the 1880s, the scientific management era brought about widespread changes in the management of the factories that had been created at an explosive rate during the Industrial Revolution. The movement was spearheaded by an efficiency engineer and inventor, Frederick Winslow Taylor, who is regarded as the father of modern scientific management. Taylor proposed a "science of management" based on observation, measurement, analysis, and improvement of work methods, along with economic incentives. He also believed that management's tasks are to plan, carefully select and train workers, find the best way to perform each job, achieve cooperation between management and workers, and separate management activities from work activities. Taylor's work was based on his idea that conflicts between labor and management occur because management has no idea how long jobs actually take. He therefore focused on time studies that evaluated work methods in great detail to identify the best way to do each job. Taylor's classic 1911 book, *The Principles of Scientific Management,* explained these guiding principles: (1) development of science for each element of work; (2) scientific selection and training of workers; (3) cooperation between management and employees; and (4) responsibility shared equally between workers and management (Taylor, 1911). Other early contributors to scientific methods of management were Frank and Gillian Gilbreth, who worked on standardization, and Henry Gantt, who emphasized the psychological effects that work conditions have on employees—he developed a time-based display chart to schedule work. Quantitative inventory management was developed by F. W. Harris in 1915. In the 1930s, W. Shewhart and associates developed statistical sampling techniques for quality control (Stevenson, 2002; p. 23). World War II prompted the growth of operations research methods, and development of project management techniques; linear programming and queuing methods followed in the 1950s. After the 1970s, the development and wider use of computers and management information systems (MIS) reshaped all these techniques because large amounts of data could be analyzed for decision making in organizations. Tools for quality improvement such as total quality management (TQM) and continuous quality improvement (CQI) became very popular in the 1980s and 1990s; then came supply chain management and productivity improvement techniques, in particular re-engineering.

THE HEALTH CARE MANAGER AND DECISION MAKING

A health care manager can be a chief executive officer (CEO) or chief operating officer (COO), or a middle-level manager to whom the duties are delegated. At the top management level, a health care manager's responsibilities include planning for capacity, location, services to be offered, and facility layout; those responsibilities are strategic. The health care manager also is ultimately responsible for overseeing service production through supply chain management, quality monitoring and improvement, and organizing health services to be either produced or outsourced. Finally, the health care manager is responsible for patient and personnel scheduling, and for optimally staffing the facility and directing job assignments and work orders. Regardless of whether health care managers are directly involved or delegate these responsibilities, their ultimate responsibility remains. Generally, operational decisions are delegated to mid- and lower-level decision makers, while strategic decisions are evaluated at the organization's top levels. With the integrated delivery systems (IDS) movement, health care organizations are becoming larger and more complex, so health care managers are in dire need of the most recent, reliable information derived from quantitative data analysis in order to make informed decisions. Information technology (IT) has become integral to management decision processes.

INFORMATION TECHNOLOGY (IT) AND HEALTH CARE MANAGEMENT

If they are to analyze their current situations and make appropriate changes to improve efficiency as well as the quality of care, health care managers need appropriate data. The data, from various sources, are collected by information technology embedded in systems either internal or external to the health care organization. For example, decisions about the location of a new health facility will require analysis of data on the communities under consideration (such as census, epidemiological data, and so on). Decisions about nurse staffing will require internal data on patient admissions and acuity that are collected routinely by the hospital. This book identifies the sources of the data for various decision-making tools and emphasizes the use of IT for informed decision making by health care managers.

THE SCOPE OF HEALTH CARE SERVICES, AND RECENT TRENDS

According to the Organization for Economic Cooperation and Development (OECD) countries, their members' total expenditures on health services constituted from 5.3 to 14.7 percent of gross domestic product (GDP) in 2002, making that a very significant sector from a public policy perspective. Moreover, the statistics in Table 1.1 show an increasing trend in health care expenditures. The countries that spent about 4.3 percent of their budgets on health care in the late-1990s are now spending 50 percent more. The United States is the country spending the highest percentage of GDP on health care. Its percentage share of GDP was stabilized from 1998 to 2000 but has been increasing again during the last few years.

Health care, especially in the United States, is a labor-intensive industry with more than fourteen million jobs, constituting 10 percent of the workforce in 2006. As shown in Table 1.2, the health care work force is expected to reach close to seventeen million in ten years. That constitutes over 21 percent growth and is the fastest job growth area, with seven out of twenty occupations in health care (U.S. Department of Labor, 2006). The aging population—as well as the proliferation of medical technology and new treatments—contributes to this growth.

The health care industry seeks to match varying medical needs in the population. Its 580,000 establishments vary in size, complexity, and organizational structure, ranging from small-town, private practice physicians with one medical assistant to urban hospitals that employ thousands of diverse health care professionals. About 1.3 percent of the health care establishments are hospitals, but they employ over 35 percent of all health care workers. While 77 percent of health care establishments are physicians, dentists, or other health practitioners, those employ 26 percent of the health care workforce (see Table 1.2).

Advances in medical technologies, new procedures and methods of diagnosis and treatment, less invasive surgical techniques, gene therapy—all these increase longevity and improve the quality of life. Similarly, advances in information technology can improve patient care. For example, handheld order entry systems such as personal digital assistants (PDAs) and bar code scanners at bedside make health workers more efficient, and also minimize errors and thus improve the quality of care.

TABLE 1.1. **Total Expenditures on Health as % GDP for 30 OECD Countries.**

	1998	1999	2000	2001	2002	2003	2004	2005
Average	7.8	7.9	7.9	8.2	8.5	8.8	8.9	9.0
Minimum	4.3	4.6	4.8	5.4	5.3	5.4	5.5	6.0
Maximum	13.1	13.1	13.2	13.9	14.7	15.2	15.2	15.3

Source: OECD Health Data 2007.

TABLE 1.2. **Distribution of Health Providers and Health Workers in Health Services: 2006, and Expected Growth.**

Provider Type	Percent of Providers	Percent of Employment	Employment (in thousands)	Percent Change, 2006–2016
Hospitals, public and private	1.3	39.9	5,438	13.0
Nursing and residential care facilities	11.5	21.3	2,901	23.7
Offices of physicians	36.7	15.8	2,154	24.8
Offices of dentists	20.7	5.8	784	22.4
Home health care services	3.3	6.4	867	55.4
Offices of other health practitioners	19.3	4.2	571	28.3
Outpatient care centers	3.4	3.6	489	24.3
Other ambulatory health care services	1.4	1.6	216	32.3
Medical and diagnostic laboratories	2.3	1.5	202	16.8

Source: U.S. Department of Labor (2006).
www.bls.gov/oco/cg/cgs035.htm#nature

These advances usually add to costs, so cost containment is a major goal in the health care industry. To accomplish it, the health care industry has shifted the care of patients from hospital care to outpatient and ambulatory care. At the same time, managed care programs have stressed preventive care to reduce the eventual costs of undiagnosed, untreated medical conditions. Enrollment has grown in prepaid managed care programs: health maintenance organizations (HMOs), preferred provider organizations (PPOs), and point-of-service (POS) programs.

The health care industry has turned to restructuring to improve financial and cost performance. Restructuring is accomplished by achieving an integrated delivery system (IDS). An IDS merges the segments of health care delivery, both vertically and horizontally, to increase efficiency by streamlining financial, managerial, and delivery functions. More hospitals expected to be part of IDS in coming years (U.S. Department of Labor, 2004).

It is fair to conclude that the changes in the health care industry will continue and will affect the delivery of health services in terms of cost and efficiency as well as the quality of care.

HEALTH CARE SERVICES MANAGEMENT

Given such complexity in both the nature and the environment of health care, managers of such establishments face challenging day-to-day decisions as well as long-term and strategic ones. Their discipline, the management and improvement of the systems and processes that provide health care, must rely on decision tools—namely, the specific methods that can help managers analyze, design, and implement organizational changes to achieve efficiency as well as high quality of care (effectiveness) for patients.

Clearly, then, management of health care establishments requires reasoned inquiry and judgment. Therefore, health care managers must use proven scientific methods drawn from such disciplines as industrial engineering, statistics, operations research, and management science. However, it must be remembered that such quantitative tools do not, alone, shape the final decision, which may have to include other, qualitative factors to arrive at the right course of action.

An increase in the number of manager positions in health care is expected during the next decade. According to the U.S. Department of Labor statistics shown in Table 1.3, the growth in health care management positions is projected to be slightly higher than that in all health care occupations. In 2006, there were 579,000 managers employed in the health care industry, a level expected to increase by 21.3 percent within ten years. More specifically, in the top and middle management levels, the three subsections shown in Table 1.3, approximately 98,000 top executives are employed, constituting approximately 0.7 percent of the health care work force.

Future health care managers, whether in top administration or in administrative or clinical operations, will be making informed decisions using state-of-the-art decision-making techniques and the latest information from management information systems. To use those techniques successfully, however, they must also understand the distinctive characteristics of health care services.

DISTINCTIVE CHARACTERISTICS OF HEALTH CARE SERVICES

Health care operations have five major distinctive characteristics: (1) patient participation in the service process; (2) simultaneity; (3) perishability; (4) intangibility; and

TABLE 1.3. **Health Services by Occupation in 2006, and Projected Growth.**

Health Services Occupation	Employment (in thousands)	Percent Change, 2006–2016
Management, business, and financial occupations	579	21.3
Top executives	98	11.6
Professional and related occupations	5,955	21.3
Service occupations	4,334	27.1
Office and administrative support occupations	2,446	14.4
All health service occupations	13,621	21.7

Source: U.S. Department of Labor (2006).
www.bls.gov/oco/cg/cgs035.htm#nature

(5) heterogeneity (Fitzsimmons and Fitzsimmons, 2004; pp. 21–25). Let us examine each of these characteristics to better understand the decision platforms in health care.

Patient Participation

In health care, as in any service industry, to evaluate performance (efficiency and effectiveness) a distinction must be made between inputs and outputs. Patients (or their health conditions) who receive care are among the inputs into the service process. On the other hand, after diagnosis and treatment, the patient's condition constitutes the effectiveness of the health care organization—that is, output. Hence, the health care organization and the patient interact throughout the delivery of care—a profound distinction of health care as compared to manufacturing industries.

Simultaneous Production and Consumption

As a service industry, health care is produced and "consumed" simultaneously. This point reflects the fact that health is not a product to be created, stored, and sold later. (Will science achieve that via gene therapy?) One of the drawbacks of that simultaneity of "production" and "consumption" is the challenge it presents for quality control—that is, ensuring the effectiveness of the service. In manufacturing, a product can be inspected and, if found defective, not be offered for sale; meanwhile the process that is producing bad outputs is corrected. However, in health care, due to simultaneity, an instance of poor quality care cannot be "recalled," even though the process resulting in poor care can be corrected for future patients.

Perishable Capacity

Health care organizations design their services to serve with certain capacity over a given time. If the designed capacity is not used during that period, the opportunity to generate revenue from that capacity is lost. For example, consider a hospital with fifteen operating rooms that are staffed and open for twelve hours. If the surgeries are not scheduled appropriately to fill the open slots, or if a large amount of time is wasted by the turnover of the cases, a portion of the available capacity, and thus of potential revenues for that day perishes. Similarly, consider a physician's office with an available ten-hour schedule for patient visits. If the office does not receive appointments to fill all those time blocks, the practice's capacity for that day will be reduced, as will the revenues.

The Intangible Nature of Health Care Outputs

The output in health care does not comprise a tangible product on hand like food bought from your favorite fast-food restaurant, where you can judge the quality of the food as much as the promptness of the service. In health care, it is not so obvious what the patient has paid for. For one thing, since a healing process takes time, the opinions of patients about the service quality of their care are formed over time. Moreover, health care is not something that can be tested or handled before deciding on it. Although health care monitoring groups, as well as health care facilities in their marketing, may provide information about the quality of an organization's services, one patient's experience may nevertheless not equal that of another receiving the same service because patients' conditions and perceptions are never identical.

The High Levels of Judgment Called Upon, and the Heterogeneous Nature of Health Care

Although some routine health care tasks can be automated (recording patient history via IT), there remain a wide range of tasks that require a high level of judgment, personal interaction, and individual adaptations, even in a given service category. For example, a surgeon and an anesthetist must make specific decisions before operating, to plan the surgery for the particular condition of patient. The heterogeneity of patients' conditions, already noted, often mandates considerable specialization in the delivery of care.

Even given these distinctive characteristics of health care, managers work together with clinicians to standardize health organizations' operations for both efficiency and effectiveness. Examples of such standardization are the diagnostic and treatment protocols developed for the care of various diseases.

SUMMARY

Contemporary health care managers must understand the distinctive characteristics of the health care services and use state-of-the-art decision-making techniques with the latest information available to plan and organize their facilities for best quality patient care. The remaining chapters of this book will discuss and show the use of state-of-the-art decision-making techniques and their applications in health care.

KEY TERMS

Health Care Manager

Decision Techniques

Health Care Providers

Perishable Capacity

CHAPTER

2

FORECASTING

LEARNING OBJECTIVES

- Describe the need for forecasting in health care operations.
- Review the various approaches to forecasting.
- Differentiate the data driven and opinion- or judgment-based forecasts.
- Recognize what type of forecasting approach should be taken for various health care forecasting situations.
- Develop accuracy checks and controls for forecasts.
- Analyze and use forecast information in operations or in strategic decisions.

Every day, health care managers must make decisions about service delivery without knowing what will happen in the future. Forecasts enable them to anticipate the future and plan accordingly. Good forecasts are the basis for short-, medium-, and long-term planning and are essential input to all types of service production systems. Forecasts have two primary uses: to help managers plan the system and also to help them plan the use of the system. Planning the system itself is long-range planning: about the kinds of services supplied and the number of each to offer, what facilities and equipment to have, which location optimizes service delivery to the particular patient population, and so on. Planning the use of the system is short-range and medium-range planning for supplies and workforce levels, purchasing and production, budgeting, and scheduling.

All of the previous plans rely on forecasts. Forecasting is not an exact science, however; its results are rarely perfect, and the actual results usually differ. For the best possible forecasts, a health care manager must blend experience and good judgment with technical expertise.

All forecasts have certain common elements regardless of the technique used. The underlying assumption is that past events will continue. It also is a given that errors will occur because of the presence of randomness and that actual results are more than likely to be different from those predicted. Forecasts of a group of items (aggregate forecasts) tend to be more accurate than those for individual items. For example, forecasts made for a whole hospital would tend to be more accurate than a departmental forecast because forecasting errors among a group tend to cancel each other. Finally, it is generally accepted that forecast accuracy decreases as the time horizon (the period covered) increases. Short-range forecasts face fewer uncertainties than longer-range forecasts do, so they tend to be more accurate. A flexible health care organization, which responds quickly to changes in demand, makes use of a shorter, more accurate forecasting horizon than do less flexible competitors, who must use longer forecast horizons.

STEPS IN THE FORECASTING PROCESS

Many forecasting methods are available to health care managers for planning, to estimate future demand or any other issues at hand. However, for any type of forecast to bring about later success, it must follow a step-by-step process composed of five major steps: (1) goal of the forecast and the identification of resources for conducting it; (2) time horizon; (3) selection of a forecasting technique; (4) conducting and completing the forecast; and (5) monitoring the accuracy of the forecast.

Identify the Goal of the Forecast

This indicates the urgency with which the forecast is needed and identifies the amount of resources that can be justified and the level of accuracy necessary.

Establish a Time Horizon

Decide on the period to be covered by the forecast, keeping in mind that accuracy decreases as the time horizon increases.

Select a Forecasting Technique

The selection of a forecasting model will depend on the computer and financial resources available in an organization, as well as on the complexity of the problem under investigation.

Conduct the Forecast

Use the appropriate data and make appropriate assumptions with the best possible forecasting model. Health care managers often have to make assumptions based on experience with a given situation, and sometimes by trial and error. In forecasting, analyzing appropriate data refers to: (a) the availability of relevant historical data, and (b) recognizing the variability in a given data set.

Monitor Accuracy

Since there is an arsenal of techniques available, appropriate for different situations and data representations, health care managers must examine their data and circumstances carefully to select the appropriate forecasting approach. Be prepared to use another technique if the one in use is not providing acceptable results. Health care managers must also be alert to how frequently the forecast should be updated, especially when trends or data change dramatically.

FORECASTING APPROACHES

In its simplest forms, forecasting includes judgments, whether individual or juries of opinions. Although this is not a sophisticated mathematical model, a brief explanation of such approaches is prudent.

Judgmental Forecasts

Judgmental forecasts rely on analysis of such subjective inputs as executive opinions, contracts, insurance, HMO, PPO, or POS company estimates, consumer surveys, mental estimates of the market, intuition, outside (consultant) opinions, and the opinions of managers and staff. A health care manager may use staff to generate a judgmental forecast or several forecasts from which to choose. Examples of judgmental forecasting include the Delphi method, jury of executive opinion, and naïve extrapolation.

The Delphi method, which obtains the opinions of managers and staff who have relevant knowledge, is frequently used. A series of questionnaires is circulated to a group of experts, with each successive questionnaire developed from the previous one, in order to achieve a consensus on a question, for example, the potential of a new high-technology health service. The Delphi method is useful for forecasting technological changes and their impacts; often the goal is to predict when a certain event will occur. Use of the Delphi method has certain advantages. It saves costs to use questionnaires rather than an assembly of many experts. Furthermore, the isolation of each participant helps to eliminate a "bandwagon effect," and since the anonymity of each participant is preserved, honest responses are likely. The Delphi is not without weaknesses, however; ambiguous questions may lead to a false consensus, anonymity may diminish the sense of accountability and responsibility by the respondents, and panel members may change if the process takes a long time (for example, one year or more) to complete. Finally, studies have not proved or disproved the accuracy of Delphi forecasts.

The jury of executive opinion model uses the consensus of a group of experts, often from several functional areas within a health care organization, to develop a forecast. It differs from the Delphi method in its reach, scope, and time horizons: opinions are sought from health care organization's members rather than from an external source, and the forecast may take much less time. The participants are far more likely to interact with each other under the jury of executive opinion model.

A naïve extrapolation involves making a simple assumption about the economic outcome of the next period, or a subjective extrapolation from the results of current events.

At the other end of the forecasting spectrum are mathematical and statistical techniques using historical data, called time series.

Time-Series Approach

A time series is a sequence of evenly spaced observations taken at regular intervals over a period of time (such as daily, hourly, weekly, monthly, or yearly). An example of a time series is the monthly admissions to a multisystem hospital. Forecasts from time-series data assume that future values of the series can be predicted from past values. Analysis of a time series can identify the behavior of the series in terms of trend, seasonality, cycles, irregular variations, or random variations. A trend is a gradual, long-term, upward or downward movement in data. Seasonality refers to short-term, relatively frequent variations generally related to factors such as weather, holidays, and vacations; health care facilities often experience weekly and even daily "seasonal" variations.

Cycles are patterns in the data that occur every several years, often in relation to current economic conditions. Such cycles often exhibit wavelike characteristics that mimic the business cycle. Irregular variations are "spikes" in the data caused by chance or unusual circumstances (examples: severe weather, labor strike, use of a new high-technology health service); they do not reflect typical behavior and should be identified and removed from the data whenever possible. Random variations are residual variations that remain after all other behaviors have been accounted for. Graphing the data provides clues to a health care manager for selecting the right forecasting method. Figures 2.1 through 2.3 illustrate these common variations in data.

Techniques for Averaging

Historical data usually contain a certain amount of noise (random variation) that tends to obscure patterns in the data. Randomness arises from a multitude of relatively unimportant factors that cannot possibly be predicted with any certainty. The optimal situation would be to completely remove randomness from the data and leave only "real" variations (for example, changes in the level of patient demand). Unfortunately, it is usually impossible to distinguish between these two kinds of variations. The best one can hope for is that the small variations are random and the large variations actually mean something. Averaging techniques smooth out some of the fluctuations in a data set; individual highs and lows are "averaged" out. A forecast based on an average shows less variability than the original data set does. The result of using averaging techniques is that minor variations are treated as random variations and essentially "smoothed" out of the data set. Although the larger variations, those deemed likely to reflect "real" changes, are also smoothed, it is to a lesser degree. Three techniques for averaging are described in this section: naïve forecasts, moving averages, and exponential smoothing.

Naïve Forecasts The simplest forecasting technique is termed the naïve method. A naïve forecast for any period simply projects the previous period's actual value. For example, if demand for a particular health service was 100 units last week, the naïve

FIGURE 2.1. *Seasonal Variation Characteristics.*

FIGURE 2.2. *Cycle Variation.*

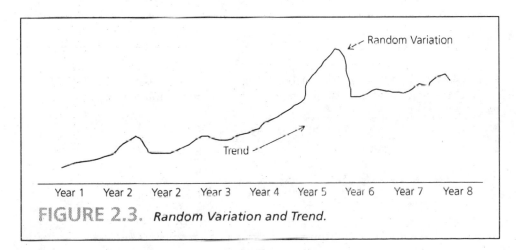

FIGURE 2.3. *Random Variation and Trend.*

forecast for the upcoming week is 100 units. If demand in the upcoming week turns out to be 75 units, then the forecast for the following week would be 75 units. The naïve forecast can also be applied to a data set that exhibits seasonality or a trend. For example, if the seasonal demand in October is 100 units, then the naïve forecast for *next October* would equal the actual demand for *October of this year.*

Although this technique may seem too simplistic, its advantages are low cost, ease of preparation, and comprehension. Its major weakness, of course, is its inability to make highly accurate forecasts. Another weakness is that it simply replicates the actual data, with a lag of one period; it does not smooth the data. However, the decision to use naïve forecasts certainly has merit if the results experienced are relatively close to the forecast (if the resulting accuracy is deemed acceptable). The accuracy of a naïve forecast can serve as a standard against which to judge the cost and accuracy of other techniques; the health care manager can decide whether or not the increase in accuracy of another method is worth its additional cost.

Moving Averages (MA) While a naïve forecast uses data from the previous period, a moving average forecast uses a number of the most recent actual data values. The moving average forecast is found by using the following equation:

$$F_t = MA_n = \frac{\sum A_i}{n} \tag{2.1}$$

where

F_t = forecast for time period t
MA_n = moving average with n periods
A_i = actual value with age i
i = "age" of the data ($i = 1, 2, 3...$)
n = number of periods in moving average

EXAMPLE 2.1

An OB/GYN clinic has the following yearly patient visits and would like to predict the volume of business for the next year for budgeting purposes.

Period(t)	Age	Visits
1	5	15,908
2	4	15,504
3	3	14,272
4	2	13,174
5	1	10,022

Solution

Using formula [2.1], the three-period moving average (MA_3) for period 6 is

$$F_6 = MA_3 = (14{,}272 + 13{,}174 + 10{,}022) \div 3 = 12{,}489$$

With the available data, a health care manager can back forecast earlier periods; this is a useful tool for assessing accuracy of a forecast, as will be explained later. Computation of three-period moving averages for the OB/GYN visits then would look like this (Figure 2.4):

Period(t)	Age	Visits	Forecast
1	5	15,908	
2	4	15,504	
3	3	14,272	
4	2	13,174	15,228
5	1	10,022	14,317
6			12,489

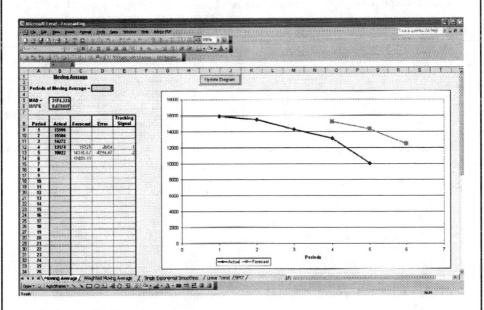

FIGURE 2.4. *Excel Template Solution: Moving Average (MA_3) for OB/GYN Clinic.*

Source: Excel template screen shots reprinted by permission from Microsoft Corporation.

This technique derives its name from the fact that as each new actual value becomes available, the forecast is updated by adding the newest value and dropping the oldest and then recalculating the average. Thus, the forecast "moves" by reflecting only the most recent values. For instance, to calculate the forecasted value of 15,228 for period 4 (F_4), the visits from periods 1 through 3 were averaged; to calculate F_5, visits from period 1 were dropped, but visits from period 4 were added to the average.

A health care manager can incorporate as many data points as desired in the moving average. The number of data points used determines the sensitivity of the forecasted average to the new values being added. The fewer the data points in an average, the more responsive the average tends to be. If a manager seeks responsiveness from the forecast, only a few data points should be used. It is important to point out, however, that a highly sensitive forecast will also be more responsive to random variations (less smooth). On the other hand, moving averages based on many data points will be smoother, but less responsive to "real" changes. The decision maker must consider the cost of responding more slowly to changes in the data against the cost of responding to what may be simply random variations.

Excel template evaluation for this problem is shown in Figure 2.4, with the example set up for three-period moving averages. Actual data and the MA_3 forecast for years 4 through 6 (as shown 3-MA) can be observed in columns B and C, respectively. (The information in the other columns and rows will be discussed later in the chapter.) In addition to tabular forecasting results, the graph in Figure 2.4 provides pictorial information on the forecast.

Determining a Reasonable Number of Periods for the Moving Average The health care manager faces the problem of selecting an appropriate number of periods for the moving average forecast. Of course, the decision depends upon the number of periods available and also on the behavior of the data that would yield the best forecast for a given situation. In general, the more periods in a moving average, the less responsive the forecast will be to changes in the data, creating a lag response. To illustrate this, an example with twenty-eight periods of historical data is described in Example 2.2, following.

EXAMPLE 2.2

A pediatric clinic manager would like to find the best moving average forecast for the next month's visits. The past data contain the last twenty-eight months.

Solution

The solution to this problem requires calculation of moving averages for various periods (for instance: MA_3 through MA_7). Two approaches can be used to identify the best MA period: (1) graph, and (2) minimum forecasting errors.

For the graph, the results of each MA_n would be graphed, and then the moving average forecast that fits or represents the original data best would be selected. The second method, which will be discussed later in the chapter, would evaluate the actual versus the forecast (errors); at this point it suffices to show how responsive the various MA_n forecasts are to the actual data.

Weighted Moving Average (WMA). Moving average forecasts are easy to compute and understand; however, all the values are weighted equally. For example, in an eight-year moving average, each value is given a weight of one-eighth. Should data that are ten years old have equal weight (importance) with data collected last year? It certainly depends on the situation that a health care manager faces, but he or she could choose to compute a weighted average to assign more weight to recent values. A weighted average is similar to a moving average, except that it assigns more weight to the most recent values in a time series. For example, the most recent data might be given a weight of 0.5, the next most recent value a weight of 0.3, and 0.2 for the next. These values are totally subjective (based on the manager's previous experiences with the data in question), with the only requirements being that the weights sum to 1.00, and that the heaviest weights are assigned to the most recent values. Trial and error is used to find an acceptable weighting pattern. The advantage of a weighted average over a simple moving average is that the weighted average is more reflective of the most recent actual results. Formally, weighted moving average is expressed as:

$$F_t = MA_n = \sum w_i A_i \qquad (2.2)$$

EXAMPLE 2.3

Continuing with Example 2.1, because there is a downward trend in visits and in period 5 there is a sharp decline, a weight of 0.5 or even higher is justified by the health care manager to calculate a weighted average for period 6.

Solution

In this analysis, a weighted average, using formula [2.2], for the OB/GYN clinic for period 6 would be:

$$F_6 = 14{,}272 \times 0.2 + 13{,}174 \times 0.3 + 10{,}022 \times 0.5 = 11{,}818.$$

Period(t)	Age	Visits	Weights	Forecast
1	5	15,908		
2	4	15,504		
3	3	14,272	0.2	
4	2	13,174	0.3	
5	1	10,022	0.5	
6				11,818

Excel template evaluation for this problem is shown in Figure 2.5, with the problem set up for three-period moving averages and the associated weights.

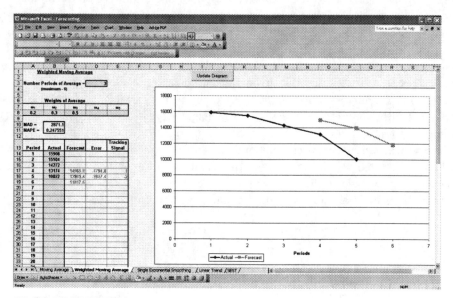

FIGURE 2.5. *Excel Template Solution: Weighted Moving Average (WMA₃) for OB/GYN Clinic.*

Source: Excel screen shots reprinted by permission from Microsoft Corporation.

Single Exponential Smoothing (SES). In a single exponential smoothing forecast, each new forecast is based on the previous forecast plus a percentage of the difference between that forecast and the actual value of the series at that point, expressed as:

New forecast = Old forecast + α(Actual value − Old forecast)

where α is the smoothing constant, expressed as a percentage. Formally, the exponential smoothing equation can be written as:

$$F_t = F_{t-1} + \alpha(A_{t-1} - F_{t-1}) \tag{2.3}$$

where

F_t = forecast for period t
F_{t-1} = forecast for period t–1
α = smoothing constant
A_{t-1} = actual value (that is, patient visits) in period t–1.

EXAMPLE 2.4

Using the data from Example 2.1, build forecasts with smoothing constant $\alpha = 0.3$.

Solution

Following the previous example and formula [2.3], we can build forecasts for periods as data become available (see Figure 2.6 for an example). After period 1 the health care manager would have the number of actual visits, which is recorded as 15,908, and with this information the best one can do for the second period is a naïve forecast. Hence, 15,908 becomes the forecast for period 2. When period 2 data become available, the data will be recorded as actual—in this case, 15,504. Now to forecast period 3, with $\alpha = 0.3$, the new forecast would be computed as follows:

$$F_3 = 15,908 + 0.3(15,504 - 15,908) = 15,786.8.$$

Then, for period 3, if the actual visits turn out to be 14,272, the next forecast would be:

$$F_4 = 15,786.8 + 0.3(14,272 - 15,786.8) = 15,332.4.$$

Similarly, F_5 and F_6 can be calculated as:

$$F_5 = 15,332.4 + 0.3(13,174 - 15,332.4) = 14,684.9$$
$$F_6 = 14,684.9 + 0.3(10,022 - 14,684.9) = 13,286.0$$

| | Smoothing constant $\alpha = 0.3$ | | Error |
Period(t)	Actual (Visits)	Forecast	(Actual – Forecast)
1	15,908	—	
2	15,504	15,908	−404.0
3	14,272	15,786.8	−1,514.8
4	13,174	15,332.4	−2,158.4
5	10,022	14,684.9	−4,662.9
6		13,268.0	

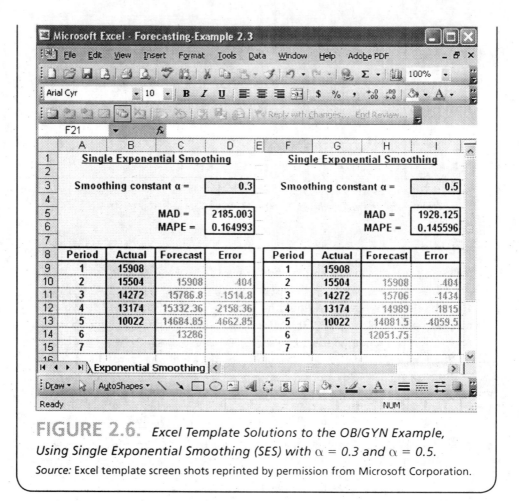

FIGURE 2.6. *Excel Template Solutions to the OB/GYN Example, Using Single Exponential Smoothing (SES) with* $\alpha = 0.3$ *and* $\alpha = 0.5$.

Source: Excel template screen shots reprinted by permission from Microsoft Corporation.

The smoothing constant α represents a percentage of the forecast error. Each new forecast is equal to the previous forecast plus a percentage of the previous error.

The closer the smoothing constant (α) is to one, the faster the forecast is to adjust using forecast errors (the greater the smoothing). Commonly used values for α range from 0.1 to 0.6 and are usually selected by judgment or trial and error. To illustrate the effect of the higher α values, the same example is shown with $\alpha = 0.5$ in Example 2.5.

Techniques for Trend

A trend is a gradual, long-term movement caused by changes in population, income, or culture. Assuming that there is a trend present in a data set, it can be analyzed by finding an equation that correlates to the trend in question. The trend may or may not

EXAMPLE 2.5

Using the data from Example 2.1, build forecasts with smoothing constant $\alpha = 0.5$.

Solution

		Smoothing constant $\alpha = 0.5$		Error
Period(t)	Visits	Forecast		(Actual – Forecast)
1	15,908	—		
2	15,504	15,908		−404.0
3	14,272	15,706.0		−1,434.0
4	13,174	14,989.0		−1,815.0
5	10,022	14,081.5		−4,059.5
6		12,051.8		

be linear in its behavior. Plotting the data can give a health care manager insight into whether a trend is linear or nonlinear.

As can be easily noticed, F_6 with $\alpha = 0.5$, with value of 12,051.8, is much less than the previous F_6, with value of 13,286, where α was 0.3. That demonstrates the faster adjustment with respect to the emphasis given recent data.

The smoothing constant value at the lower extreme $\alpha = 0.0$, does not account for errors in predictions and places heavy emphasis on the aged data from old periods (no adjustment to the latest forecast), while at the other extreme, $\alpha = 1.0$, it puts emphasis on the most recent data (greatest adjustment to the latest forecast), thus basically providing a naïve forecast, as shown in Example 2.6 below.

Forecasting Techniques Based on Linear Regression By minimizing the sum of the squared errors, which is called the least squares method, regression analysis can be used to create a representative line that has the form:

$$Y = a + bx \tag{2.4}$$

where
  y = the predicted (dependent) variable
  x = the predictor (independent) variable
  b = the slope (rise/run) of the data line
  a = the value of y when x is equal to zero.

Consider the regression equation example $y = 20 + 5x$. The value of y when $x = 0$ is 20 and the slope of the line is 5. Therefore, the value of y will increase by five

EXAMPLE 2.6

Using the data from Example 2.1, build forecasts with smoothing constants $\alpha = 0.0$ and $\alpha = 1.0$. (See Figure 2.7.)

Solution

Period (t)	$\alpha = 0.0$		Error	$\alpha = 1.0$		Error
	Visits	Forecast	(Actual – Forecast)	Visits	Forecast	(Actual – Forecast)
1	15,908	—		15,908	—	
2	15,504	15,908	–404.0	15,504	15,908	–404.0
3	14,272	15,908.0	–1,636.0	14,272	15,504.0	–1,232.0
4	13,174	15,908.0	–2,734.0	13,174	14,272.0	–1,098.0
5	10,022	15,908.0	–886.0	10,022	13,174.0	–3,152.0
6		15,908.0			10,022.0	

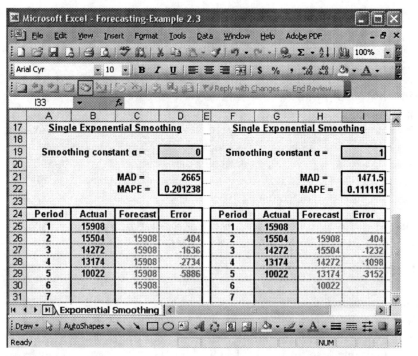

FIGURE 2.7. *Excel Template Solutions to the OB/GYN Example, Using Single Exponential Smoothing (SES) with $\alpha = 0.0$ and $\alpha = 1.0$.*

Source: Excel template screen shots reprinted by permission from Microsoft Corporation.

units for each one-unit increase in x. If $x = 15$, the forecast (y) will be $20 + 5(15)$, or 95 units. This equation could be plotted on a graph by finding two points on the line. One of those points can be found in the way just mentioned, putting in a value for x. The other point on the graph would be a (that is, y_x at $x = 0$). The coefficients of the line, a and b, can be found (using historical data) with the following equations:

$$b = \frac{n\left(\sum xy\right) - \left(\sum x\right)\left(\sum y\right)}{n\left(\sum x^2\right) - \left(\sum x\right)^2} \tag{2.5}$$

$$a = \frac{\sum y - b \sum x}{n} \tag{2.6}$$

The graph in Figure 2.8 illustrates the regression line concept, showing the errors that are minimized by the least square method by positioning the regression line using the appropriate slope (b) and y-intercept (a).

Example 2.7 illustrates the linear regression forecast.

FIGURE 2.8. Linear Regression.

EXAMPLE 2.7

A multihospital system (MHS) owns twelve hospitals. Revenues (x, or the independent variable) and profits (y, or the dependent variable) for each hospital are given following. Obtain a regression line for the data and predict profits for a hospital with $10 million in revenues. All figures are in millions of dollars.

| Multihospital System Revenues and Profits Data | | | | |
Hospital	Revenue (x)	Profit (y)	xy	x^2
1	7	0.15	1.05	49
2	2	0.10	0.2	4
3	6	0.13	0.78	36
4	4	0.15	0.6	16
5	14	0.25	3.5	196
6	15	0.27	4.05	225
7	16	0.24	3.84	256
8	12	0.20	2.4	144
9	14	0.27	3.78	196
10	20	0.44	8.8	400
11	15	0.34	5.1	225
12	7	0.17	1.19	49
Total	132	2.71	35.29	1,796

Solution

After calculating $\Sigma x, \Sigma y, \Sigma xy, \Sigma x^2$, substitute into the Equations [2.5] for a and [2.6] for b, respectively.

$$b = \frac{n\left(\sum xy\right) - \left(\sum x\right)\left(\sum y\right)}{n\left(\sum x^2\right) - \left(\sum x\right)^2} = \frac{12(35.29) - 132(2.71)}{12(1796) - 132(132)} = 0.01593.$$

$$a = \frac{\sum y - b\sum x}{n} = \frac{2.71 - 0.01593(132)}{12} = 0.0506.$$

Hence, the regression line is:

$$y_x = 0.0506 + 0.01593x.$$

To predict the profits for a hospital with $10 million in revenue, simply plug 10 in as the value of x in the regression equation:

$$\text{Profit} = 0.0506 + 0.01593(10) = .209903$$

Multiplying this value by one million, the profit level with $10 million in revenue is found to be $209,903.

We can observe the same solution from Excel as shown in Figures 2.9 and 2.10. After data entry (Figure 2.9A), by clicking on "Tools" the user can chose "Data Analysis" then "Regression" from the pop-up menu, which is shown on the overlay. In the next step, the user identifies Y and X ranges as well as output range on a pop-up menu, shown in Figure 2.9B.

FIGURE 2.9A

FIGURE 2.9B. *Excel Setup – Linear Regression for the Multihospital System Example.*

Source: Excel screen shots reprinted by permission from Microsoft Corporation.

Clicking OK will result in regression output as shown in Figure 2.9, where reader can verify *y*-intercept (0.0506) and slope (0.01593) values. Placing these values into the equation shown earlier will yield:

$$\text{Profit} = 0.0506 + 0.01593(10) = .209903.$$

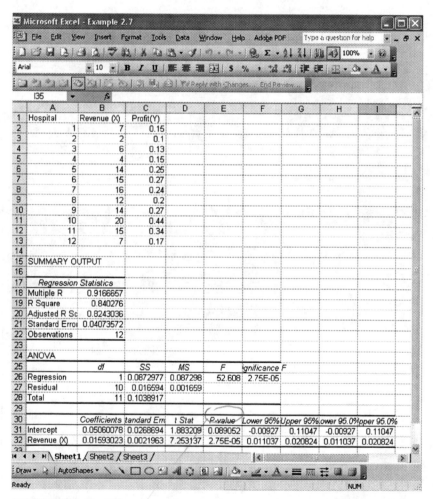

FIGURE 2.10. *Excel Solution to the Multihospital System Example.*

Source: Excel screen shots reprinted by permission from Microsoft Corporation.

Shows revenue is highly correlated to profit since p-value is so small

Linear Regression as a Trend Line Linear regression often is used to describe trends in health care data. The only difference in this application is that the independent variable *x* takes a value in time and is shown as *t*, and the equation is represented as:

$$y = a + bt \qquad (2.7)$$

where

 y = the predicted (dependent) variable
 t = the predictor time variable
 b — the slope of the data line
 a = value of *y* when *t* = 0

Graphic illustration of a negative trend line (when *b* < 0) is shown in Figure 2.11. If the trend were positive (*b* > 0), it would have looked like that in Figure 2.8.

FIGURE 2.11. *Linear Regression as a Trend.*

EXAMPLE 2.8

Referring back to the OB/GYN example, the health care manager can estimate the trend line by using regression analysis.

Solution

Figures 2.12 and 2.13 show the visit data and the regression analysis conducted through Excel as well as Excel template. The health care manager can observe that the strong R^2, coefficient of determination, value coupled with significant *F* statistics ($p < 0.015$) provides good predictor confidence for this model. The *y*-intercept (*a*) is at 18,006.6, and the slope of line is declining at a yearly rate of 1,410.2 visits (negative value). With this model the health care manager predicts that visits will be at 9,545 (Visits = 18,006.6 + 0.015(6) = 9545) in the next period, which is closer to reality than are the results from the other methods predicted so far.

Graphical illustration of the results is shown in Figures 2.12 and 2.13, where both actual and predicted values can be observed. This graph in Figure 2.12 can be generated by checking the "Line Fit Plots" option on "Regression" pop-up menu.

FIGURE 2.12. *Excel Linear Trend Graphic Solution to the OB/GYN Example.*

Source: Excel screen shots reprinted by permission from Microsoft Corporation.

FIGURE 2.13. *Excel Template Solution to the OB/GYN Example.*

Source: Excel screen shots reprinted by permission from Microsoft Corporation.

Trend-Adjusted Exponential Smoothing A variation of simple exponential smoothing can be used when a time series exhibits a trend. This method is called trend-adjusted exponential smoothing, to differentiate it from simple exponential smoothing. If a data set exhibits a trend, simple smoothing forecasts will reflect it accurately. For example, if the data are increasing, each forecast will be too low. Decreasing data will result in trends that are too high. If the health care manager detects a trend in the data after plotting it on a graph, trend-adjusted smoothing would be preferable to simple smoothing.

A single exponential smoothing with trend (SEST) forecast has two components: smoothed forecast (SF) and trend (T). Thus, the formula for SEST for the next period, $t + 1$, can be written as:

$$SEST_t = SF_{t-1} + T_{t-1} \qquad (2.8)$$

where

$$SF_{t-1} = F_{t-1} + \alpha\,(A_{t-1} - F_{t-1}) \qquad (2.9)$$

previous period's forecast + smoothed error, and

$$T_t = T_{t-1} + \beta\,(F_t - F_{t-1} - T_{t-1}) \qquad (2.10)$$

previous period's trend + smoothed error on trend.

In order to use this set of formulas, the health care manager must decide on the values of smoothing constants of α, β—each would take values between 0 and 1—with the initial forecast and obtain an estimate of trend. The values of smoothing constants can be determined with experimentation. However, a health care manager who experiences relatively stable visits (demand) would want to lessen random and short-term effects by using a smaller α; but if visits (demands) are rapidly changing, then larger α values would be more appropriate to capture and follow those changes. Using small versus larger β values to incorporate the effect of a trend follows the same logic. In the absence of a known trend, the health care manager can compute this from available historical data. The SEST model is illustrated in Example 2.9.

EXAMPLE 2.9

Historical data on receipts for a physician office for health insurance billings of the previous 15 months are as follows:

T	Receipts
1	13,125
2	13,029
3	14,925
4	10,735

5	11,066
6	11,915
7	15,135
8	13,484
9	14,253
10	11,883
11	12,077
12	12,857
13	12,162
14	11,600
15	11,480

Using smoothing constant values for $\alpha = 0.4$ and $\beta = 0.3$, construct an appropriate SEST model to predict billings for period 16.

Solution

We will use the first half of the data to develop the model ($t = 1$ through 7), and the second half ($t = 8$ through 14) to test the model. Then we will attempt to predict next period ($t = 16$). Two of the unknowns in the model are the trend estimate and the starting forecast. The trend estimate (T_0) can be calculated by averaging the difference between periods $t = 1$ through 7, using $T_0 = (A_1 - A_n)/(n - 1)$—or for our example, $T_0 = \dfrac{13,125 - 15,135}{7 - 1} = -\dfrac{2,010}{6} = -335$ (a downward trend). The starting forecast (SF_0) for the model test period is the naïve forecast using the seventh period plus the trend estimate (T_0). Hence, the eighth period can be written as:

$$F_8 = SF_0 + T_0, \text{ or}$$
$$F_8 = 15,135 - 335.5 = 14,800.$$

Calculation of SF_8 and T_8 using smoothing constant values for $\alpha = 0.4$ and $\beta = 0.3$, the ensuing forecast values for model testing during periods of 8 through 15 using formulas: [2.8], [2.9], and [2.10]; and the final forecast for period 16 are shown below. An Excel template solution is shown in Figure 2.14.

t	A_t	F_t	$SF_t = F_t + \alpha (A_t - F_t)$ $\alpha = 0.4$	$T_t = T_{t-1} + \beta (F_t - F_{t-1} - T_{t-1})$ $\beta = 0.3$
8	13,484	14,800.00	14,273.60	−335.00
9	14,253	13,938.60	14,064.36	−492.92
10	11,883	13,571.44	12,896.06	−455.19

11	12,077	12,440.87	12,295.32	−657.80
12	12,857	11,637.52	12,125.31	−701.47
13	12,162	11,423.84	11,719.10	−555.13
14	11,600	11,163.97	11,338.38	−466.55
15	11,480	10,871.83	11,115.10	−414.23
16		10,700.87		

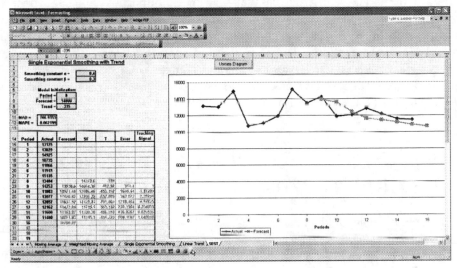

FIGURE 2.14. *Excel Template – SEST Solution to Example 2.9.*

Source: Excel screen shots reprinted by permission from Microsoft Corporation.

Techniques for Seasonality

Knowledge of seasonal variations is an important factor in demand planning and scheduling. Seasonality is also useful in planning capacity for systems that must be designed to handle peak loads. **Seasonal variations** in a data set consistently repeat upward or downward movements of the data values that can be traced to recurrent events. The term can also mean daily, weekly, monthly, or other regularly recurring patterns in data. Seasonality in a data set is expressed in terms of the amount that actual values deviate from the average value of a series. Seasonality is expressed in two models: additive and multiplicative. In the **additive** model, seasonality is expressed as a quantity (example: 5 units), which is added or subtracted from the series average in order to incorporate seasonality. In the **multiplicative** model, seasonality is expressed as a percentage of the average amount (example: 1.15), which is then multiplied by the value of a series to incorporate seasonality. The multiplicative model is used much more often than the additive model.

The seasonal percentages in the multiplicative model are referred to as seasonal indexes. Suppose that the seasonal index for the number of heart bypass surgeries at a hospital in October is 1.12. This indicates that bypass surgeries for that month are 12 percent above the monthly average. A seasonal index of 0.88 indicates that surgeries in a given month are at 88 percent of the monthly average.

If time series data contain trend and seasonality, the health care manager can remove (decompose) the seasonality by using seasonal indexes to discern a clearer picture of the trend. Removing seasonality in the multiplicative model is done by dividing each data point by its seasonal index (relative). Calculation of a seasonal index depends upon the period being considered which identifies the index (such as: quarterly indexes, monthly indexes, or daily indexes). In each case, the health care manager must collect enough seasonal data to calculate averages for the season, and then divide that by the overall average to find the seasonal index or relative. In Example 2.10, the indexes for various seasonal values are illustrated.

EXAMPLE 2.10

To prepare plans and budgets, "HEAL-ME" Hospital management wants to forecast the inpatient demand for the coming year. But, they would like to know what kind of seasonal variations are exhibited in the data shown in Table 2.1, which depict the average daily patient count for the past 28 months (from July, Year 1 to October, Year 3).

Solution

Quarterly Indexes Technique. The data in Table 2.1 can be reorganized in quarters by combining averages for the values January–March (Q1), April–June (Q2) July–September (Q3), and October–December (Q4), as shown in Table 2.2. As can be observed, two values of Q1, Q2, and Q4 are averaged over Years 2 and 3; Q3 had three values in its average. Then quarterly averages are divided by the overall average (529), yielding the quarterly index. Here, the index values do not differ much from each other, so for these data seasonal adjustment on a quarterly basis is not justified.

Monthly Indexes Technique. In the absence of quarterly variation, a health care manager may want to investigate monthly variation in the historical data. The data are organized in similar manner in Table 2.3, where index values exhibit more variation than the quarterly indexes showed in Table 2.2. The health care manager now can divide each of the monthly values by monthly indexes to discern the trend in the data.

TABLE 2.1. Heal-Me Hospital Average Daily Patient Days.

	MONTHS	Saturday	Sunday	Monday	Tuesday	Wednesday	Thursday	Friday	Average per Day
1	JULY	493	478	500	506	520	534	517	507
2	AUGUST	489	471	507	542	542	542	521	521
3	SEPTEMBER	499	480	499	526	536	550	543	519
4	OCTOBER	502	480	501	533	547	550	527	520
5	NOVEMBER	478	468	496	530	535	530	519	508
6	DECEMBER	503	484	499	523	533	537	533	516
7	JANUARY	532	530	535	550	558	567	557	547
8	FEBRUARY	514	491	514	537	541	552	554	529
9	MARCH	483	461	484	507	525	528	512	500
10	APRIL	500	475	493	524	537	540	536	515
11	MAY	483	459	470	508	519	525	529	499
12	JUNE	491	479	499	526	529	535	511	510
13	JULY	487	470	504	533	541	528	528	513
14	AUGUST	502	476	503	534	540	545	554	522

(continued)

TABLE 2.1. *(Continued)*

	MONTHS	Saturday	Sunday	Monday	Tuesday	Wednesday	Thursday	Friday	Average per Day
15	SEPTEMBER	540	509	527	545	566	573	555	545
16	OCTOBER	537	516	546	573	587	587	595	563
17	NOVEMBER	508	503	532	557	555	546	537	534
18	DECEMBER	509	480	505	517	523	535	529	514
19	JANUARY	528	517	538	565	558	568	576	550
20	FEBRUARY	541	516	539	558	575	575	574	554
21	MARCH	537	522	549	572	576	584	566	558
22	APRIL	530	510	529	550	564	572	567	546
23	MAY	512	487	504	531	538	552	558	526
24	JUNE	530	510	532	563	582	584	556	551
25	JULY	503	489	516	559	564	558	549	534
26	AUGUST	514	496	528	560	567	562	539	538
27	SEPTEMBER	532	512	514	548	563	564	554	541
28	OCTOBER	516	490	514	556	574	575	562	541
	Grand Means	511	491	514	541	550	554	545	**529**

TABLE 2.2. Quarterly Indexes for Heal-Me Hospital.

Quarter	Year 1	2	3	Quarterly Average	Quarterly Index
1		525	554	540	1.020
2		519	541	530	1.001
3	516	527	538	527	0.996
4	515	537		526	0.994
Overall Average				529	

TABLE 2.3. Monthly Indexes for Heal-Me Hospital.

Month	Year 1	2	3	Monthly Average	Monthly Index
JANUARY		547	550	549	1.036
FEBRUARY		529	554	542	1.023
MARCH		500	558	529	0.999
APRIL		515	546	531	1.002
MAY		499	526	513	0.968
JUNE		510	551	531	1.002
JULY	507	513	534	518	0.979
AUGUST	521	522	538	527	0.996
SEPTEMBER	519	545	541	535	1.011
OCTOBER	520	563	541	541	1.023
NOVEMBER	508	534		521	0.984
DECEMBER	516	514		515	0.973
Overall Average				529	

TABLE 2.4. **Daily Indexes for Heal-Me Hospital.**

Days	Daily Average	Daily Index
Monday	513.5	0.971
Tuesday	540.5	1.022
Wednesday	549.8	1.039
Thursday	553.5	1.046
Friday	544.9	1.030
Saturday	510.5	0.965
Sunday	491.4	0.929
Overall Average	529.0	1.000

For example, the seasonal (monthly) effect removed from July year 1 data by dividing the historical value for that period (507) by the monthly index of July (0.979), yields a nonseasonal July demand for year 1 of 518 (507 ÷ 0.979 = 518). The remaining periods can be similarly calculated and then the appropriate forecasting technique (such as trend analysis) can be employed to predict the trend more accurately.

Daily Indexes Technique Daily variation in hospitalization, especially in an emergency department, is a very common occurrence in the health care industry. Daily indexes for HEAL-ME Hospital are calculated similarly, this time by dividing daily averages by the overall average, as shown in Table 2.4. As can be observed, there is even greater variation within the week (for instance, Sundays versus Thursdays) in this particular example.

Employing Seasonal Indexes in Forecasts

Earlier, in the discussion of the monthly indexes technique (Example 2.10), it was noted that indexes may be used to remove or decompose the seasonal variations in order to discern trends and other effects in the data. If a trend is detected, the health care manager can use historical data with the seasonal effect removed in the forecasting model. That will improve its forecasting accuracy. (The next section discusses the problem of accuracy.) In Example 2.10, after the seasonal effect is removed, the twenty-eight-month data have an upward linear trend, as seen in Figure 2.15.

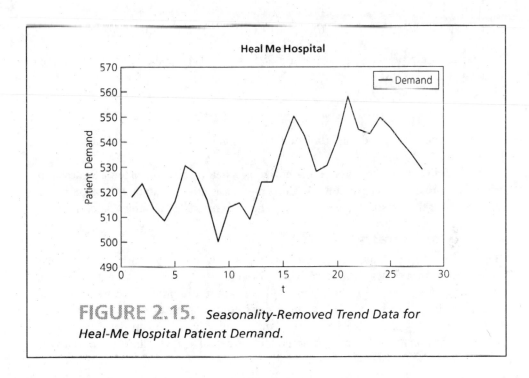

FIGURE 2.15. *Seasonality-Removed Trend Data for Heal-Me Hospital Patient Demand.*

A forecast for these data based on linear regression yields the following trend equation:

$$\text{Demand } (Y_t) = 511.06 + 1.259\ t.$$

Hence, the forecast of demand for the next three months would be:

$$Y_{29} = 511.06 + 1.259\,(29) = 547.6$$
$$Y_{30} = 511.06 + 1.259\,(30) = 548.8$$
$$Y_{31} = 511.06 + 1.259\,(31) = 550.1.$$

Having forecast the next three months, the health care manager needs to incorporate seasonality back into those forecasts. The periods $t = 29$, 30, and 31 represent the months of November, December, and January, respectively, with corresponding monthly indexes 0.984, 0.973, and 1.036. Monthly adjustments to those forecasts are calculated:

$$\text{Monthly Adjusted Forecast (t): Forecast} \times \text{Monthly Index.} \qquad (2.11)$$

for the HEAL-ME hospital example:

Period 29 (November): $547.6 \times (0.984) = 538.8$
Period 30 (December): $548.9 \times (0.973) = 534.1$
Period 31 (January): $550.1 \times (1.036) = 569.9.$

The next step in adjustment of the forecasted demand would be for daily fluctuations. As was shown in Table 2.4, HEAL-ME Hospital experiences daily variation in demand. Thus, the monthly index adjusted forecasts should be further adjusted for daily variations.

Daily Adjusted Forecast = Monthly Adjusted Forecast (t) × Daily Index $\qquad$ (2.12)

For example, for November (period 29), the adjusted forecasts for Monday and Tuesday are:

Monday, November: 538.8 × (0.971) = 523.2
Tuesday, November: 538.8 × (1.022) = 550.7.

The remaining periods and days for the complete adjusted forecasts are shown in Table 2.5.

Depending upon the forecasting horizon, a health care manager can develop a printed calendar of forecasts for care units and disseminate it so that division managers can adjust their resources according to the forecasted daily patient demand.

Accuracy of Forecasts

The complex nature of most real-world variables makes it nearly impossible to regularly forecast the future values of those variables correctly. Errors may be caused by an inadequate forecasting model, or the technique may be used improperly. Errors also result from irregular variations beyond the manager's control, such as severe weather, shortages or breakdowns, catastrophes, and so on. Random variations in the data, too, may create forecasting errors. Forecast error equals the actual value minus the forecast value:

$$Error = Actual - Forecast \qquad (2.13)$$

Forecast values that are too low result in a positive error value; forecast values that are too high result in negative error values. For example, if the actual demand for a week is 200 patients and the forecast demand was 220 patients, the forecast was too

TABLE 2.5. **Monthly and Daily Adjusted Forecasts for Heal-Me Hospital.**

Week Days	Daily Index	November	December	January
Monday	0.971	523.2	518.6	553.4
Tuesday	1.022	550.7	545.9	582.4
Wednesday	1.039	559.8	554.9	592.1
Thursday	1.046	563.6	558.7	596.1
Friday	1.030	555.0	550.1	587.0
Saturday	0.965	519.9	515.4	550.0
Sunday	0.929	500.5	496.2	529.4

high; the error was $200 - 220 = -20$. The issue of forecast errors influences two important decisions: making a choice among the forecasting alternatives, and evaluating the success or failure of a technique in use.

Two aspects of forecast accuracy have the potential to influence a choice among forecasting models. One aspect is the historical error performance of a forecast model, and the other is the ability of a forecast model to respond to changes. Two commonly used measures of historical errors are the **mean absolute deviation (MAD)** and the **mean absolute percent error (MAPE)**. MAD is the average absolute error, and MAPE is the absolute error as a percentage of actual value. The formulas used to compute MAD and MAPE are:

$$MAD = \frac{\sum |Actual - Forecast|}{n} \qquad (2.14)$$

$$MAPE = \frac{\sum |Actual - Forecast|}{\sum Actual} \qquad (2.15)$$

MAD places equal weight on all errors; thus the lower the value of MAD relative to the magnitude of the data, the more accurate the forecast. On the other hand, MAPE measures the absolute error as a percentage of actual value, rather than per period. That avoids the problem of interpreting the measure of accuracy relative to the magnitudes of the actual and the forecast values. Using Example 2.4 from SES with $\alpha = 0.3$, we observe the necessary error calculations in Table 2.6. Here sums are calculated over only four periods ($t = 2$ through 5) where both actual and forecast have values.

TABLE 2.6. Error Calculations.

Period T	Smoothing Constant $\alpha = 0.3$ Actual	Forecast	Error (Actual – Forecast)	Absolute Error |Actual – Forecast|
1	15,908	—		
2	15,504	15,908	−404	404.0
3	14,272	15,786.8	−1,514.8	1,515.0
4	13,174	15,332.4	−2,158.4	2,158.0
5	10,022	14,684.9	−4,662.9	4,662.9
6		13,286		
Sum Σ	52,972			8,740.1

Using the data from Table 2.6,

$$\text{MAD} = 8,740.1 \div 4 = 2,185.03, \text{ and}$$
$$\text{MAPE} = 8,740.1 \div 5,2972 = 0.165 \text{ or } 16.5 \text{ percent.}$$

A health care manager can use these measures to choose among forecasting alternatives for a given set of data by selecting the one that yields the lowest MAD or MAPE. Another decision health care managers have to make, however, is whether a forecast's responsiveness to change is more important than error performance. In such a situation, the selection of a forecasting method would assess the cost of not responding quickly to a change versus the cost of responding to changes that are not really there (but simply random variations).

To illustrate the influence of MAD and MAPE on the selection of a forecasting method appropriate for a given situation, a summary of the Excel template evaluation of Example 2.9 (a physician office's health insurance receipts) is shown in Figure 2.16, which includes MA_3, MA_5, SES (with $\alpha = .3$, $\alpha = .5$), and linear regression.

Examination of the MAD and MAPE errors across the forecasting techniques in Figure 2.16 reveals that the lowest errors are provided by linear regression (MAD = 977.15, MAPE = 7.7 percent), followed by single exponential smoothing with $\alpha = 0.5$ (MAD = 1,129.9, MAPE = 8.9 percent).

Forecast Control

Whatever the forecasting method used, the health care manager must ensure that it provides consistent results or continues to perform correctly. Forecasts can go out of control

FIGURE 2.16. *Alternative Forecasting Methods and Accuracy, Measured by MAD and MAPE.*

Source: Screen shots reprinted by permission from Microsoft Corporation.

for a variety of reasons: changes in trend behavior, cycles, new regulations that affect demand, and so on. Thus, a statistical control methodology should monitor the results of the forecast as more periods are added to the data. A method of constructing such statistical control on forecasts is the tracking signal. A tracking signal measures whether forecasts keep pace with up-and-down changes in actual values. A tracking signal is computed for each period, with updated cumulative forecast errors divided by MAD.

$$Tracking\ signal = \frac{\Sigma(Actual - Forecast)}{MAD} \qquad (2.16)$$

Although it can range from ±3 to ±8, the acceptable limits for tracking signal are in general within ±4, which corresponds roughly to three standard deviations. A statistical control chart can be built to monitor the performance of forecasts. If the tracking signal is positive, it indicates that the actual value is greater than the forecast; if negative, that the actual is less than the forecast. As the gap between actual and forecast gets larger, the tracking signal increases (gets closer to or beyond the control limits). When the tracking signal goes beyond acceptable limits, the health care manager should re-evaluate the forecasting methodology and investigate why it is not performing well, and perhaps try other forecasting methods. Figure 2.17 shows the solution and tracking signals of regression based forecast for "HEAL-ME" Hospital data, and Figure 2.18 displays the tracking signal in a control chart format. As can be observed, during periods 12 through 15 the tracking signal went beyond the acceptable control limits (down

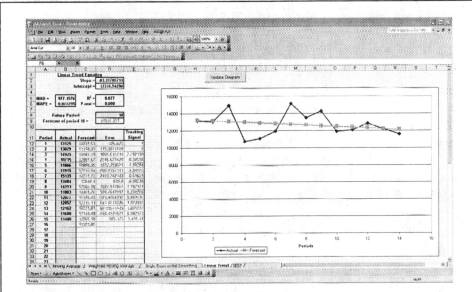

FIGURE 2.17. *Linear Trend with Tracking Signal for Patient Visit Forecast, Heal-Me Hospital.*

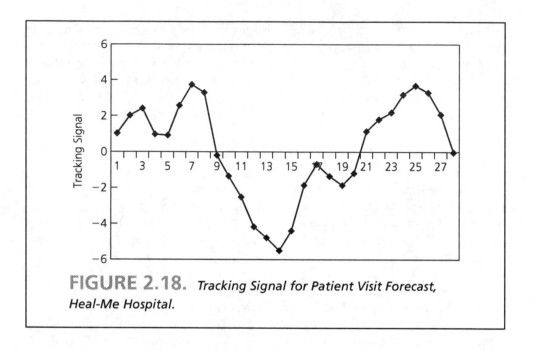

FIGURE 2.18. *Tracking Signal for Patient Visit Forecast, Heal-Me Hospital.*

to –5.5), but recovered at period 16 and stayed within acceptable limits after that. Another observation can be made from Figure 2.18, whether the forecast values are consistently higher or lower than the actual ones. Until period 8 the predicted values were below the actual. That changed from period 9 to period 20, when forecasts were higher than actual data. At the period 21 a return to under-forecast occurred.

SUMMARY

Forecasting is a basic tool for planning in health care organizations. For example, in hospitals, forecasting is applied to number of patient hospitalizations by department or nursing care units, number of outpatient visits, or visits to therapy units. In physician offices, similarly, visits and collections from insurers are examples of forecasting applications. These forecasts can be from short-horizon, a few months ahead, to medium-horizon, for one or two years. The health care manager should keep in mind that the longer the horizon of the forecast, the more prediction errors are likely.

KEY TERMS

Time Horizon
Naïve Forecast
Moving Average
Time-Series
Trend

Exponential Smoothing
Seasonal Variation
Seasonal Indexes
Forecast Accuracy

EXERCISES

2.1 The monthly ambulatory visits shown in Table EX 2.1 occurred in an outpatient clinic.

TABLE EX 2.1

Months	Visits
July	2,160
August	2,186
September	2,246
October	2,251
November	2,243
December	2,102

a. Predict visits for January, using the naïve forecast method.

b. Predict visits for January, using a three-period moving average.

c. Predict visits for January, using a four-period moving average.

2.2 Patient days in a hospital were recorded as shown in Table EX 2.2.

TABLE EX 2.2

Month	Patient Days
January	543
February	528
March	531
April	542
May	558
June	545
July	543
August	550
September	546
October	540
November	535
December	529

a. Predict naïve forecasts of patient days for February and June.

b. Predict the patient days for January, using a four-period moving average.

c. Predict the patient days for January, using the six-period moving average.

6-period won't graph

*d. Plot the actual data and the results of the four-period and the six-period moving averages. Which method is a better predictor?

2.3 Using patient days data from Exercise 2.2:

*a. Predict the patient days for January, using a four-period moving average with weights 0.1, 0.2, 0.3, and 0.4.

b. Predict the patient days for January, using a five-period moving average with weights 0.1, 0.1, 0.2, 0.2, and 0.4.

2.4 Using the visit data from Exercise 2.1:

a. Prepare a forecast for January visits, using the simple exponential smoothing method with $\alpha = 0.3$.

b. If $\alpha = 0.5$, what is the predicted value for January visits?

c. If $\alpha = 0.0$, what is the predicted value for January visits?

d. If $\alpha = 1.0$, what is the predicted value for January visits?

e. What other forecasting methods yield results similar to the exponential smoothing forecasts with $\alpha = 1.0$ and $\alpha = 0.0$?

2.5 An urgent care center experienced the average patient admissions shown in Table EX 2.5 during the weeks from the first week of December through the second week of April.

a. Predict forecasts for the admissions from the third week of April through the fourth week of May, using linear regression.

b. Forecast admissions for the periods from the first week of December through the second week of April. Compare the forecasted admissions to the actual admissions; what do you conclude?

2.6 A hospital pharmacy would like to develop a budget for allergy medications that is based on patient days. Cost and patient days data were collected over a 17-month period as shown in Table EX 2.6.

TABLE EX 2.5

Week	Average Daily Admissions
1–Dec	11
2–Dec	14
3–Dec	17
4–Dec	15

1 – Jan	12
2 – Jan	11
3 – Jan	9
4 – Jan	9
1 – Feb	12
2 – Feb	8
3 – Feb	13
4 – Feb	11
1 – Mar	15
2 – Mar	17
3 – Mar	14
4 – Mar	19
5 – Mar	13
1 – Apr	17
2 – Apr	13

TABLE EX 2.6

Period	Cost	Patient Days
October: Year 1	32,996	516
November: Year 1	34,242	530
December: Year 1	27,825	528
January: Year 2	29,807	517
February: Year 2	28,692	500
March: Year 2	34,449	514
April: Year 2	33,335	515
May: Year 2	38,217	509
June: Year 2	36,690	524
July: Year 2	35,303	524
August: Year 2	33,780	539
September: Year 2	32,843	551
October: Year 2	37,781	543
November: Year 2	27,716	528
December: Year 2	31,876	531
January: Year 3	31,463	542
February: Year 3	29,829	558

   a. Develop a linear-regression-based forecasting model to predict costs.

   b. Predict costs when patient days are 520, 530, 540, and 550.

2.7 Using hospital pharmacy data from Exercise 2.6, develop a trend-adjusted exponential smoothing forecast with a 5 0.3 and b 5 0.4 to predict costs for the March, Year 3 period (eighteenth month). Use the first nine periods to develop the model, and use the last eight periods to test the model.

2.8 In an ambulatory care center the average visits per each weekday for each month are shown in Table EX 2.8:

TABLE EX 2.8

Month	Day				
	Monday	**Tuesday**	**Wednesday**	**Thursday**	**Friday**
April	2,356	2,245	2,213	2,215	1,542
May	2,427	2,312	2,279	2,281	1,588
June	2,309	2,200	2,169	2,171	1,511
July	2,299	2,191	2,160	2,162	1,505
August	2,328	2,218	2,186	2,188	1,523
September	2,391	2,279	2,246	2,248	1,565
October	2,396	2,283	2,251	2,253	1,568
November	2,388	2,275	2,243	2,245	1,563
December	2,302	2,193	2,162	2,164	1,507
January	2,402	2,289	2,256	2,258	1,572
February	2,372	2,261	2,228	2,231	1,553
March	2,382	2,270	2,237	2,239	1,559

   a. Develop a linear regression trend forecast based on the average visits in each month.

   b. Predict the visits for April through June.

   c. Develop monthly and daily indexes for ambulatory care center visits.

   d. Using "Daily Indexes Technique," adjust predictions for April through June as well as Monday through Friday for these months, and present adjusted predictions in 3-by-5 table format.

2.9 Using the forecasting results from Exercise 2.1, calculate MAD and MAPE for naïve, three-period and four-period forecasts. Which forecast appears more accurate?

2.10 Using the forecasting results from Exercise 2.2, calculate MAD and MAPE for naïve, four-period, and six-period forecasts. Which forecast appears more accurate?

2.11 Using the data from Exercise 2.1, calculate MAD and MAPE for exponential smoothing forecasts with a 5 0.3 and with a 5 0.5. Does varying the values of a provide a more accurate forecast?

2.12 Using the forecasting results from Exercise 2.2, calculate and graph tracking signal for four-period and six-period forecasts.

CHAPTER

3

DECISION MAKING IN HEALTH CARE FACILITIES

LEARNING OBJECTIVES

- Evaluate the decision-making framework in health service organizations.
- Describe the techniques that apply to decision making under uncertainty.
- Describe the techniques that apply to decision making under risk.
- Develop and interpret the expected value of perfect information.
- Design a decision tree and solve a health care problem.
- Analyze sensitivity on outcomes and probabilities in analysis.
- Describe the multi-attribute decision making.

Managers in health care organizations must make frequent decisions, using collected data. They must decide how to direct and organize others, and also how to control processes within the system. Moreover, health care managers must also help others to reach their own decisions. Decision making, the act of selecting a course of action from among alternatives, can be quite stressful in today's dynamic and complex health care industry. Health care managers can reduce their stress somewhat if they understand how to deal with decision making and how to avoid common errors that lead to poor decisions.

THE DECISION PROCESS

Making and implementing decisions is a central function of management, and it is where health care managers concentrate their efforts. To facilitate making decisions, health care managers need to rely on the statistical and mathematical tools of management science. To implement decisions, leadership, influence, and other important behavioral skills come into play. Success depends on whether or not enough right decisions are both made and implemented. Although decisions don't always turn out as planned, a plan of action that improves the chances of a successful decision will include the following steps:

1. Identify the problem and its nature.

2. Specify objectives and decision criteria.

3. Develop alternatives.

4. Analyze and compare the alternatives.

5. Select the best alternative.

6. Implement the selected alternative.

7. Control and monitor the results.

Correctly identifying the problem is the most important part of the process. It has often been said that a well-defined problem is half solved. An improperly identified problem will cause all remaining steps to be misdirected. Often, health care managers focus on the symptoms of an underlying problem, allowing it to surface again later. Solutions must tackle the underlying problem, not the symptoms.

Early on, the health care manager must identify the criteria by which the solution will be formulated. Some examples of the criteria include costs, profits, return on investment, increased productivity, risk, company image, and the impact on demand.

The chances of finding an adequate solution to a problem increase when suitable alternatives are developed. Because virtually limitless alternatives exist for any given problem, a health care manager always runs the risk of ignoring superior alternatives. It is extremely difficult to recognize and investigate every possible outcome of the complex interrelationships that are influenced by a decision. Compiling a realistic mix of suitable alternatives often depends on the health care manager's level of experience as well as on the nature of the situation. The chances of developing a satisfactory solution are enhanced by developing a holistic view of the problem and then taking the time to carefully identify promising alternatives. The objective is to select the best one after considering the total set carefully. It should be borne in mind that the best alternative may be to do nothing at all.

Analyzing and comparing alternatives can usually be facilitated by computer programs that give a skilled health care manager the mathematical and statistical techniques for doing so. Such tools aid managers in making decisions, although they should not be treated as substitutes for the art of management. A mathematical model is an abstract representation of some real-world health care process, system, or subsystem. Selecting the best alternative depends on the objectives set by the decision maker and the criteria set for evaluating the alternatives offered by the mathematical model. In the end, the astute health care manager should ask the following question: Which alternative best fits my established objectives within reasonable time and cost constraints and will benefit the health care organization as a whole? Deciding that can be a perplexing challenge and of course is just as important as first carefully identifying the problem. Then implementing the chosen alternative is simply a matter of putting it into action.

Effective decision making requires monitoring the results of the decision to make sure that they occur as desired. If they have not, the health care manager may choose to repeat the entire process. On the other hand, investigation may uncover an error in the implementation or the calculations, or perhaps a false assumption that affected the entire process. The latter situations can often be remedied quickly and at much less cost than starting over.

Decisions are not always made in a concise and sequential way. A health care manager will often have to backtrack to uncover errors, as well as to solicit feedback from other managers and employees, especially in terms of developing and analyzing alternatives. To ensure that the organization benefits from the best solution, it is essential to involve the persons who will be affected by the decisions a manager makes.

What Causes Poor Decisions?

Despite the best efforts of a health care manager, a decision occasionally turns out poorly because of uncontrollable events. Such eventualities are not prevalent, however. Usually, failures can be traced to some combination of mistakes in the decision process. In many cases, health care managers fail to appreciate the importance of each step in the process. A common reason for that oversight is that they grow accustomed to making quick decisions, and also tend to assume that previous successes guarantee success in the current situation. Then too, health care managers often are unwilling to admit their mistakes or that they don't understand the processes involved. Other managers have trouble making decisions and wait far too long before making one.

In any case, health care managers facing a decision must deal with the phenomenon known as **bounded rationality**, or the limits imposed on decision making by costs, human abilities and errors, time, technology, and the tractability of data. Those limits are a primary reason that a manager is assigned to direct only part of a total system. The manager must contend with the recognition that it is not always possible to come up with a decision that will have the very best possible outcome. Rather, managers may often have to resort to achieving simply a satisfactory solution to the problem (Stevenson, 2002; p. 198).

Another phenomenon in poor decision making is **sub-optimization**. In a highly competitive environment, decisions are often departmentalized as separate organizational units compete for scarce resources. Individual departments often seek solutions that benefit their own department but not necessarily the health care organization as a whole. When making a decision, a health care manager should try to maintain a perspective that is broad enough so that the decision will not seriously sub-optimize the health care organization's overall goals (Stevenson, 2002; p. 198). For example, a departmental goal of minimizing the surgery department's costs could impair the facility's quality of medical care.

The Decision Level and Decision Milieu

The level of decisions and the settings in which managers must make decisions are classified according to (a) the strategic level of the decision, and (b) the level of certainty surrounding the situation, or states of nature. The strategic level of a decision can vary from low to high depending on the situation. For example, the strategic nature of daily operational decisions (such as staffing adjustments) is generally low, whereas decisions about new service offerings are more strategic. The management level making the decisions rises with the strategic importance of these decisions. Usually top-level managers make strategic decisions.

Decision makers operate in varying milieus, which require differing approaches to their evaluations. The decision milieu may be one of **uncertainty** or one of **risk;** each setting requires distinctive decision-making tools to evaluate the alternatives. In general, decisions involving an uncertain milieu are strategic in nature and occur at top levels; decisions in risk settings can occur at any management level.

Uncertainty exists in any scenario when insufficient information makes it impossible to assess the likelihood of possible future events; for example, you know the profit level per unit but are uncertain of what demand levels are probable. Risk exists when you do not know which events will occur but can estimate the probability that any one state will occur. For example, the profit per unit is known, but there is a 60 percent chance that the demand is 200 units and a 40 percent chance that demand will be 400 units. Remember, the percentages for all possible outcomes must add up to 1.0 (100 percent).

Decision Making Under Uncertainty

Under uncertainty, there are five possible decision strategies: maximin, maximax, Laplace, minimax regret, and Hurwitz criterion. A brief description of these strategies follows.

Maximin. This strategy identifies the worst possible scenario for each alternative, and aims to select the alternative that will give the largest payoff in the worst circumstances. It is regarded as pessimistic strategy.

Maximax. This strategy identifies the alternative with the best payoff (highest maximum return). It is regarded as an extremely optimistic strategy.

Laplace. This strategy calculates the average payoff for each alternative and selects the one with the highest average.

Minimax Regret. This strategy calculates the worst regret (or opportunity loss) for each alternative and chooses the one that yields the least regret, or that the health care manager can "live with" best.

Hurwitz. This strategy allows for adjusted weighting between maximin and maximax, or allows the health care manager to choose a platform on the continuum of pessimist versus optimist.

Payoff Table

A tool that is frequently used to select the best alternative given different possible outcomes is called a payoff table. The payoff table shows the expected payoffs for each alternative under various possible conditions—states of nature. A payoff table can be constructed using the outcome for alternative $i(A_i)$, and state of nature $j(S_j)$ as O_{ij}. Outcomes can be expressed in profits, revenue, or cost. A general presentation of a payoff table with m number of alternatives and n number of states is shown in Table 3.1.

It is useful to illustrate the concepts being discussed with an example. The example below develops a specific payoff table, using profits. Revenue, income, and profit outcomes follow the same directions in decision making. However, cost payoffs require reverse logic and will be discussed later in the chapter.

TABLE 3.1. **Payoff Table.**

Alternative State of Nature	S_1	S_2	....	S_n
A_1	O_{11}	O_{12}	....	O_{1n}
A_2	O_{21}	O_{22}	....	O_{2n}
...	...	...	....	.....
A_m	O_{m1}	O_{m2}	....	O_{mn}

EXAMPLE 3.1

A major imaging center is not able to meet the increased demand from patients for magnetic resonance imaging studies (MRIs). The administration is willing to explore the possibilities by evaluating such alternatives as adding one or two additional units or outsourcing to other image centers and earning a commission of $30 per MRI.

A feasibility analysis showed that three major demand chunks could occur in the future, summarized as 500, 750, and 1,000 additional MRI requests. The financial analysis of the potential business summarizes profits and losses under additional MRI demand chunks in a payoff table shown in Table 3.2.

To evaluate this case in the absence of further information about demand, we turn to tools of decision making under uncertainty. Here the health care manager can be a pessimist, an optimist, or anything on that continuum. Let's examine how, under various behavioral patterns of health care managers, their decisions would vary.

Maximin Case

Suppose the health care manager is a pessimist decision maker, who would consider the worst possible outcomes and then choose the best alternative among them, thus maximizing the minimum payoffs. To evaluate this situation, the health care manager would scan through each row of the payoff table and find the worst outcome for each alternative. In this case, the worst possible outcomes for each decision alternative are loss of $15,000 for buying one MRI unit, loss of $150,000 for buying two MRI units, and profit of $15,000 for outsourcing. As shown in Table 3.3, among these three, the best outcome is $15,000 profit, so the decision under maximin would be "Outsource." That option gives the pessimist decision maker a guaranteed minimum payoff.

TABLE 3.2. Demand for Additional MRIs.

Alternatives	500 Cases	750 Cases	1,000 Cases
Buy One MRI Unit	−15*	200	300
Buy Two MRI Units	−150	100	725
Outsource	15	22.5	40

*In thousands of dollars.

Maximax Case

Here the decision maker is an optimist, considering the best possible outcomes and then choosing the best alternative among them, hence maximizing the payoffs. To evaluate the situation in this way, the health care manager would scan through each row of the payoff table and find the best outcome for each alternative. In this case, the best possible outcomes for each alternative are profit of $300,000 for buying one MRI unit, profit of $725,000 for buying two MRI units, and profit of $40,000 for outsourcing. Among these three the best payoff, as shown in Table 3.4, is $725,000, hence the decision under maximax would be "Buy Two MRI Units." For the optimist health care manager, that option gives the maximum payoff.

Hurwitz Case

Here the health care manager's behavior can fluctuate from pessimism to optimism, depending upon recent experiences with similar situations. Hurwitz provides a measure for assigning a weight toward optimism and the remainder of the weight to pessimism. Hurwitz optimism weight would vary $0 \leq \alpha \leq 1$. When the weight $\alpha = 1$, the decision becomes optimistic and when $\alpha = 0$, the decision is pessimistic. Selection of

TABLE 3.3. Maximin Solution.

Alternatives	500 Cases	750 Cases	1,000 Cases	Worst
Buy One MRI Unit	−15*	200	300	−15
Buy Two MRI Units	−150	100	725	−150
Outsource	15	22.5	40	15

*In thousands of dollars.

TABLE 3.4. Maximax Solution.

Alternatives	500 Cases	750 Cases	1,000 Cases	Best
Buy One MRI Unit	−15*	200	300	300
Buy Two MRI Units	−150	100	725	725
Outsource	15	22.5	40	40

*In thousands of dollars.

α value other than zero, the optimistic value, also produces a weight, which can be named the pessimistic value, denoted as $1 - \alpha$. The Hurwitz criterion is in fact a weighted average of optimist and pessimist outcomes, and the decision, therefore, is a byproduct of the magnitude of weight chosen. To evaluate the situation on hand, the health care manager would scan through each row of the payoff table and find the best outcome and the worst outcome for each alternative. Then for each alternative she or he would calculate Hurwitz Value (HV) as follows:

$$HV(A_i) = \alpha\,(\text{row maximum}) + (1 - \alpha)\,(\text{row minimum}) \qquad (3.1)$$

In the example, recall that the best possible outcome for the decision to buy one MRI unit ($i = 1$) is a profit of \$300,000 and the worst outcome is a \$15,000 loss. Let's assume that the health care manager would like to stay in the middle of the road to optimism with a value of 0.5. Then the HV value for the three alternatives would be:

HV(Buy One MRI Unit) = 0.5(300,000) + (0.5) (− 15,000) = 142,500
HV(Buy Two MRI Units) = (0.5)(725,000) + (0.5) (− 150,000) = 287,500
HV(Outsource) = 0.5(40,000) + (0.5)(15,000) = 27,500.

Hence, with α value of 0.5 the decision would be, "Buy Two MRI Units," which provides the highest payoff and is the same decision as full optimistic behavior. One can check the sensitivity of this decision by changing α values (in this case downward) to see when the choice of alternative changes. When α value goes down to 0.24, the decision switches to "Buy One MRI Unit"—a middle-of-the-road decision—and finally, with α value of 0.1, the decision switches to "Outsource," the alternative that is equivalent to full pessimistic behavior. Table 3.5 summarizes the sensitivity analysis, using the Hurwitz optimism parameter.

Minimax Regret Case

Another way to evaluate decisions under uncertain situations is from the perspective of opportunity loss. Regret refers to the opportunity loss that occurs when an alternative is chosen and a particular state of nature occurs. More specifically, the regret is the difference between the best possible outcome under a state of nature and the actual outcome from choosing a particular alternative.

In order to evaluate minimax regret decisions, the health care manager must develop a regret table, which converts the payoff table to opportunity losses. Computation of a regret starts with the state of nature—a column in a payoff table— and is formulated as:

$$\text{Regret}(R_{ij}) = \text{maximum payoff for column } j - \text{payoff}_{ij} \qquad (3.2)$$

In the MRI example, consider the first state of nature—an additional MRI demand of 500. In this column of the payoff table ($j = 1$) the maximum payoff is \$15,000. Therefore, a health care manager who had chosen the alternative of "Outsource" would

TABLE 3.5. **Sensitivity Analysis Using Hurwitz Optimism Parameters.**

α	HV	Decision Alternative
1.0	725,000*	Buy Two MRI Units
0.5	287,500	Buy Two MRI Units
0.4	200,000	Buy Two MRI Units
0.3	112.500	Buy Two MRI Units
0.24	60,600	Buy One MRI Unit
0.2	48,000	Buy One MRI Unit
0.1	17,500	Outsource
0.0	15,000	Outsource

*In dollars.

TABLE 3.6. **Opportunity Losses (Regrets).**

Alternatives	500 Cases	750 Cases	1,000 Cases	Worst
Buy One MRI Unit	30*	0	425	425
Buy Two MRI Units	165	100	0	**165**
Outsource	0	177.5	685	685

*In thousands of dollars.

regret nothing when such demand becomes the actuality; here zero is defined as no regret. However, if the first alternative had been chosen then $15,000 − (−$15,000) = $30,000 would be the amount of regret. Similarly, the regret for the second alternative would be $165,000 [$15,000 − (−$150,000) = $165,000]. Proceeding to the two other columns in a similar way, the opportunity loss table is completed, as shown in Table 3.6.

Once the opportunity loss table is created, the minimax rule can be applied. This time the health care manager would try to minimize worst opportunity losses. To evaluate the situation in this way, the health care manager would scan through each row of the opportunity loss table and find the worst regret for each alternative. The worst possible regrets for the alternatives are $425,000 for buying one MRI unit, $165,000 for buying two MRI units, and $685,000 for outsourcing. Among these three, the minimum regret is $165,000, so the decision under minimax regret would be "Buy Two MRI Units," the option that gives the health care manager the least opportunity loss.

Laplace Case

Also known as the principle of "insufficient reason," Laplace strategy is the first, though very simplistic, way of introducing the probability concept into decision making. Since under uncertainty no known probabilities exist, the health care manager can assume equally likely probabilities for each state of nature, there being no reason to assign differently (insufficient reason principle). For n states of nature, the probability for each state under the Laplace strategy would be $1/n$. Thus, each state of nature is represented by a uniform probability distribution (is equally probable). To evaluate the situation in the example, the health care manager would assign $1/3$ probability for each state of nature—each level of additional demand for MRI. In order to reach a decision, now the health care manager must calculate expected outcomes, or weighted payoffs. For each alternative i, expected outcome is calculated using the following formula:

$$E(A_i) = \Sigma_j \, p_j O_{ij} \tag{3.3}$$

For the MRI example, the calculation for "Buy One MRI Unit" would be:

$$E(\text{Buy One MRI Unit}) = (1/3) \times (-15,000) + (1/3) \times (200,000) + (1/3) \times (300,000) = \$161,666.$$

Similarly, other alternatives' expected values are calculated as shown in Table 3.7. Using the Laplace criterion, the health care manager would then choose the alternative with the highest expected payoff, in this case "Buy Two MRI Units."

TABLE 3.7. Laplace Strategy.

Probability Alternatives	1/3 500 Cases	1/3 750 Cases	1/3 1,000 Cases	Expected Value
Buy One MRI Unit	−15*	200	300	161.67
Buy Two MRI Units	−150	100	725	**225**
Outsource	15	22.5	40	25.83

*In thousands of dollars.

Decision Making Under Risk

Between the two extremes of certainty and uncertainty lies the state of risk. The scenarios considered here hold that the probability of any type of outcome can be estimated. The risk environment is the most common decision-making environment for health care managers. As said, the health care manager may have past data—objective probabilities—from similar circumstances, or subjective estimates of the probabilities. Objective probabilities can be obtained through theory, or empirically. Theoretical objective probability uses mathematical theory and a logical framework. For example, the probability of rolling six on a die is theoretically one-sixth and should converge to this value over repeated experiments. Similarly, a coin toss experiment would yield 0.50 probability that the outcome will be "heads." A variety of well-known probability distributions would provide the health care manager with objective information (probability) to assign to various states of nature, if the situation fits the conditions for a given probability distribution. Another way to obtain objective probabilities is to conduct controlled empirical studies to estimate the probability of a given situation. Then the empirical distributions can be used or converted/approximated to one of the known probability distributions using the statistical "goodness-of-fit" test.

Real-world problems, however, especially of a strategic nature, do not always lend themselves to objective probability estimation in a short time. And as discussed earlier, for certain decisions bounded rationality limits the health care manager's time, ability, or resources to collect objective probabilities in a reasonable time. In the absence of objective probabilities that are reliable, subjective probability becomes prominent. Laplace strategy, discussed earlier, provides that under the principle of insufficient reason—if no reliable objective probabilities can be determined for the time being—all states of nature may be equally probable. That is, it is better to assign equal probabilities than to have none. When more time and information become available, health care managers can modify the probability information subjectively. Of course, objective assessments, especially empirical ones, would take much longer. Generally, health care decision makers have some knowledge, or can obtain it, that applies to the decision at hand. Such knowledge includes the environment surrounding the decision and the states of nature. That knowledge (partly intuition) provides processing and quantification of the likelihood of events (states of nature) for that problem. For example, the health care manager intuitively rank-orders the likelihood of events.

To take advantage of this evolving thought process, one can easily establish a subjective probability distribution. Let us consider the additional MRI demand case, and suppose that the health care manager thinks that the most likely event is an additional demand of 750 cases per month. To start the process, assign an arbitrary weight to this event, say 1. In the next step, the health care manager thinks that the additional demand for MRIs at 500 cases per month is three times less likely than the most likely event just identified, and so gives it a weight of 1/3. The health care manager thinks that the last event, demand for 1,000 MRI cases, as compared to the most likely event is about 1/3 also. Using the same common denominator, we can express these weights as:

Event	Weight	Sum
750 cases	1	3/3
500 cases	1/3	1/3
1,000 cases	1/3	1/3
Overall		5/3

Then divide each weight by the overall sum (5/3) to standardize and derive the subjective probability distribution as shown below:

Event	Weight	Sum	Standardization	Subjective Probability
750 cases	3/3	3/3	1/(5/3)	= 0.6
500 cases	1/3	1/3	(1/3)/(5/3)	= 0.2
1,000 cases	1/3	1/3	(1/3)/(5/3)	= 0.2
Overall		5/3		1.00

Whether derived objectively or subjectively, having the probabilities on hand equips the health care manager to evaluate situations under risk. Expected value model and decision tree are some of the tools that provide structured evaluation of such decision-making situations.

Expected Value Model

If the outcomes are measured in monetary value, as in this case, the expected value model is generally named as expected monetary value, or EMV. Once the health care manager has assessed the probability distribution, computation of the expected values for each alternative is straightforward, using the same formula (3.3) shown previously in Laplace strategy as follows:

$$EMV(A_i) = \Sigma_j p_j O_{ij}.$$

If the outcomes represent regrets (opportunity losses), then one can calculate expected opportunity losses, or EOL. Following the same MRI example with assessed probabilities as in the previous section, the payoff table for EMV is shown in Table 3.8. For example, the expected value calculation for "Buy One MRI Unit" would be $(-15 \times 0.2) + (200 \times 0.6) + (300 \times 0.2) = 177$. Other alternatives calculated in similar fashion are shown in Table 3.8.

In this case the health care manager would choose the first alternative "Buy One MRI Unit." However, since two expected monetary values (EMV) are so close, a sensitivity analysis and other factors might be considered to make the final decision.

TABLE 3.8. Payoff Table for EMV.

Probability Alternatives	0.2 500 Cases	0.6 750 Cases	0.2 1,000 Cases	Expected Value
Buy One MRI Unit	−15*	200	300	**177**
Buy Two MRI Units	−150	100	725	175
Outsource	15	22.5	40	24.5

*In thousands of dollars.

TABLE 3.9. Expected Opportunity Loss.

Probability Alternative	0.2 500 Cases	0.6 750 Cases	0.2 1,000 Cases	Expected Opportunity Loss
Buy One MRI Unit	30*	0	425	**91**
Buy Two MRI Units	165	100	0	93
Outsource	0	177.5	685	243.5

*In thousands of dollars.

Expected Opportunity Loss

The probabilities can also be incorporated into the regrets (or opportunity losses) calculated earlier. In this way the health care manager can assess the expected losses and try to minimize them with a proper decision. Table 3.9 shows the opportunity loss table that incorporates this idea. Calculations of expected opportunity loss follow the formula:

$$\text{EOL}(A_i) = \Sigma_j p_j R_{ij} \qquad (3.4)$$

In this case, the health care manager would choose the same alternative, "Buy One MRI Unit" to minimize the potential opportunity losses. Using either EMV or EOL, the decision by the health care manager would be the same; why?

Expected Value of Perfect Information (EVPI)

You may recall that the probability distribution used in the EMV and the EOL models was subjectively derived and that as time passes on and more information becomes available either for purchase or to be collected, the probabilities can be updated so that the health care manager can make more informed decisions. However, under bounded rationality, one has to assess how much of the resources can be spent to gather more appropriate information. Collecting information incurs expenses, so the dilemma the health care manager faces is how much to spend to make a better decision. Note that additional information is not restricted to updating the probability distribution, but may relate to more accurate outcomes as well. Here, the concept of expected value of perfect information (EVPI) provides an avenue for assessing the situation and determining the level of resources the health care manager would be willing to commit for this situation. Of course information can be obtained more cheaply than by EVPI, but its quality may not be good or reliable. However, the health care manager would like to know the upper limit, or maximum price, that can be spent to obtain the information.

In order to evaluate this situation, first consider the case in which one had perfect information about the state of nature or which event would occur. Then it would be very simple (certainty condition) for the health care manager to choose the alternative yielding the best outcome. For example, if 500 cases are sure to occur, then the health care manager would choose the "Outsource" alternative to secure $15,000. Similarly, for 750 and for 1,000 cases, the decisions would be "Buy One MRI Unit" and "Buy Two MRI Units," yielding $200,000 and $725,000, respectively. But all the health care manager knows at the time are the probabilities of these events (risk), none being known to be certain. However, we know how the manager would have decided if any event was certain to occur. The outcomes of those certainty decisions are summarized in Table 3.10. Using known probabilities at the time, one can calculate the expected value under certainty (EVUC). For this case

$$EVUC = \Sigma_j p_j (Best\, O_{ij}\, given\, S_j) \qquad (3.5)$$

EVUC for this case, then, simply is $(0.2 \times 15,000) + (0.6 \times 200,000) + (0.2 \times 725,000) = 268,000$.

However, the health care manager is currently operating under risk and would like to achieve certainty conditions to make the best decision. The expected value of perfect information then would be the difference between expectations under certainty ($268,000) and under risk or EMV ($177,000). Formally,

$$EVPI = EVUC - EMV \qquad (3.6)$$

In the ongoing example, EVPI = $268,000 - $177,000 = $91,000. Readers should note that this value is equivalent to the minimum expected opportunity loss presented in Table 3.9. Hence, EVPI = minimum {EOL}. EVPI formula holds only when event probabilities are the same for all alternatives.

TABLE 3.10. Best Outcomes Under Certainty.

Probability	0.2	0.6	0.2
Alternatives	500 Cases	750 Cases	1,000 Cases
Buy One MRI Unit	−15*	**200**	300
Buy Two MRI Units	−150	100	**725**
Outsource	**15**	22.5	40

*In thousands of dollars.

TABLE 3.11. Total Cost of Alternatives Under Various Demand Conditions.

Alternatives	500 Cases	750 Cases	1,000 Cases
Buy One MRI Unit	2,050*	2,075	2,100
Buy Two MRI Units	4,050	4,075	4,100
Outsource	5	10	15

*In thousands of dollars.

What If Payoffs Are Costs?

Information on various decision situations does not always come in the context of revenue or profit. Often the information collected represents the costs associated with the decision situation and can be organized in the payoff table as such. The techniques discussed above can easily be applied to cost payoff tables by reversing the logic. For example, the pessimist decision maker who used the maximin criterion on profit/revenue would reverse the logic by using minimax cost. That is, one would search for the maximum costs of each alternative and then choose the alternative with minimum cost. Similarly, the optimist decision maker would use the minimin cost by choosing the minimum among the minimum cost alternatives.

Minimax regret works similarly to the revenue/profit situation; however, a cost regret table has to be constructed. To illustrate decisions based on cost payoffs, follow the Table 3.11, where the cells in the payoff matrix are given costs in thousands of dollars.

TABLE 3.12. Regret Table Using Costs.

Alternatives	500 Cases	750 Cases	1,000 Cases
Buy One MRI Unit	2,050 – 5 = **2,045***	2,075 – 10 = **2,065**	2,100 – 15 = **2,085**
Buy Two MRI Units	4,050 – 5 = **4,045**	4,075 – 10 = **4,065**	4,100 – 15 = **4,085**
Outsource	5 – 5 = **0**	10 – 10 = **0**	15 – 15 = **0**

*In thousands of dollars.

The pessimist health care manager using minimax cost would decide to outsource. Here the maximum costs for each alternative are identified (in thousands of dollars) as $2,100, $4,100, and $15, respectively. The minimum of these maximums is $15, which yields outsourcing as the best alternative. On the other hand, the optimist health care manager would use the minimin cost criterion, where the row minimums are $2,050, $4,050, and $5, respectively. The decision for this case is, however, again outsourcing, showing the decision is insensitive to a health care manager's behavior (or risk-taking attitude) because of the big gap in costs.

To complete the example with minimax, a regret (opportunity loss or cost avoidance) table has to be created. To do that, in each column identify the lowest cost and subtract that from the other alternative's cost. Table 3.12 shows the results: each alternative shows zero regrets under the outsourcing alternative.

Searching row-wise, we observe that the maximum regrets for alternatives are $2,085, $4,085, and $0, respectively. Hence the decision using minimax regret would be outsourcing.

THE DECISION TREE APPROACH

Decision tree is another way to visualize and solve problems of this nature. The tree is drawn from left to right, with square and circle nodes that are connected by lines (branches). The initial square node is the starting point (root of the tree), and branches emanating from it identify the alternatives—rows in the payoff table. The branches are connected to circle nodes, which represent the future events, or the states of nature—columns in the payoff table. The circle nodes also are called event nodes, which require probabilities. Payoffs are assigned to the terminating branches coming out of event nodes. Note that the probabilities on branches coming from the same event node must add up to one. The decision tree version of the payoff table shown in Table 3.8 is depicted in Figure 3.1.

Analysis of the Decision Tree: Rollback Procedure

To analyze the problem using the decision tree format, starting from the left, the expected values are calculated for every event node. The calculations use the expected monetary

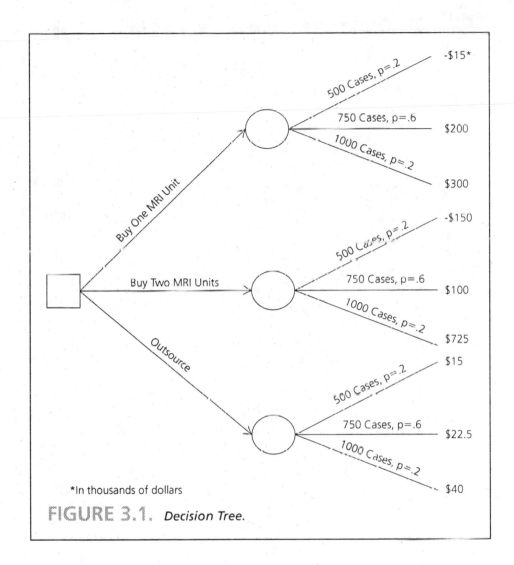

*In thousands of dollars

FIGURE 3.1. *Decision Tree.*

value formula (3.3), $\text{EMV}(A_j) = \Sigma_j p_j O_{ij}$, explained earlier. These expected values are then placed on the event nodes to compare the alternatives. For example, the expected value calculation for "Buy One MRI Unit" would be $(0.2 \times -15) + (0.6 \times 200) + (0.2 \times 300) = 177$ (in $000s). The other nodes yield 175 and 24.5, respectively. Among these monetary values, the highest expected return is 177; hence the decision is "Buy One MRI Unit." The other decision branches of the tree should no longer be considered, thus they are truncated—shown by placing the "‖" symbol on them. The final decision's expected value, 177, is then placed on the initial decision node, showing what monetary value the health care manager can expect with this decision. Figure 3.2 illustrates the results of the rollback method.

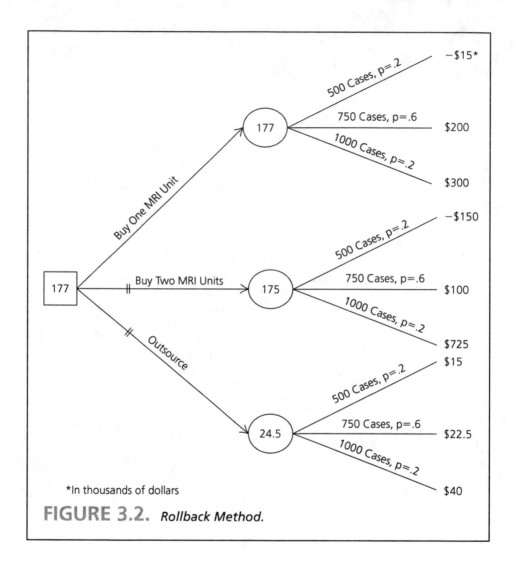

FIGURE 3.2. *Rollback Method.*

Excel Illustration of Payoff and Decision Tree Methods

Excel template for "Decision Analysis" provides an easy platform for analyzing decision problems by using either the payoff table or the rollback procedure for the decision tree. Figure 3.3 displays the payoff table and the analysis results. Figure 3.4 shows the decision tree and the results of the rollback procedure.

DECISION ANALYSIS WITH NONMONETARY VALUES AND MULTIPLE ATTRIBUTES

Often, available data on various measures are in other than monetary terms, so the situation may not lend itself to quantification in monetary values. Furthermore, there

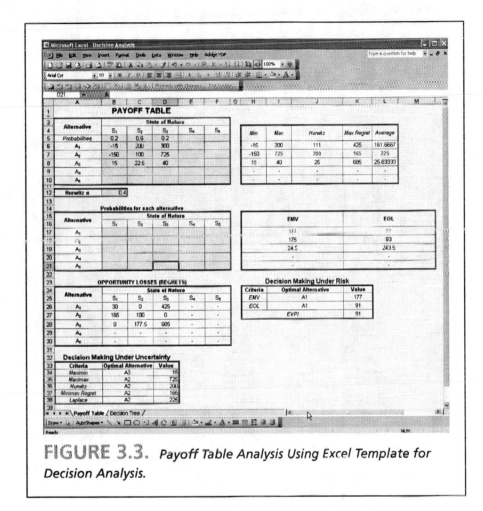

FIGURE 3.3. *Payoff Table Analysis Using Excel Template for Decision Analysis.*

Source: Excel, screen shots reprinted by permission from Microsoft Corporation.

may be multiple measurements on various attributes of the problem. Under those conditions, the health care manager must resort to other techniques to evaluate or assess outcomes. The selection of the appropriate alternative when decisions are conceptualized by more than one attribute can be illustrated by the following example:

EXAMPLE 3.2

After evaluating responses to a request for proposals (RFPs), a hospital supply chain manager, along with the task committee on procurement, summarized the major components of the proposals from suppliers for a group of surgical supplies, as shown in Table 3.13.

FIGURE 3.4. *Decision Tree and Rollback Procedure Using Excel Template for Decision Analysis.*

Source: Excel, screen shots reprinted by permission from Microsoft Corporation.

As it can be depicted from the table, the nonmonetary attributes of this procurement and potential contract are more important, as highlighted in the importance rankings. In addition, there are minimum acceptable levels for each attribute that may play a role in the decision. In such situations, the health care manager has to employ decision-making procedures incorporating those factors. Multi-attribute decisions can use procedures to simplify the process. The three simple procedures that can be used either independently or in combination are dominance, minimum attribute satisfaction, and most important attribute.

Dominance Procedure. If an alternative (X) is at least as good as another alternative (Y) on all attributes and strongly the choice on at least one attribute, then alternative

TABLE 3.13.   **Summary of Supplier Proposals.**

Alternative→ Attributes*	Supplier A	Supplier B	Supplier C	Importance Ranking	Minimum Acceptable Level
Availability	7	7	7	1	≥ 7
Reliability of Information Technology	7	5	7	2	≥ 6
Quality of Products	8	9	8	3	≥ 7
Cost in $000 per Year	23,749	24,195	23,688	5	≤ 25,000
On-Time Delivery	97%	95%	97%	4	≥ 95%

*Attributes are scored on a 1–10 scale (with the exception of those associated with costs and on-time-delivery percentage), with a score of 10 being most favorable.

X dominates alternative Y. Evaluation of the alternatives using dominance procedure is conducted by considering a pair of alternatives at a time. If there are many alternatives, there might be many pair-wise comparisons that have to be completed. In Example 3.2, there are three alternatives, so three pair-wise comparisons will be made. If there were four alternatives, the number of pair-wise comparisons would be six; why? To illustrate dominance, let's take the first pair of alternatives: Supplier A versus Supplier B. Here, on the first attribute, "Availability," both vendors score equally, so we move on to the second attribute, "Reliability of Information Technology," where Supplier A has the better score, and on this attribute is the stronger choice. However, to complete the dominance evaluation, the health care manager must make sure the remaining attributes are at least equal or favorable to Supplier A. For "Quality of Products," however, those distributed by Supplier B are preferred to those from Supplier A. Therefore, Supplier A, which scores better than Supplier B on the remaining attributes, does not dominate Supplier B. The next comparison would be between Supplier A and Supplier C. On the first three attributes, both distributors have the same scores, and on "Cost" Supplier C is preferred to Supplier A for its lower cost. On the last attribute, "On-Time Delivery," Supplier A is no better than Supplier C. Thus, Supplier C dominates Supplier A. Using the dominance procedure, then, the health care manager can eliminate Supplier A from further consideration. That leaves the last pair, Supplier B and Supplier C, for evaluation. Supplier C is the preferred choice on the first two attributes, but on "Quality of

Products" Supplier B scores better; hence there is no dominance between these two vendors. It should be reiterated that the dominance process is best for reducing a number of inferior alternatives from consideration, but may not find a unique solution for the decision—as in this case, where two alternatives survived the process. Other procedures may be applied next to select an alternative.

Minimum Attribute Satisfaction Procedure. When evaluating alternatives, especially in contract proposals, minimum acceptable standards may be considered. When requests for proposals are developed, therefore, they often specify the acceptable standards, or minimum attributes. Evaluation of alternatives in those terms is conducted differently from the dominance procedure; pair-wise comparisons are not used. Instead, all alternatives are considered simultaneously for each minimum attribute. If any alternative is not satisfactory for a given minimum attribute, that alternative is eliminated. In Example 3.2, starting with the first attribute, "Availability," one can observe that all vendors satisfy the minimum acceptable level of 7. However, on "Reliability of Information Technology," Supplier B scores 5, which is less than the minimum acceptable level of 6, so Supplier B must be eliminated. The health care manager should complete the evaluation by checking the minimum attributes on the remaining alternatives. In this case, the remaining alternatives satisfy the minimum acceptable levels, so both Supplier A and Supplier C remain as choices, but once more no unique solution (single selection) emerges. That is a weakness of this procedure, as well. Again, another procedure may then be applied to find the unique solution.

Most Important Attribute Procedure. If neither of the above procedures yield a solution, this procedure in most instances will. In Example 3.2, a ranking in importance of the attributes developed by the vendor selection team is shown. Applying that ranking is done as in minimum attribute satisfaction, by simultaneously considering all alternatives, first for the highest-ranking attribute and then, if no solution is obtained, for the next attribute. The top-ranking attribute is "Availability," for which all three vendors have the same score, so the health care manager moves on the second-highest-ranked attribute, "Reliability of Information Technology." There Supplier A and Supplier C have the same highest score of 7; Supplier B scores only 5 and is eliminated. Still searching for the unique solution, the health care manager next considers the third-ranked attribute, "Quality of the Products," with a score of 8 for each vendor; both vendors survive. Moving on to the fourth-ranked attribute, "On-Time Delivery," again finds both vendors with the same score, 97 percent. The last-ranking attribute, "Cost," however, clearly breaks this tie in favor of Supplier C, which has lower cost than Supplier A. Hence the unique solution to this particular decision is Supplier C.

Although the most important attribute procedure can find unique solutions, it often can do so without evaluating all attributes. In the example above, if scores were not equal, the vendor with the highest score would be the choice.

SUMMARY

To facilitate making decisions, health care managers need to rely on the statistical and mathematical tools of management science. To implement decisions, leadership, influence, and other important behavioral skills come into play. When making a decision, a health care manager should try to maintain a perspective that is broad enough so that the decision will not seriously sub-optimize the health care organization's overall goals. This chapter examined decision techniques under various platforms to help health care managers.

KEY TERMS

Decision Making
Bounded Rationality
Sub-optimization
Risk
Uncertainty
Payoff Table

Expected Monetary Value
Expected Value of Perfect Information
Decision Tree
Rollback Procedure
Multiple Attributes
Dominance.

EXERCISES

3.1 WECARE, a newly formed primary care group practice, is seeking a location among five possible sites. For these practices, which are largely unregulated for their locations, the location decisions are influenced mainly by market forces and the personal preferences of the key physicians. The data on potential profit for the demand levels at each possible site are shown in Table EX 3.1.

TABLE EX 3.1

states of nature

Physician Preferred Sites	Payoff: Profit (in $1,000) for Demand Levels		
	High	Medium	Low
A	350	150	(250)
B	590	350	(500)
C	600	225	(250)
D	550	400	(250)
E	475	325	(200)

alternatives

a. Some members of the practice are pessimists; which location would they choose?

b. There also are very optimistic members in the group; which location would they choose?

c. What would be the Laplace strategy solution for the site? $p = 0.33$

d. What is the minimax regret solution to this problem? Best outcome - particular outcome

e. What is the solution for a Hurwitz optimism value of 0.4?

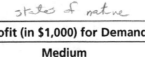

$$0.4 (\text{Row max}) + (1 - 0.4)(\text{Row min})$$

3.2 WECARE group practice hired an analyst who estimated the probability for each demand level at each site as shown in Table EX 3.2.

TABLE EX 3.2

Physician Preferred Sites	Probability for Given Level of Potential Demand		
	High	Medium	Low
A	0.10 D	0.55	0.35
B	0.20 D	0.50	0.30
C	0.10 D	0.60	0.30
D	0.15 D	0.40	0.45
E	0.30 D	0.40	0.30

Using data from Exercise 3.1 and the above probabilities, what is the EMV solution to the site selection?

3.3 A CEO of a multihospital system is planning to expand operations into various states. It will take several years to get certificate of need (CON) approvals so that the new facilities can be constructed. The eventual cost (in millions of dollars) of building a facility will differ among states, depending upon finances, labor, and the economic and political climate. An outside consulting firm estimated the costs for the new facilities as based on declining, similar, or improving economies, and the associated probabilities as shown in Table EX 3.3.

TABLE EX 3.3

State	Declining .25	Same .40	Improving .35
Kentucky	22	19	15
Maryland	19	19	18
North Carolina	19	17	15
Tennessee	23	17	14
Virginia	25	21	13

a. The CEO remembered the Decision Support Systems class from graduate studies (a long time ago) and decided to use that information for the company's decision process. The first action was to draw a decision tree and calculate the EMV for each event node; then the best site would be selected for the next hospital for the system.

0.7 of #1m!
= 700,000

b. However, feeling uneasy with the limited data, the CEO wanted to collect more information about economic conditions and to allocate money in the budget for that purpose. The CEO remembered that there is a way to calculate how much the company can tolerate for the additional information. $EVPI = EVUC - EM/$

3.4 The health care manager is quite concerned about the recent deterioration of a section of the building that houses her urgent care operations. According to her analyst assistant, four options merit her consideration: (A) a new building, (B) major structural renovation, (C) moderate renovation, and (D) minor renovations. Moreover, three possible weather conditions could affect the costs of fixing the building within the next six months. Good weather condition has a probability of 0.40; moderate weather with rain has a probability of 0.35, and bad weather has a probability of 0.25.

If good weather materializes, (A) will cost $215,000; (B) will cost $120,000, (C) will cost $90,000; and (D) will cost $56,000. If moderate weather materializes, the costs will be $255,000 for (A); $145,500 for (B); $98,000 for (C); and $75,000 for (D). If bad weather materializes, the costs will be $316,000 for (A); $214,000 for (B); 123,000 for (C); and $119,000 for (D).

a. Build a payoff table.

b. Draw a decision tree for this problem. (Show cost outcomes, probabilities, and EMV for each event node.)

c. Using expected monetary value (rollback procedure), which alternative should be chosen?

d. Calculate and interpret the expected value of perfect information.

3.5 A health care supply chain manager is considering signing a contract with one of three major distributors. The decision is based strictly on cost minimization, and the cost of each contract varies according to the discount negotiated (deep, moderate, or low). The payoff table depicting costs and probabilities (of discount negotiation levels) is shown in Table EX 3.5.

TABLE EX 3.5

Distributor	Cost (in million $) and probability of discounts		
	Deep	Moderate	Low
Alliance/BBMC	68	70	78
	0.20	0.60	0.20
General Medical	69	71	78
	0.30	0.50	0.20
Owens/Minor	71	73	80
	0.40	0.55	0.05

a. Assuming that the health care supply manager is an optimist, which distributor would be chosen?

b. What would be the opportunity loss (cost avoidance) approach to the solution (hint: regrets)?

c. What would be the selection using EMV?

3.6 Draw a decision tree for Exercise 3.5, and use the roll back procedure to solve this problem.

3.7 Given the decision tree in the figure below, which alternative should be chosen?

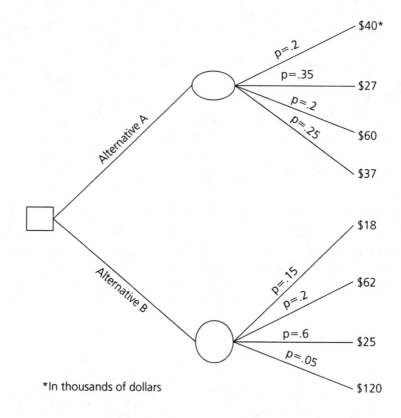

*In thousands of dollars

3.8 The payoff table (Table EX 3.8) shows alternatives for three new product line decisions: Gamma Knife, daVinci Heart Procedure, Prostate Seed Implants, and two states of nature for the demand for these products. Payoffs (revenue) are given in millions of dollars. The health care facility can afford to implement only one of the product lines in the near future.

TABLE EX 3.8

Product Line	State of Nature	
	Medium	High
Gamma Knife	10	40
daVinci Surgical Robot	24	36
Prostate Seed Implants	20	35

a. What is the pessimistic strategy for the new product line?

b. What is the optimistic strategy for the new product line?

c. What would be the Laplace strategy for the new product line?

d. What is the minimax regret solution to this problem?

e. What is the solution for a Hurwitz optimism value of 0.6?

3.9 Probabilities for the state of nature in Exercise 3.8 are estimated as in Table EX 3.9.

TABLE EX 3.9

Product Line	State of Nature	
	Medium	High
Gamma Knife	0.65	0.35
daVinci Surgical Robot	0.60	0.40
Prostate Seed Implants	0.85	0.15

a. Draw a decision tree for the product line decision.

b. Using rollback procedure and EMV, what is the solution to product alternatives?

3.10 The vice president for human resources of a Fortune 500 company located in Richmond, Virginia is about to decide on health benefit options for the employees. The attributes and alternative matrix (Table EX 3.10) has been compiled from responses to a request for proposal (RFP).

a. Use the dominance procedure to select the HMO contract.

b. Use the minimum-attribute-satisfaction procedure to select the HMO contract.

c. Use the most-important-attribute procedure to select the HMO contract.

TABLE EX 3.10

Attributes/ Alternative	HMO Contract #1	HMO Contract #2	HMO Contract #3	HMO Contract #4	Importance Ranking	Minimum Satisfaction Level
Average speed of answer for member/provider calls in seconds	52	45	45	49	3	≤ 45
Percent of calls that are abandoned	5.5%	6.2%	4.5%	5%	10	≤ 5%
Percent of calls getting busy signal (blocked)	13%	11%	9%	10%	11	≤ 10%
Number of workdays it takes to finalize 80% of the claims submitted in a given day	13	10	10	14	7	≤ 10
Percent of claims processed without error (overall, error free for any reason)	97%	98.3%	98.1%	95.6%	8	≥ 98%
Percent of the claims free of financial errors (without under or over payment)	95%	97.9%	98.2%	97%	9	≥ 98%
Percent of response to written inquiries	91%	92%	97%	89%	12	≥ 97%
Medical costs per covered life	390	360	360	425	1	≤ 400
Administrative costs per covered life	105	121	95	98	5	≤ 100
Network breadth (number of providers)	4,700	5,500	5,500	4,500	4	≥ 4,000
Network depth (number of specialty providers)	1,350	1,100	1,400	950	6	≥ 1,000
NCQA Accreditation	Yes	Yes	Yes	Yes	2	Yes
HMO offices locally operated	No	Yes	Yes	Yes	13	Yes

3.11 To guide the decision for buying a new color ultrasound for the radiology department, the attribute/alternative matrix (Table EX 3.11) has been compiled from responses to a request for proposal (RFP).

TABLE EX 3.11

Attributes/ Alternative	Supplier #1	Supplier #2	Supplier #3	Supplier #4	Importance Ranking	Minimum Satisfaction Level
Cost (in $000)	20	18	17	18	10	⩽ 18
Delivery time in weeks	4	3	3	3	7	⩽ 3
Past performance	8	6	7	9	8	⩾ 6
Integration ability	7	8	8	7	5	⩾ 7
Capacity	8	5	7	8	4	⩾ 7
Product's market share	18%	22%	24%	20%	3	⩾ 20%
Reliability	7	9	9	9	1	⩾ 9
Ease of maintenance	8	6	8	8	9	⩾ 8
Ease of use	7	7	9	7	6	⩾ 7
Supplier's financial status	5	7	7	5	2	⩾ 7

Attribute scores reflect ratings of 1 through 10 (10 being best) with the exception of cost, delivery time, and product's market share.

   a. Use the dominance procedure to select the supplier.

   b. Use the minimum-attribute-satisfaction procedure to select the supplier.

   c. Use the most-important-attribute procedure to select the supplier.

3.12 A hometown dialysis center is not able to meet the increased dialysis demand from patients with renal failure. The administration is exploring possibilities by evaluating different alternatives: opening an additional dialysis unit, outsourcing with other dialysis centers, or having some patients do their own dialysis at home after training.

A feasibility analysis showed that opening a new dialysis unit is expected to have a fixed cost of $400,000 and a variable cost of $150 per session. In the case of contracting out with another dialysis center, the cost was found to be $270 per session. The fixed and variable costs of placing patients on self-dialysis, including the training and the equipment, amount to $120,000 and $180, respectively. Patients are charged, according to the Medicare-allowable payment, $350 per session, for an annual total of 104 sessions (52 weeks at two sessions per week). The feasibility study also gave the probabilities for different demand levels. The probability for a monthly average demand of 50 patients is $p = 0.1$; for a monthly average of 75 patients is $p = 0.4$; for a monthly average of 100 patients is $p = 0.3$; and for a monthly average of 125 patients is $p = 0.2$.

The administrator of the center would be expected to evaluate the three alternatives with regard to those demand options, according to the criteria in Table EX 3.12.

TABLE EX 3.12

| | Possible Future Demand | | | |
Alternatives	50 patients	75 Patients	100 Patients	125 Patients
Expansion	640*	1,160	1,680	2,200
Outsourcing	416	624	832	1,040
Self Dialysis Program	764	1,206	1,648	2,090

*in $ 000s.

The monetary payoffs are shown in the body of the table. All the values are displayed in present value terms to make the alternatives comparable. If an expansion is considered, the payoff will vary from $640,000 to $2,200,000 across the four possible states of nature. For outsourcing, low demand will have a present value of $416,000 and higher demand of over $1,040,000. A self-dialysis program would bring in from $764,000 to $2,090,000. The selection of an option depends on the level of certainty with which demand can be estimated. Such certainty rarely exists, especially in health care decisions. But if it does exist, simply choose the best available option (highest profit/least cost) under that state of nature. For example, if the manager is certain that the demand level for the new facility will be low, then the small facility should be built; under moderate demand conditions, a medium facility should be built; and if demand is expected to be high, a large facility should be built. Although complete certainty is rare in such situations, the payoff table offers some perspective for the analyses.

    a. What is the EMV decision?

    b. What is the minimax regret decision?

    c. What is the EVPI?

CHAPTER

FACILITY LOCATION

LEARNING OBJECTIVES

- Recognize the need for location analysis.
- Evaluate alternative location methods and their application to health care facilities.
- Review the Geographic Information Systems (GIS) and their use in health care facility location.
- Develop a facility location using appropriate location analysis.

Locating health services in a community is not an everyday decision for health care managers. However, it is important to study this problem, not so much simply because of its strategic nature, but because, in addition, today's health care facilities are operating in competitive markets, which means that building or relocating new facilities is a strategic decision that cannot tolerate mistakes. A health care facility must not be built where demand is mediocre or will be so. Similarly, the facility must be sized to meet both current and future demand accurately, or the location must have expansion opportunities.

Many complex factors, including an area's population, currently available services, and present and future demand, must be considered in locating health care facilities. For example, R. Timothy Stack, President and CEO of Piedmont Medical Center in Atlanta, Georgia, has stated that Atlanta has a population of 4.2 million living in twenty counties around the city center. Many of these counties are expected to grow by as much as 20 percent over the next five years. By 2025, demand for hospital beds in greater Atlanta is projected to increase by 60 percent, one of the fastest growth rates in the United States.

Equally important to consider, the Atlanta health care market is fragmented. There is no predominant referral hospital and no clear market leaders overall in offering various specialized services. Currently, greater Atlanta has sixty-one hospitals, including a Veterans Affairs Hospital. Furthermore, the city is headquarters of both the federal Centers for Disease Control and the American Cancer Society. In such a growing but complex health care market, the larger facilities are planning to build new hospitals or expand existing ones, as well as adding tertiary programs (R. T. Stack, 2004).

In health care, facility construction faces the hurdle of first obtaining a certificate of need (CON). Deciding on a location does not guarantee a quick start-up, as in retail or fast-food industries. In the health care industry, then, sound forecasting of current and potential demand is indispensable for location decisions. Usually that means examining the primary, secondary, and tertiary markets for the proposed facility, especially for hospitals, whose managers must examine population characteristics such as age, sex, education, employment, and prevailing epidemiological outcomes (Virginia Atlas of Community Health, 2004). The many factors in demand analysis delineate the kind of facility that should be built or relocated to the location(s) under consideration. Examples are the service mix (young population needing OB/GYN and pediatric specialties), technology (extensive cardiac technologies for aged populations), and size.

A market shift of population to other localities (for example, the suburbs) is a major reason for location decisions. As part of marketing strategy, health care facilities want to expand their services to new suburbs by opening satellite locations. Multiple-campus health care facilities are now almost the norm in many markets for hospital chains, IDS, or strategic health care alliances. They also serve to feed complicated cases to the main hospital.

If demand for the current health care facility is strong and growing, and there is enough land and capability to expand it, the facility need not move to a new location unless other factors (such as high operational costs, traffic congestion, and parking facilities) have become significant. On the other hand, a new location decision does become necessary when a facility cannot be expanded because no more land is available to it. If the demand is strong in the current location, facility managers would seek new, additional sites to distribute the supply of health care for the strong demand by opening satellite facilities. However, if the demand has shifted to the suburbs and the current facility is very old, a more appropriate decision would be to build a new facility at a new location.

In all cases, location decisions are strategic, requiring a long-run commitment of the health care organization's resources. To identify acceptable alternatives, both for the physical location and for the method of expansion, using appropriate decision tools as well as analytical skill is necessary.

A location decision for health care managers is generally arrived at through this process: (1) an agreement on the decision criteria for evaluations of alternatives (profit, market share, and community considerations); (2) identification of important factors; (3) development of location alternatives; (4) evaluation of the alternatives; and (5) final selection. Decision criteria should include factors related to the region, the community, and the site that encompass both cost and nonfinancial concerns.

Regional factors include availability of markets or market stakeholders (patients, physicians, payers, and employers). Community factors include the attitudes of citizens to new developments, the availability of and proximity to supporting services (for example, medical staff offices, social services, security, and allied health services), and environmental regulations specific to that community. Site-related factors include land, size and usable area, acquisition costs; existing facilities on the land if they indicate any renovation or demolition costs; access to public and other transportation, roads, and parking; zoning; and CON (Stevenson, 2002; pp. 358–366).

LOCATION METHODS

Various quantitative methods are available to aid location decisions, depending upon the nature of the problem. In this chapter, we present cost-profit-volume analysis, factor rating methods, multi-attribute methods, and the center-of-gravity method; one or more can be used to make an informed decision. No one method may be right for all facility location problems; however, cost analysis is always part of the solution package.

Cost-Profit-Volume (CPV) Analysis

In this method, also known as break-even analysis, health care managers evaluate the fixed costs and the variable costs of building and operating a facility in each of the alternative locations. Of course, the revenues and resulting profits expected to be generated by volume (demand) help to justify the selection of a site. In general, the cost structures of each site, especially the fixed cost, will differ from each other, as will volume. Besides hospitals, examples of facilities that can face location decisions and hence use CPV analysis would be nursing homes, assisted living facilities, independent laboratories, imaging centers (MRI, CAT scan), physician practice (group) offices, and small to medium-size clinics. The CPV analysis assumes one product line at a time for simplicity. For multiple product lines such as hospitals, CPV analysis may be based on Diagnosis Related Groups (DRGs) or on each product; then the analysis can be aggregated to the hospital level. For simplicity, we will examine the use of this method for an imaging facility.

In CPV analysis, the following relationships define the costs and profits:

$$\text{Profit} = \text{Revenue (R)} - \text{Total cost (TC), where}$$
$$\text{Revenue} = \text{Unit Price (p)} \times \text{quantity (Q),}$$
$$\text{Total cost} = \text{Fixed cost (FC)} + \text{variable cost (VC),}$$
$$\text{Variable cost} = \text{variable cost per unit (v)} \times \text{quantity (Q).}$$

More formally,

$$\text{Profit} = R - TC \tag{4.1}$$
$$R = pQ \tag{4.2}$$
$$TC = FC + VC \tag{4.3}$$

and

$$VC = vQ \tag{4.4}$$

or

$$\text{Profit} = (pQ) - [FC + vQ] \tag{4.5}$$

and

$$\text{Profit} = (p - v)Q - FC. \tag{4.6}$$

Analysis may first consider the total cost outcomes; then one performs profitability analysis using possible charges (price) per unit. The above formula can be used to determine the volume for an assumed level of profit:

$$Q = \frac{\text{Profit} + FC}{p - v} \tag{4.7}$$

EXAMPLE 4.1

Imaging using electron beam computed tomography (EBCT) is a technology for diagnosing and evaluating the presence of coronary artery heart disease and diseases of the lung. Keep-Me-Healthy Imaging Company (KMHIC) provides services in fifteen locations across the country and is interested in expanding its centers to other locations. KMHIC expects to collect $300 per unit of service from patients' insurance. The cost information is determined for the next East Coast location with three alternative sites as follows:

Site	Fixed Cost/Year (in Million $)	Variable Cost per Unit	Expected Demand/Year
Baltimore	1.6	$30	15,000
Norfolk	1.5	$40	10,000
Richmond	1.25	$80	8,000

What would be the ideal location based on CPV analysis?

Solution

Calculation of total cost for each of the three sites using formula (4.3) yields the lowest cost for the Richmond site.

Site	$TC = FC + vQ$
Baltimore, MD	$1{,}600{,}000 + 30 \times 15{,}000 = \$2{,}050{,}000$
Norfolk, VA	$1{,}500{,}000 + 40 \times 10{,}000 = \$1{,}900{,}000$
Richmond, VA	$1{,}250{,}000 + 80 \times 8{,}000 = \$1{,}890{,}000$

A sensitivity analysis for involved parameters will further aid decision making. One of the parameters in this case is volume (quantity). Hence, a graphical solution to this problem can provide a comfort zone for the health care manager, based on expected volumes, in deciding which site is more plausible. Figure 4.1 depicts the best sites on the basis of patient volume. If annual volume is fewer than 5,000 patients, from the total cost perspective Richmond is the best site. If the annual expected volume is between 5,000 and 10,000 patients, the lowest costs would occur at the Norfolk site. Baltimore is the best location for patient volumes higher than 10,000 per year. Figure 4.1 traces the lowest total cost curves for each of the volume zones.

When profit is the immediate consideration, using formula (4.6), Profit $= (p - v)$ $Q - FC$, for the same sites, we obtain:

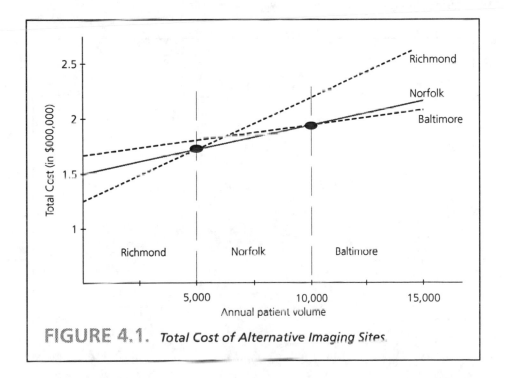

FIGURE 4.1. *Total Cost of Alternative Imaging Sites.*

Site	Profit = $(p - v)\,Q - FC$
Baltimore, MD	$[(300 - 30) \times 15{,}000] - 1{,}600{,}000 = \$2{,}450{,}000$
Norfolk, VA	$[(300 - 40) \times 10{,}000] - 1{,}500{,}000 = \$1{,}100{,}000$
Richmond, VA	$[(300 - 80) \times 8{,}000] - 1{,}25{,}000 = \$\ 510{,}000$

The Baltimore site is almost five times as profitable as the Richmond one. Clearly, two different choices emerge based respectively on total cost and on profit. Although the decision may seem very clear to open the site in Baltimore, if the expected volumes are not realized as forecast, the profit-based decision may not prove to be the best one. To illustrate this graphically, Figure 4.2 imposes the revenue line to the existing total cost for each site. Clearly, no site makes a profit before reaching annual patient volume of 5,770. From this point to 10,000 patients, Norfolk is the most profitable site (has the largest gap between the revenue and the cost line). With over 10,000 patients, Baltimore becomes the more profitable site.

Factor Rating Methods

Factor rating methods are used when site alternatives have to be evaluated on attributes (factors) other than costs (money). Such attributes may be measured on a common scale (scoring from 1–100) or by multiple scales, some of which are not numeric (acceptable, medium, good, and excellent). Thus, this method for evaluating alternative sites varies with information availability and scoring metric.

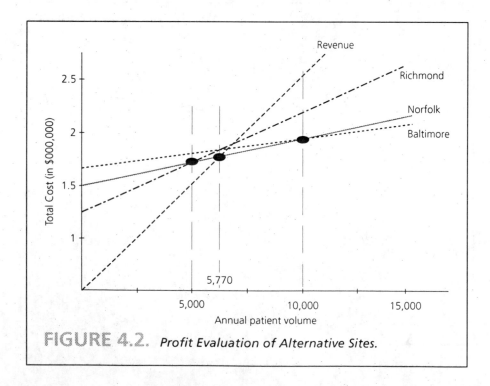

FIGURE 4.2. *Profit Evaluation of Alternative Sites.*

The first step in this methodology is to identify the relevant factors. The next step is to check whether all the factors can be evaluated by the same metric. Third, determine whether for this particular site decision any of the factors are more important than others; if so, either each factor can be ranked, or weights can be assigned to each factor according to its relative importance. Then an analysis of the scores (ranks and weights if applicable) is carried out to identify the best alternative. These analyses may be simple or weighted summations of assigned scores.

EXAMPLE 4.2

A medical center would like to establish a satellite clinic to provide medical care for residents living in recently developed suburbs. Four potential sites are under consideration. Land acquisition, building, and equipment costs have been evaluated, as have population, education level, median household income, and percentage insured. As can be observed from Table 4.1, the factors are reported in different measurement units (metric), so they must be either converted to the same metric or analyzed using the multi-attribute procedures discussed in Chapter Three.

TABLE 4.1. **Factors to be Considered in Establishing a Satellite Clinic.**

	Zip Codes of Potential Sites			
Factors	23059	23233	23112	23832
Land	$350,000	$390,000	$245,000	$200,000
Building	$450,000	$450,000	$435,000	$425,000
Operating	$235,000	$240,000	$220,00	$205,000
Population Size	15,683	50,296	38,660	25,775
Elderly	7%	12%	6%	5%
Education	92%	96%	93%	90%
Income	$73,668	$67,917	$63,519	$61,738
Insured	88.2%	88.6%	88.5%	88.1%

Source for noncost factors: Virginia Atlas of Community Health, 2004.

One way to convert the different scores to the same metric is to rate each site's value for a given factor, relative to each of the others. For example, the most desirable value in land cost is $200,000, at site 23832. In comparison, site 23059, with $350,000, has a score of 57. The score is calculated using formula:

$$Relative\ score = \frac{Most\ desirable\ outcome}{Evaluated\ outcome} \qquad (4.8)$$

and

$$Relative\ score = \frac{\$200,000}{\$350,000} \times 100 = 57.$$

In this example, lower costs; higher population size; higher percentages of those 65 and older, of high school graduates, and of those insured; and higher median income are considered desirable. If the most desirable outcome has the highest value (compared to the lowest, as in costs), the relative score is obtained by reversing the formula as:

$$Relative\ score = \frac{Evaluated\ outcome}{Most\ desirable\ outcome}. \qquad (4.9)$$

For example, the median household income score for site 23233 is:

$$Relative\ score = \frac{\$67,917}{\$73,668} \times 100 = 92.$$

A preliminary evaluation can be done by summing all the relative scores for each site. The site with the highest total score becomes the primary candidate for selection. In this case (shown in Table 4.2), site 23233, with a score of 723, is the best choice.

In this example, all factors, including costs and community, received the same treatment or equivalent weights. However, the relative values of the factors can differ for different decision makers who are choosing sites. For example, cost factors might be considered more important than community factors. Similarly, the importance of the percentage of insured in the community might affect the survival of a clinic more than the percentage of high school graduates (implication of employability) would. In such cases, health care managers may want to assign relative weights to the individual factors. To do so, the least important factor is assigned a score of 1, and the other factors are compared relative to that factor. Let us suppose that the percentage of high school graduates is the least important factor and gets a score of 1. Compared to that factor, median household income is, say, fifteen times as important; the percentage sixty-five and older is five times as important; the percentage of insured is twenty-five times as important; population size is nine times as important; land acquisition and building costs are each twenty times as important; and operating costs are twenty-five times as important. The relative factor scores and weights are displayed in Table 4.3. To calculate their relative weights (importance), each score is divided by the total relative score, in this case 120. As shown in Table 4.3, for example, the

TABLE 4.2. Relative Scores on Factors for a Satellite Clinic.

Factors	Zip Codes of Potential Sites			
	23059	23233	23112	23832
Land	57	51	82	100
Building	94	94	98	100
Operating	87	85	93	100
Population Size	31	100	77	51
Elderly	58	100	50	42
Education	96	100	97	94
Income	100	92	86	84
Insured	100	100	100	99
Sum of Relative Scores	624	723	682	670

TABLE 4.3. Relative Factor Scores and Weights.

Factors	Relative Scores	Weights
Land	20	0.167
Building	20	0.167
Operating	25	0.208
Population Size	9	0.075
Elderly	5	0.042
Education	1	0.008
Income	15	0.125
Insured	25	0.208
Sum of Relative Scores	120	1.00

TABLE 4.4. Composite Scores.

Zip Codes of Potential Sites

Factors	Weights	23059	23233	23112	23832
Land	0.167	57 × 0.167 = 9.5	51 × 0.167 = 8.5	82 × 0.167 = 13.6	100 × 0.167 = 16.7
Building	0.167	94 × 0.167 = 15.7	94 × 0.167 = 15.7	98 × 0.167 = 16.3	100 × 0.167 = 16.7
Operating	0.208	87 × 0.208 = 18.2	85 × 0.208 = 17.8	93 × 0.208 = 19.4	100 × 0.208 = 20.8
Population Size	0.075	31 × 0.075 = 2.3	100 × 0.075 = 7.5	77 × 0.075 = 5.8	51 × 0.075 = 3.8
Elderly	0.042	58 × 0.042 = 2.4	100 × 0.042 = 4.2	50 × 0.042 = 2.1	42 × 0.042 = 1.7
Education	0.008	96 × 0.008 = 0.8	100 × 0.008 = 0.8	97 × 0.008 = 0.8	94 × 0.008 = 0.8
Income	0.125	100 × 0.125 = 12.5	92 × 0.125 = 11.5	86 × 0.125 = 10.8	84 × 0.125 = 10.5
Insured	0.208	100 × 0.208 = 20.8	100 × 0.208 = 20.8	100 × 0.208 = 20.8	99 × 0.208 = 20.7
Composite Score		82	87	90	92

percentage of insured has a weight of .208 (25/120), and land cost has a weight of 0.167 (20/120).

The next step would be to calculate a weighted aggregated score (a composite score) for each site. This is carried out by multiplying factor weights to site scores for each factor and then taking the sum. Table 4.4 illustrates these calculations.

Of the composite scores (weighted sums), site 23832 has the best score. This example demonstrates that weighted scores versus raw scores make a marked difference in site selection decisions.

Multi-Attribute Methods

As was discussed in Chapter Three, this method allows for metric-free selection decisions using dominance, minimum attribute (factor) satisfaction, and—most important—attribute procedures. To illustrate an application of these procedures to site selection, Table 4.5 lists importance rankings and minimum acceptable levels for each factor for the satellite clinic problem presented earlier in the chapter. A health care manager would make the assessments for each factor, together with his or her analytical team.

Dominance Procedure. Dominance is defined as follows: If an alternative site (X) is at least as good as another alternative (Y) on all attributes and strongly the choice at least on one attribute, then alternative X dominates alternative Y.

TABLE 4.5. Satellite Clinic Factor Rankings and Minimum Acceptable Levels.

Factors	Zip Codes of Potential Sites				Importance Ranking	Minimum Acceptable Levels
	23059	23233	23112	23832		
Land	$350,000	$390,000	$245,000	$200,000	3	≤ $350,000
Building	$450,000	$450,000	$435,000	$425,000	4	≤ $450,000
Operating	$235,000	$240,000	$220.00	$205,000	2	≤ $225,000
Population Size	15,683	50,296	38,660	25,775	6	≥ 25,000
Elderly	7%	12%	6%	5%	7	> 5%
Education	92%	96%	93%	90%	8	≥ 90%
Income	$73,668	$67,917	$63,519	$61,738	5	≥ $60,000
Insured	88%	88%	88%	88%	1	≥ 85%

As noted earlier, evaluation of alternatives using dominance procedure views one pair of alternatives at a time, so for many alternatives, many pair-wise comparisons have to be completed. In this example, there are four alternatives, so there will be six pair-wise comparisons. To illustrate the dominance, let's take the first pair of alternatives, 23059 versus 23233. Here, on the first factor, "Land," 23059 is better (lower cost); moving on to the second factor, "Building," both alternatives have equal cost ($450,000); thus we move to the next factor, "Operating," for which 23059 is again better than 23233. "Population Size," however, is greater for 23233 than for 23059; hence, 23059 is no longer better than 23233. There is no need to evaluate the remaining factors for this pair.

The next pair comparison can be made between 23059 and 23112. This pair has similar results: on the first four factors 23112 is better, but on the fifth factor, elderly, 23059 is better, so we stop the comparison of this pair at this point. Moving to the next pair, 23059 versus 23832, our conclusion is the same; on the fifth factor 23832 loses its dominant position.

The comparison of 23233 and 23112 breaks up on the fourth factor, population size. Similarly, in the 23233 versus 23832 comparison, the advantage of 23832 is lost on the fourth factor. The last pair-wise comparison is of 23112 and 23238, where 23112 breaks the advantage of 23832 on the fourth factor.

Hence, using dominance procedure, we cannot select a site. We cannot even eliminate a site as inferior relative to the others.

Minimum Attribute Satisfaction Procedure. Evaluation of alternatives, especially in site selection, often considers minimum acceptable standards. Therefore, when developing site alternatives, analysts and managers often specify these acceptable standards. Evaluation of alternatives, though, is conducted differently than those in dominance procedure. Here, as we saw in the supplier selection example in Chapter Three, pair-wise comparisons are not used; instead, for each factor all alternatives are considered simultaneously. If any alternative does not meet the minimum acceptable standard satisfactory for a given factor, that alternative is eliminated.

In the ongoing satellite site example, starting with the first factor in Table 4.6, "Land," the 23233 site is eliminated since its costs are over $350,000. For the next factor, all remaining sites are satisfactory. For the third factor, site 23059 is eliminated since its operating cost is higher than $225,000. For the remaining factors, both sites have satisfactory scores, so both 23112 and 23832 remain as candidates. Hence, again, there is no unique solution and other procedures can be applied to obtain one.

Most Important Attribute Procedure. When the previous procedures yield no solution, this procedure in most instances will. For our site selection example, the importance of the factors (attributes), as developed by the selection team, is shown in Table 4.7.

Like the minimum attribute satisfaction procedure, this one considers all alternatives simultaneously, beginning with the highest-ranking attribute. If the site's scores for that attribute do not point to a solution, analysis moves to the next ranked attribute. The top ranking attribute here is "Insured." Since all four sites have the same score, the health care manager moves on to the second-highest-ranked factor, "Operating," where 23832 has the lowest cost. Now the others are eliminated and site 23832 is the choice.

TABLE 4.6. Satellite Clinic Factor Minimum Acceptable Levels.

Zip Codes of Potential Sites

Factors	23059	23233	23112	23832	Minimum Acceptable Level
Land	$350,000	$390,000	$245,000	$200,000	≤ $350,000
Building	$450,000	$450,000	$435,000	$425,000	≤ $450,000
Operating	$235,000	$240,000	$220,00	$205,000	≤ $225,000
Population Size	15,683	50,296	38,660	25,775	≥ 25,000
Elderly	7%	12%	6%	5%	≥ 5%
Education	92%	96%	93%	90%	≥ 90%
Income	$73,668	$67,917	$63,519	$61,738	≥ $60,000
Insured	88%	88%	88%	88%	≥ 85%

TABLE 4.7. Satellite Clinic Factor Importance Rankings.

Zip Codes of Potential Sites

Factors	23059	23233	23112	23832	Importance Ranking
Land	$350,000	$390,000	$245,000	$200,000	3
Building	$450,000	$450,000	$435,000	$425,000	4
Operating	$235,000	$240,000	$220,00	$205,000	2
Population Size	15,683	50,296	38,660	25,775	6
Elderly	7%	12%	6%	5%	7
Education	92%	96%	93%	90%	8
Income	$73,668	$67,917	$63,519	$61,738	5
Insured	88%	88%	88%	88%	1

Center-of-Gravity Method

This method is useful when the geographic position of a location is important in terms of distribution of the services or materials. For instance, a multihospital system may want to locate their supply warehouse in a community or region that will minimize the distribution distance based on the volume of transactions from this warehouse to each hospital or clinic. Similarly, locating a specialty laboratory, a blood bank, or an ambulance service may use this method, which is based on minimum distribution costs. The method works with coordinates on a map and shows existing facilities or communities with respect to the proposed new facility.

Figure 4.3 displays the map of the Richmond metropolitan area with seven hospitals of interest, using a coordinate system. Using the map coordinates, their positions are identified in Table 4.8.

Let us locate a blood bank supply center that will serve all seven hospitals. First let us assume that the quantities of blood supplies shipped to each hospital (or the number of shipments) are equal. The center-of-gravity location is calculated by taking the average of x and y coordinates, using the following formulas.

FIGURE 4.3. *Richmond Metropolitan Area Hospitals.*

Source: Street Atlas USA 8.0, DeLorme, Two DeLorme Drive, P.O. Box 298 Yarmouth, ME 04096.

TABLE 4.8.   Selected Richmond Metropolitan Area Hospitals.

		Coordinates	
Hospital ID	Hospital Name	x	y
H1	Bon Secours-St. Francis	1.0	1.0
H2	HCA/CJW Medical Center-Johnston Willis	3.3	2.7
H3	HCA/Henrico Doctors	5.1	6.2
H4	HCA/CJW Medical Center-Chippenham Campus	5.5	2.9
H5	Bon Secours-St. Mary's	5.9	5.4
H6	VCU Medical Center	8.3	3.8
H7	Children's Hospital	7.8	4.9

$$\bar{x} = \frac{\sum x_i}{n} \quad \text{and} \quad \bar{y} = \frac{\sum y_i}{n}$$

where

$\bar{x}$ = x coordinate of blood bank

$\bar{y}$ = y coordinate of blood bank

x_i = x coordinate of hospital i

y_i = y coordinate of hospital i

n = number of hospitals

x = x coordinate of blood bank

y = y coordinate of blood bank.

For the blood bank example:

$$\bar{x} = \frac{1.0 + 3.3 + 5.1 + 5.5 + 5.9 + 8.3 + 7.8}{7} = \frac{36.9}{7} = 5.3$$

$$\bar{y} = \frac{1.0 + 2.7 + 6.2 + 2.9 + 5.4 + 3.8 + 4.9}{7} = \frac{26.9}{7} = 3.8$$

Hence, the blood bank can be located at coordinates 5.3, 3.8, north of H4 (CJW-Chippenham campus).

In reality, of course, the blood bank's interactions with each hospital will not be the same. In Table 4.9 yearly shipments from the blood bank to each hospital are identified as Q.

Inclusion of the frequency of activity between the blood bank and hospitals can be formulated using a weighted average formula as follows:

$$\bar{x} = \frac{\sum x_i Q_i}{\sum Q_i} \quad \text{and} \quad \bar{y} = \frac{\sum y_i Q_i}{\sum Q_i}.$$

Weighted average solution for blood bank would be:

$$\bar{x} = \frac{1.0(460)+3.3(470)+5.1(250)+5.5(480)+5.9(320)+8.3(700)+7.8(120)}{460+470+250+480+320+700+120}$$

$$= \frac{14560}{2800} = 5.2$$

$$\bar{y} = \frac{1.0(460)+2.7(470)+6.2(250)+2.9(480)+5.4(320)+3.8(700)+4.9(120)}{460+470+250+480+320+700+120}$$

$$= \frac{9647}{2800} = 3.4.$$

TABLE 4.9. Selected Richmond Metropolitan Area Hospitals and Their Interaction with the Blood Bank.

| Hospital ID | Hospital Name | Coordinates | | Yearly Shipments |
		x	y	Q
H1	Bon Secours-St. Francis	1.0	1.0	460
H2	HCA/CJW Medical Center-Johnston Willis	3.3	2.7	470
H3	HCA/Henrico Doctors	5.1	6.2	250
H4	HCA100/CJW Medical Center-Chippenham Campus	5.5	2.9	480
H5	Bon Secours-St. Mary's	5.9	5.4	320
H6	VCU Medical Center	8.3	3.8	700
H7	Children's Hospital	7.8	4.9	120

When the number of shipments is considered, the location of the blood bank moves slightly southwest. Figure 4.4 depicts both nonweighted and weighted solutions to the blood bank location.

Geographic Information Systems (GIS) in Health Care

Geographic information systems are valuable tools for storing, integrating, and displaying data for specific geographic areas. Health care managers can use color-coded map systems indicating the levels and types of disease and analyze the associated data on utilization and the potential for health care business in the area. GIS are excellent starting points to identify potential markets for new product lines and are used by other service industries such as banks, retailers, and restaurants.

Health services researchers have been studying and applying GIS for a decade. The Dartmouth Atlas of Health Care, developed by Dartmouth Medical School, provides information helpful to health care businesses of many sorts, including primary care (Goodman and others, 2003). Most notably, National Cancer Institute provides customizable maps at state and county levels for various cancer mortality rates by gender and age-specific groups. The Web site http://www3.cancer.gov/atlas also provides

FIGURE 4.4. *Richmond Metropolitan Area Blood Bank Locations.*

Source: Street Atlas USA 8.0, DeLorme, Two DeLorme Drive, P.O. Box 298 Yarmouth, ME 04096.

comparative geographic analysis in five-year slices. As an example, Figure 4.5 displays county-level cancer mortality rates for the entire United States for white males of all ages, from 1970 to 1994 (http://cancercontrolplanet.cancer.gov/atlas/index.jsp).

Using this information, health care managers can develop new service lines or adjust the current offerings for their service areas.

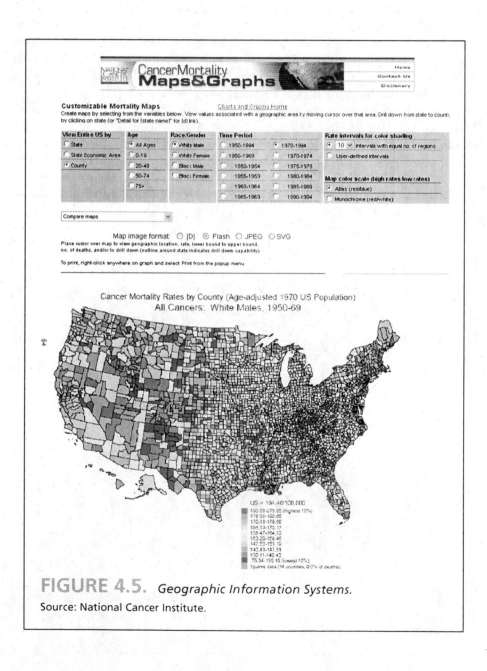

FIGURE 4.5. *Geographic Information Systems.*

Source: National Cancer Institute.

SUMMARY

In this chapter, a discussion of reasons that prompt health care managers to consider new locations for health care facilities is provided. The methodology of location site selection depends on a particular problem and available data. A portfolio of site selection methods—cost-profit-volume analysis, factor rating methods, and center-of-gravity method—and their use were offered as potential tools to health care managers.

KEY TERMS

Cost-Profit-Volume Analysis
Factor Rating
Multi-Attribute Methods

Center of Gravity
GIS.

EXERCISES

4.1 An independent MRI services company wishes to expand their present operation by adding another center. Four locations have been studied. Each potential site would have the same labor and materials costs, of $200 per procedure. The MRIs generate revenue of $375 irrespective of location. Rental and equipment costs per year for the four sites are as follows:

Location A: $525,000

Location B: $585,000

Location C: $480,000

Location D: $610,000.

    a. Determine the volume necessary at each location to realize $2,000,000 in profits, and which location is the most likely candidate.

    b. If the expected volumes of MRIs are, respectively, 15,500; 20,200; 18,300; and 19,200 for locations A, B, C, and D, which location should be chosen?

4.2 A Doc-in-a-Box office, a group of family practitioners, is looking for a new location to expand their services. Three locations are identified with fixed costs. Because of diverse population profiles in each location, patient visits, variable costs, and revenues vary in each location as shown in Table EX 4.2.

TABLE EX 4.2

	A	B	C
Average Revenue Per Patient	60	60	60
Average Variable Cost Per Patient	44	47	45
Average Number of Visits	13,500	12,000	11,500
Fixed Costs in $	120,000	145,000	140,000

   a. Determine the location based on total cost.

   b. Determine the location based on revenue.

   c. Determine the location based on profit.

   d. Determine the sensitivity of the decision in (c) for varying values of visits. (Hint: Draw a graph of cost, revenue, and profit.)

4.3 Urology Associates (UA), a group practice, is seeking expansion of their services to other regions. A health care analyst evaluated six factors to be considered by UA for three locations, as shown in Table EX 4.3.

TABLE EX 4.3

Factors	Weight	Location I	II	III
Access	0.15	80	70	60
Parking	0.25	90	76	72
Building	0.15	88	90	89
Population Density	0.25	94	94	80
Operating Costs	0.10	98	90	82
Proximity of Other Health Care Offices	0.10	96	75	75

Factor scores are based on 0–100 points.

Determine the new UA location based on the three possibilities' composite factor scores.

4.4 WE RESCUE, Inc., a firm providing nationwide ambulance services, intends to expand its service range through a new branch in the suburbs of the mid-Atlantic region. The data were gathered to evaluate three different possible sites: Suburb A, Suburb B, and Suburb C, for the new location. The data include factor ratings, minimum satisfactory level, and importance rankings of each factor (attribute), as shown in Table EX 4.4.

TABLE EX 4.4

Attributes (factors)	Weights	Suburb A	Suburb B	Suburb C	Minimum Satisfaction Level	Importance Ranking
Contracting and land cost	0.1	65*	76	45	70	3
Labor availability and costs	0.15	50	65	60	65	5
Transportation and road network	0.15	60	70	75	80	4

Suppliers/ supporting service companies	0.13	75	60	65	85	6
Average time per emergency trip	0.22	95	75	70	95	2
Accessibility to hospital	0.18	85	80	65	90	1
Employee preferences	0.07	60	50	55	75	7
Total	1.00					
Average revenue per patient visit		50	40	45		
Patient volume		20,000	20,000	20,000		
Fixed cost		200,000	300,000	250,000		
Avg. variable cost per patient		25	18	20		

Factor scores are based on 0–100 points.

   a. Decide which location should be chosen for a new ambulance service location on the basis of the alternatives' maximum composite score.

   b. Determine whether any location dominates the others.

   c. Choose a location based on the minimum satisfaction procedure alone.

   d. Choose a location based on the most important attribute procedure alone.

   e. Choose a location based on cost-volume analysis.

   f. After all the analyses above, which location would you support, and why?

4.5 A contract dispute with the landlord prompted a multichain hospital to reconsider and optimize the location of their regional warehouse for medical supply materials to minimize the time for deliveries to their twelve hospitals in the region. The current warehouse is located at (x 5 3, y 5 3). The coordinates of the hospitals in the region are given in Table EX 4.5.

TABLE EX 4.5

Hospitals	x	y
H1	3	7
H2	9	4
H3	6	9

(Continued)

TABLE EX 4.5 (Continued)

Hospitals	x	y
H4	3	9
H5	8	2
H6	4	1
H7	6	4
H8	5	7
H9	1	8
H10	4	6
H11	10	5
H12	12	3

a. Draw a map showing the positions of the current warehouse and hospitals.

b. Determine the new location of warehouse by using the center-of-gravity method.

4.6 The hospitals identified in Exercise 4.5 vary in size, so the need for medical supplies varies, which affects the number of deliveries for each. The health care supply chain manager determined the number of trips per year to each hospital, as shown in Table EX 4.6.

TABLE EX 4.6

Hospitals	Number of Deliveries
H1	230
H2	280
H3	345
H4	112
H5	235
H6	405
H7	90
H8	370
H9	189
H10	405
H11	109
H12	130

Determine the new location of the warehouse by using the weighted center-of-gravity method.

CHAPTER

FACILITY LAYOUT

LEARNING OBJECTIVES

- Review the importance of layout and its relationship to health care productivity.

- Describe the various layout methodologies and their applications to health care facilities.

- Analyze simple health care layout problems and evaluate their cost effectiveness.

Whenever an existing facility is renovated or a new facility designed, the chance exists to develop a layout that will improve process flow and minimize wasted space. When a new facility is designed, the facility layout should be integrated into the architectural design. Limitations on building lot size and shape, however, may heavily influence the layout configurations available. In other situations, a new layout is achieved simply by renovating an existing area, in which case the size and shape of the area are set, and the limitations relate to the funds available.

Planning facility layout is important for many reasons. The amount of capital invested in new construction or renovation is usually substantial. The results are long-term: While minor modifications may be possible, the overall layout will last well into the future. Furthermore, layout has an enormous effect on daily operations. Not only does layout dictate the distance a patient must travel from one department to another; it also influences which staff members are likely to interact and communicate.

The basic goals in developing a facility layout should be functionality and cost savings. Functionality includes placing the necessary departments, such as the operating and recovery rooms, close together. Functionality also includes keeping apart those departments that should not be together. Overall, functionality includes aspects of a layout that may not be immediately quantifiable, such as facilitating communication and improving staff morale.

Cost savings include reduction in travel times between areas, reduced construction costs by minimizing the space required, and allowing for reduced staffing by placing similar job functions close together. Two key elements of these goals are saving space and reducing the travel distance and time between departments. The amount of space allocated to a given department often is set by factors beyond the control of the facility planner, whose job it then is to make the most of that space. A poorly designed workspace harms both productivity and quality. Another aspect, the travel distance between departments, is a cost that can reach enormous proportions long-term. What may seem a short walk to a designer may add up, over the life of a facility, to days lost to travel. That not only adds to costs but also weakens staff morale.

Facility layout is a complex process with many variables. Given unlimited time, space, and funding, it would be possible to develop and create the optimal layout. Given the constraints on any project, though, layout planning should still provide the best layout possible in any situation—one that can save money, improve the quality of care, and improve staff morale. A good layout will draw on the experiences of the planner, the technical knowledge of the staff who will be using the facility, a strong understanding of how to minimize wasted space and movement, and the forecasts of future needs. Although a planner usually acquires most of these skills, certain technical knowledge of a field is something the facility layout planner may never acquire. A strong understanding of the tools needed to minimize wasted space and movement, however, is readily taught and provides a good background from which to begin a facility layout (Stevenson, 2002; p. 232).

The three basic types of layouts are the product layout, the process layout, and the fixed-position layout. These layouts may be applied to either a single department or an entire facility (group of departments). Therefore, the elements of the layout may be either whole departments or individual pieces of equipment (hospital beds, cafeteria equipment). An actual facility layout is almost always a mixture of the three basic types. A hospital may have an overall process layout as all the departments are grouped (intensive care, nursing units, administration). At the department level, there may be some product layouts (cafeteria, labs), and fixed-position layouts (an operating room).

PRODUCT LAYOUT

The product layout arranges equipment (departments) in the order of product process flow. This type of layout is generally used in a production setting, where services (processes) are standardized and there is little variation, such as an assembly line. A product layout is generally less flexible and requires higher initial equipment cost, but minimizes process cycle time and increases equipment utilization. The product layout might be used for a hospital cafeteria.

The specifics of a product layout are generally determined by the product or service itself. Most of the decisions involve balancing the line so that each station has approximately the same cycle time, the time for one item to pass through that workstation. If one workstation takes much longer than the next, then the second workstation is likely to spend much time waiting for parts from the first. Conversely, if the second workstation takes longer than the first, then the first is likely to spend much time waiting to move parts to the second (Stevenson, 2002; pp. 232–235). Since variability is inherent in patient care, the product layout is rarely useful in health care other than for supporting activities. Although the processes involved in patient care may be common among a group of patients with a similar diagnosis, the amounts of time that patients spend in each process must of necessity vary greatly. A cafeteria line is a common example of a health service industry product layout.

PROCESS LAYOUT

The process layout groups types of processes (departments, equipment, and so on) together to provide the most flexibility. Examples of a process layout can be found in physician offices (group practice), clinics, or hospitals. The hospital groups together functions such as intensive care, surgery, emergency medicine, and radiology as separate departments. This arrangement allows one patient entering through the emergency room to be seen in radiology, possibly surgery, and then intensive care, and another to be admitted directly for elective surgery and then to intensive care. The variability among patients makes such flexibility necessary. Another complicating factor is that it is often not clear when a specific bed will become open, so that scheduling a particular patient for a particular bed may not be possible. The downside of a process layout is high material handling costs. While it is necessary to have the flexibility to move patients from one department to any other department, it saves time to move the patient through adjacent departments along a common path.

Process Layout Tools

The many tools for designing a process layout generally weigh both quantitative and qualitative factors in deciding which departments should be placed closer together. The number of trips that employees make between two departments is a quantitative measure that can approximate the cost of having the two departments far apart. Hazards such as supplemental oxygen and open flames (as in a kitchen) are qualitative factors to consider.

Qualitative factors are easily analyzed in a closeness rating chart, developed by Richard Muther (1962), named systematic layout planning (SLP). The closeness rating chart is essentially a grid that qualitatively assesses the desired closeness between departments. For some departments, closeness may be undesirable. The grid of a closeness rating chart resembles the mileage chart on a map; the rating for department A relative to B is the same as the rating for B relative to A. Codes denote the desired closeness, according to the relative strength of the closeness: A—absolutely necessary, E—very important, I—important, O—ordinary importance, U—unimportant, and X—undesirable. The codes take these factors into consideration: (a) whether similar equipment or facilities are used, or similar work performed; (b) sharing the same personnel, records, and communication; (c) sequence of workflow; and (d) unsafe or unpleasant conditions (Muther and Wheeler, 1962). Different colors for the codes may make the chart more visually effective but are not necessary to the tool. The closeness rating chart may be used to create a block diagram for an effective layout. The chart may also be used to check the effectiveness of a layout that was created using another method or computer tool.

Using a heuristic rule, the first step in assigning departments to available spaces according to desired closeness relationships is to identify the absolutely necessary and the undesirable relationships. That is, all departments with A and X coded relationships would be identified and their workplaces laid out on the available space. Then other departments with E, I, and O ratings would fit in. Let us develop a layout to illustrate this method.

EXAMPLE 5.1

A long-term care facility will be constructed with total available area of 200 × 400 feet, as shown in Figure 5.1. The dimensions of each department and the desired relationships among the departments are depicted in Figure 5.2. A functional layout with the given parameters is desired.

200 ft

400 ft

FIGURE 5.1. *Available Space for Layout of Long-Term Care Facility.*

As can be observed from Figure 5.2, it is important that the patient room area and the ambulance entrance be close to each other. On the other hand, the main entrance is not desired to be close to the laundry facilities or to the ambulance entry. The next parameter is the size of each department (also shown in Figure 5.2), so an algorithm can be applied to provide a solution to the layout, using the closeness rating method. It should be noted that the patient room area will be the space left after other departments are logically laid out according to the closeness ratings algorithm.

Following the heuristic algorithm suggested above, the following A and X relationships are identified: Namely, in A relationships, the nurses' station and the ambulance center, as well as the nurses' station and patient areas, must be adjacent. On the other hand, in X relationships, the main entrance must be away from the ambulance entrance, laundry, and dietary department.

A	X
1–2	2–5
1–3	4–5
	5–6

The next step is to identify the most frequent department in each relationship. In A relationships, the nurses' station (1) appears twice, and in X relationships

Area in feet	Department
40 * 80	1. Nurse's station
40 * 40	2. Ambulance entrance
Remaining space	3. Patient room area
40 * 80	4. Laundry
80 * 80	5. Main entrance
40 * 80	6. Dietary department

A absolutely necessary
E very important
I important
O ordinary importance
U unimportant
X undesirable

FIGURE 5.2. *Closeness Rating Chart for Long-Term Care Facility.*

the main entrance (5) appears three times. Using these departments as a starting base, we can show a draft of the desirability on a layout drawn to scale, as underlined by the A and X relationships. Figure 5.3 displays this start. We should note that the patient room area and the ambulance entrance have E ratings, so they can be close each other. Similarly, the dietary department can be close to the nurses' station. Although there is no unique solution to this problem, a layout solution can be conceived as shown in Figure 5.4.

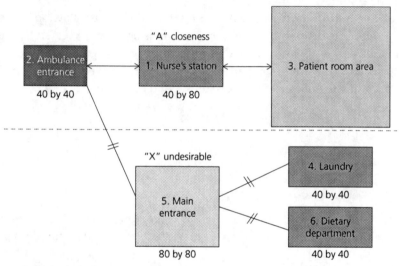

FIGURE 5.3. *A and X Closeness Representation.*

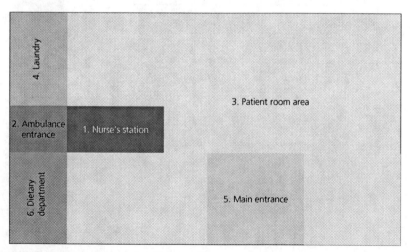

FIGURE 5.4. *Layout Solution.*

Method of Minimizing Distances and Costs

If the objective of the layout is to create efficiencies in functional areas where repetitive processes (nurses walking in hallways to fetch supplies or delivering care for patients) occur, then minimizing the costs or repetitive distances traveled becomes a goal. Data representing such traffic can be summarized in a from-to chart. A from-to chart is generally a table listing the departments to be considered and the number of trips (or flow) between them in a given period. Once such traffic information is identified, those areas with the most frequent interaction may be assigned adjacent to each other, and an initial layout can be generated. However, there may be many possible assignments. If three departments are to be assigned three spaces, there are six possible layouts. This is calculated by factorial formulation, $n!$, where n represents departments. Increasing the number of departments dramatically increases the number of possible solutions. For example, for four departments, $4!$, there are 24 possible assignments.

More formally, D_{ij}, W_{ij}, and C_{ij} represent the distance, interdepartmental traffic, and cost, respectively, between departments i and j. The objective of the layout is to minimize total cost (TC) function, and the problem can be specified as:

$$Minimize\ TC = \sum_{ij} D_{ij}\ W_{ij}\ C_{ij} \qquad (5.1)$$

As with any quantitative tool, however, the layout developed is only as good as the quantitative data used. Care should be taken to make sure that current data are used, though without incurring data acquisition costs greater than the savings to be generated by the design effort. The time period chosen should be long enough to account for fluctuations over time, so that the data represent long-term travel between the departments. This method rarely, if ever, develops an optimal layout, so that may be implemented as the lowest cost that can be obtained by trying different assignments of the departments to the available spaces according to the frequency of interactions (flow), W_{ij}. Almost always, the initial layout will require modification to accommodate qualitative factors that do not show up using the from-to chart. Exhibit 5.1 illustrates a from-to chart for a small hospital, displaying daily interactions, W_{ij}, among six departments.

As noted earlier, for this particular problem there may be $6!$, or 720 possible solutions. If we obtain the distances between departments and assume equal costs (C_{ij}) of flow (for example, nurses' travel times can be converted to cost by using wage information), which layout solution provides the minimal total cost? Let us illustrate this with a simple example.

Computer-Based Layout Programs

Several computer programs can generate the initial possible layouts, using both the from-to chart method and the closeness rating chart. Some of these programs also allow the user to consider travel costs associated with movement between different departments. Most of the programs start with departments in random positions, calculate some relative cost measure, and then move departments in pairs or triplets until the layout with a lower relative cost is found. It is important to note that depending on which method is used, some programs may not necessarily generate an optimal solution. Although computer programs generate only an initial layout from which to start, that is an excellent starting point that may lead to a layout that might not otherwise have been developed.

The most widely used program in this area is Computerized Relative Allocation of Facilities Technique (CRAFT) (Muther and Wheeler, 1962). Excel template provides a CRAFT-based layout where distance, flow, and costs are part of the required inputs. The two most commonly used distance measures between departments can be straight line, also called Euclidian distance or squared Euclidian; and rectilinear distance, known as Manhattan distance, which emulates the streets of Manhattan in New York City. Manhattan distance means that, to go from one place to another, one has to travel up or down, right or left through the streets, rather than crossing to the buildings. Most real-life problems have similar conditions: in order to go from one department to another, one has to walk through corridors, take elevators, and so on, emulating travel in Manhattan. Hence, the rectilinear distance measure will be used in our computerized layout solutions.

The solution to the example of the small hospital problem presented in Exhibit 5.1 is generated using Excel template. For simplicity, we assume that the space available is rectangular and that all departments are equal in size. The available space can hold two departments widthwise and three departments lengthwise. Figure 5.6 shows the data entry, total cost, and alternative layouts that can be generated by user for the problem. After few trials of various assignment scenarios, the best layout with the minimum total cost (TC) of 641 is obtained. This final layout (with assignment of 2, 3, 1, 4, 5, 6) provides 84 units of savings compared to the initial layout (with assignment of 1, 2, 3, 4, 5, 6) at total cost of 725. If this is converted to dollars per year, one can add up the savings to compare against the costs of the layout (being changed from the existing one).

Fixed-Position Layout

The fixed-position layout consists of the fixed service positions where personnel and materials come together to perform the service. In industry, this type of layout is generally used when the product being processed is either too bulky or too delicate to move (such as airplane assembly or spacecraft assembly). In health care, consider that in an operating room the service position is the operating table. In an inpatient hospital room (especially in an intensive care unit) the service position is the patient bed. Generally, designing a fixed-position layout entails positioning several service positions within a given area, each of which may require an adjacent but separate support area (such as a scrub room with an operating room). Developing a fixed-position layout may not be as simple as it seems. Often, conflicts about space constraints and even timing have to be resolved. For example, in an operating room a suspended x-ray machine and overhead lighting may have to be used in the same space.

EXHIBIT 5.1. From-To Chart for a Small Hospital.

A = operating room
B = emergency room
C = outpatient clinic
D = intensive care unit
E = nursing units
F = dietary dept

From \ To	A	B	C	D	E	F
A	-	10	3	42	12	1
B	23	-	0	31	15	2
C	11	1	-	3	5	0
D	38	7	0	-	39	21
E	19	6	4	27	-	36
F	0	3	0	23	35	-

Note that this chart may be condensed to:

	A	B	C	D	E	F
A	-	33	14	80	31	1
B	-	-	1	38	21	5
C	-	-	-	3	9	0
D	-	-	-	-	66	44
E	-	-	-	-	-	71
F	-	-	-	-	-	-

EXAMPLE 5.2

Consider the departments A, B, and C of a small hospital. Assume the distance between the locations 1 and 2 to be 100 feet, between 1 and 3 to be 200 feet, and between 2 and 3 to be 100 feet. Assign these departments to locations 1, 2, and 3 in a rectangular space.

Assuming that on average a nurse can walk 100 feet in 30 seconds and earns $48.00 per hour including fringe benefits, what is the total initial cost of the initial layout? A summary of the information for this problem is shown in Table 5.1. Since there are three departments to be assigned three locations, there are 3! = 6 possible assignment configurations, as shown in Table 5.2.

To make a proper assignment, locations can be organized in pairs based on the minimum distance and the highest departmental flows. Then the highest total departmental flow for department pairs can be calculated as shown in Table 5.3. The department pair A-B/B-A has the highest total flow, at 33 interactions. Hence, it is convenient and logical to place departments A and B to locations 1 and 2, and department C to location 3. So we would choose to implement assignment configuration #1 from Table 5.2.

The next step would be calculation of the total cost (TC) for this configuration. If a nurse can walk 100 feet in 30 seconds, the cost of that walk is 40 cents. (In one hour, there are 3,600 seconds. Hence, 3,600/30= possible 120 such walks; $48/120 = $0.40 per 100-foot walk.)

Table 5.4 summarizes the TC for this configuration. We used a heuristic approach to find this solution. Other configurations (for example, 2 through 6) can be can be calculated, and then the minimum TC among the configurations would be the best solution.

TABLE 5.1. **Distance and Flows Among Three Hospital Departments.**

| | Distance Among Locations | | | Flow Among Departments | | |
| | | Location | | | | Department | |
From/To	1	2	3	From/To	A	B	C
1	–	100	200	A	–	10	3
2	100	–	100	B	23	–	1
3	200	100	–	C	11	1	–

As can be seen, calculating each configuration is computation-intensive, and enormously so when the number of departments increases. For that reason, computer-based solutions for the minimum total cost are desirable. An Excel template solution to this problem is provided in Figure 5.5. The best solution that minimizes total cost is provided by layout arrangement at $2,040.

TABLE 5.2. Possible Assignment Configurations of Departments to Three Locations.

Assignment Configurations	Locations 1	Locations 2	Locations 3
1	A	B	C
2	A	C	B
3	B	A	C
4	B	C	A
5	C	A	B
6	C	B	A

TABLE 5.3. Ranking Departments According to Highest Flow.

Trips Between Locations	Distance in Feet	Department Pair	Workflow	Total Flow
1–2	100	B–A	23	33
2–1	100	A–B	10	
2–3	100	C–A	11	14
3–2	100	A–C	3	
1–3	200	C–B	1	2
3–1	200	B–C	1	

TABLE 5.4. Total Cost of a Layout.

Department	To	Flows	Location	Distance	Distance x Flow $D_{ij} W_{ij}$	Combined $D_{ij} W_{ij}$	Total Cost $D_{ij} W_{ij} C_{ij}$
A	B	10	1–2	100	$10 \times 100 = 1{,}000$	1,600	$1{,}600 \times .4 = 640$
	C	3	1–3	200	$3 \times 200 = 600$		
B	A	23	2–1	100	$23 \times 100 = 2{,}300$	2,400	$2{,}400 \times .4 = 960$
	C	1	2–3	100	$1 \times 100 = 100$		
C	A	11	3–1	200	$11 \times 200 = 2{,}200$	2,300	$2{,}300 \times .4 = 920$
	B	1	3–2	100	$1 \times 100 = 100$		
Total						6,300	$2,520

FIGURE 5.5. *Excel Template Solution.*

Source: Screen shots reprinted by permission from Microsoft Corporation.

FIGURE 5.6. *Excel Template Solution and Final Layout for a Small Hospital.*

Source: Screen shots reprinted by permission from Microsoft Corporation.

SUMMARY

This chapter explored concepts and methods for layout decisions. Improving the layout of a health care facility is one of the methods referred to by reengineering and productivity that are discussed in Chapters Six and Nine. Health care managers should keep in mind that improved layouts that save costs will pay the one-time layout-change costs over the years. A cost-benefit analysis showing such cost recovery is an essential part of justifying such changes as well as making the facility more efficient.

KEY TERMS

Product Layout
Process Layout
Fixed Position Layout

Closeness Rating
From-To Chart
Flow

EXERCISES

5.1 Figure EX 5.1 shows the relationship diagram among the seven sections of a PPO office. The dimensions of the OB/GYN, orthopedics, family practice, pediatrics, and radiology departments each are 200 3 200 feet; the reception area and supply room each are 200 3 400 feet. Arrange these seven departments in a space given as 600 3 600 feet, so that the layout meets the conditions specified in the relationship diagram matrix.

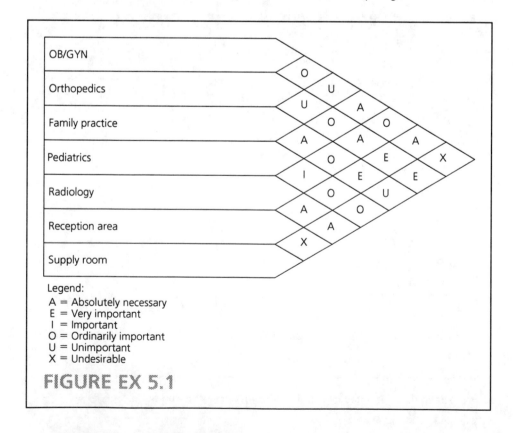

Legend:
A = Absolutely necessary
E = Very important
I = Important
O = Ordinarily important
U = Unimportant
X = Undesirable

FIGURE EX 5.1

5.2 A relationship diagram among nine equal-size sections of a small clinic was developed by the building committee of the organization, as shown in Figure EX 5.2.

Arrange the clinic's sections so they satisfy the rating conditions. The final layout should be arranged as three-by-three equal-size sections where the mechanical room is at the lower right corner of the building, as shown below:

		Mechanical room

5.3 Develop a relationship rating for the nine departments of a new clinic, plus its reception area. The storage and mechanical area has no role in clinical operations, and its location is predetermined.

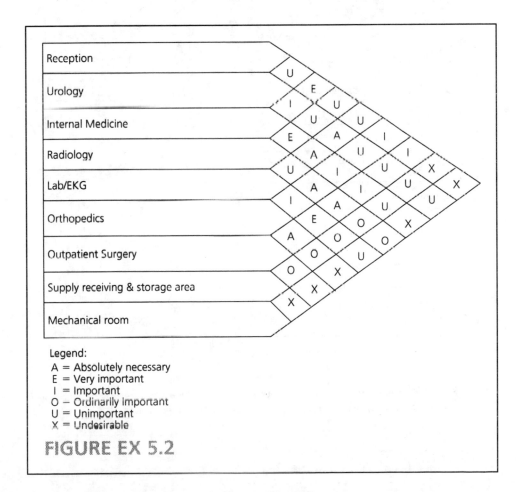

Legend:
A = Absolutely necessary
E = Very important
I = Important
O = Ordinarily important
U = Unimportant
X = Undesirable

FIGURE EX 5.2

Place the clinical departments in the following layout according to the conditions developed in Figure EX 5.3.

	Reception and Waiting Area	
		Storage & Mechanical

Reception & Waiting Area

Neurology

Internal Medicine

Rheumatology

Cardiology

Orthopedics

Outpatient Surgery

OB/GYN

Radiology

Lab/EKG

Legend:
A = Absolutely necessary
E = Very important
I = Important
O = Ordinarily important
U = Unimportant
X = Undesirable

FIGURE EX 5.3

5.4 Table EX 5.4 shows the current and proposed layouts for a group practice. The cost of travel per 1,000 feet is estimated to be $4. Moving departments costs $17,500 each.

TABLE EX 5.4

Current Layout

| Waiting room | Exam room area | Procedure room | Lab/EKG |

Total transportation cost (flow × distance) = 3,225,000

Proposed Layout

| Procedure room | Exam room area | Waiting room area | Lab/EKG |

Total transportation cost (flow × distance) = 2,381,100.

a. What are the efficiency savings of the proposed layout?

b. What is the cost of the proposed layout?

c. In how many years can the cost of the new layout be recovered?

5.5 Determine which placement of departments for a newly designed urgent care center will minimize transportation costs. Assume that it costs $1 to travel a meter. Flow and distance matrices are shown in Table EX 5.5.

TABLE EX 5.5

Distances (in meters) From/To	Women's Center	Behavioral Health	Cardiac Care	Day Surgery	Lab/EKG	Radiology
Women's Center	–	60	120	150	180	210
Behavioral Health		–	60	90	120	180
Cardiac Care			–	30	60	100
Day Surgery				–	30	60
Lab/EKG					–	60
Radiology						–
Trips (per month)	Women's Center	Behavioral Health	Cardiac Care	Day Surgery	Lab/EKG	Radiology
From/To						
Women's Center	–	0	0	2,400	600	1,200
Behavioral Health	10	–	2,650	90	650	800
Cardiac Care	1,260	5	–	30	60	100
Day Surgery	920	0	1,550	–	30	60
Lab/EKG	1,900	300	3,000	930	–	60
Radiology	320	10	1,750	575	60	–

5.6 The administrator of the Vacationers Hospital (VH) recognized the amount of traffic in the corridors. This prompted her to think about possible problems with the current layout. The core work of the patient care is performed in an area 300 3 150 feet, as shown in Table EX 5.6.1.

TABLE EX 5.6.1.

Entrance/Initial Processing	Waiting Room	Exam Room I	150 feet
Exam Room 2	X-Ray	Lab/EKG	↑
Operating Room	Recovery Room	Cast Setting Room	↕ ↓

300 feet

←———————————————————————————→

All rooms (departments) measure 100 feet (length) by 50 feet (width). Walking distance from one department to another is completed by rectangular working patterns. Assuming that a trip originates from the center of a department and terminates at the center of an adjacent department, a person would walk 150 feet (25 feet from the center of the originating department to the hallway, 100 feet on the hallway to an adjacent department, and 25 feet from the hallway to the center of the adjacent department). The results of a six-month-long work sampling study analyzing the movement of VH patients and staff between the departments, averaged per month, are presented in a from-to chart, as shown in Table EX 5.6.2.

TABLE EX 5.6.2. From-To Chart: Monthly Traffic Between Departments (Number Of People in Motion).

	Department	1	2	3	4	5	6	7	8	9
1	Entrance/Initial Processing	.	.	.	.	.	.	.	.	.
2	Waiting Room	1,900	.	.	.	.	.	.	.	.
3	Exam Room 1	1,750	250	.	.	.	.	.	.	.
4	Exam Room 2	1,600	300	900	.	.	.	.	.	.
5	X-Ray	500	675	750	1,005	.	.	.	.	.
6	Lab/EKG	800	650	880	870	400	.	.	.	.
7	Operating Room	375	0	225	300	325	650	.	.	.
8	Recovery Room	0	0	0	0	0	0	1,125	.	.
9	Cast-Setting Room	0	0	0	0	985	525	0	0	.

A consultant informed the administrator that every 1,000 extra feet walked (by either patients or staff) cost $5.50 a month in terms of lost productivity (assuming flows and costs are symmetrical among departments). The objective is to minimize unnecessary walking by changing the location of each department on the basis of traffic data. To move a department costs $20,000 per room, except for lab/EKG, operating room, and x-ray, which cost $75,000 each.

    a.   Determine whether it would be worthwhile to change the layout of the hospital.

    b.   How many years would it take to recover the cost of layout changes?

(Hint: Total transportation costs of this problem can be calculated by using Excel template).

CHAPTER

6

REENGINEERING

LEARNING OBJECTIVES

■ Describe the scope of reengineering applications in health care.

■ Review the work design concepts in health care.

■ Differentiate and apply job enlargement and job enrichment in health care.

■ Develop work measurement by using time standards.

■ Evaluate the design and development of a work sampling study.

■ Analyze bottlenecks by using work simplification tools for health care reengineering.

Adequate organizational performance is a major concern for health care managers. Performance issues generally come to the surface in terms of the financial situation and of market share in competitive health markets. Health care institutions can be classified into three groups in terms of their performance: (1) those that perform adequately with no imminent risk in their finances or market share, (2) those whose performance is marginally adequate, and (3) those whose performance is less than expected. Irrespective of their category, health care institutions must pay close attention to their performance. Declining profit margins, shrinking market shares, high patient dissatisfaction—all are certain indicators of performance problems. Especially, poor performers operating with negative margins are in great need of improvement. Yet, at the other end of the continuum, the benchmark institutions cannot afford to lose their market leadership in either efficiency or effectiveness, which can occur unless they continuously improve their operations.

Health care managers use various methods to improve institutional performance in terms of finances and productivity, but also in the quality of care they provide. To improve financial performance, health care managers have often sought organizational change, restructuring, and downsizing. Although those methods may improve the financial base of the organization or productivity at least temporarily by "cutting the fat," namely by reducing the staff across the board, they create other problems. In particular, reducing staff can lead to major problems in the quality of care. These methods not only violate the basic premise of optimality (they create suboptimal solutions), but also fail to follow the known Pareto principle: "While improving a part of the organization, one should not make other parts of the organization worse off."

Two other contemporary and popular methods that aim to improve both performance and quality are total quality management (TQM) and continuous quality improvement (CQI) (discussed further in Chapter Twelve), which are geared to make incremental changes over time. Thus, realization of their performance gains may take a long time (often five to six years), and success lies with management's commitment to and persistence in this gradual change. During the long implementation processes, management's commitment can become diluted and TQM and CQI can lose their initial lure, ending up in failure. Another reason for TQM and CQI program failures is that responsibility for carrying out its tasks is assigned to only a limited number of people, without organizational commitment across the board (Bergman, 1994).

Reengineering is a methodology intended to overcome the difficulty in realizing TQM and CQI performance over a long duration, as well as the myopic conduct of organizational change, restructuring, and downsizing. Hammer and Champy (1993), who launched the reengineering movement in the early 1990s, suggest a radical redesign of business processes to achieve dramatic improvements in performance measures: quality and cost, service and speed. They urge that conventional wisdom and familiar assumptions be discarded in favor of fresh forward rethinking to design contemporary business processes. In health care, reengineering conceptualizes the delivery process differently, from financing to delivery of the care. Specifically, a strategic view of arranging, delivering, and managing care with new methods is the essence of reengineering health care—change is required across departmental, organizational, operational, and administrative procedures.

An early example of applying reengineering in health care is patient-focused (or patient-centered) care. Think about a hospital that offers patient-focused cardiac care for a patient recuperating from a heart attack or bypass surgery. Caregivers (nursing staff) are trained to perform EKGs and draw blood, so fewer staff care for the patient. That enhances the consistency of patient care and makes the stay as comfortable as possible—elements of the quality of care. Patients also are given one-on-one education about heart disease and cardiac rehabilitation exercise, and their families receive education about their health.

To accomplish patient-focused care, the provider melds cross-departmental functions to address patients' immediate medical care, recovery, and health education. That is a new way of thinking and organizing the health care delivery process, from a set of functional departmental processes to a comprehensive, integrated, and seamless process that is centered on the patient.

Reengineering should eliminate delays and duplications in health care delivery, so recovery is speeded and costs are reduced. New health care delivery processes have to be designed with the cooperation of systems engineers, clinical care professionals, and administrators alike, to eliminate unnecessary tasks and automate any tasks that lend themselves to automation. The new processes may require new skill sets for employees who must handle automation or other information technology components of the new system. Thus employees must be retrained if they are to provide the comprehensive, undisruptive care described in the cardiac care example above. The assumption is that highly technically specialized caregivers can also perform informational and educational tasks of patient care; that with the help of technology, tasks can be redefined with no additional burden. The goal is to break down "silo" mentality among the departments by examining such common processes as admissions, scheduling, and discharge plans to serve patients in a less fragmented and more comfortable way. This aim is especially important in reengineering the processes of such ancillary departments as housekeeping, foodservice, pharmacy, and supply chain.

To reengineer the system, health care managers must be able to understand work-design, jobs, job measurement, process activities, and reward systems, all well-known concepts of industrial engineering. With that knowledge, they can recognize the bottlenecks in the old system, identify unnecessary and repetitive tasks, and eliminate them in the reengineered system of care. Beyond those skills, however, the structure of the health care organization, the roles of managers and the people in processes, and especially their culture, beliefs, and values must be taken into account, as these factors, too, influence the chances of success for a reengineering project. One can conceptualize this as adding value to service process without adding additional resources to achieve waste-free health care delivery system. This is also known as "Lean in Health Care."

Note, moreover, that once processes are reengineered, health care managers must continue reengineering to lead their organizations in the market.

WORK DESIGN IN HEALTH CARE ORGANIZATIONS

As part of reengineering, administrators of health care organizations must recognize the power of human resources management. Considering that more than 40 percent of a health care organization's expenses are expenditures for manpower, the need to manage that resource is obvious. Furthermore, with the aging population and the resulting intensity of tertiary care, the overall proportion of a health care facility budget devoted to labor is likely to grow.

Management of human resources can be difficult. However, ensuring the productivity and satisfaction of clinical staff is not guided only by the ability to deal effectively with employees. Human resources management must start by understanding the work environment and particularly the design of the work itself. An operations perspective emphasizes that the work design must be such that employees are satisfied, organizational productivity is high, and costs are minimal.

Work Design

Work design consists of job design, work measurement, work simplification, and worker compensation (see Figure 6.1). The remainder of this chapter discusses these components, with particular emphasis on work measurement.

Work design is influenced by other areas of the organization. For instance, regulatory requirements, such as reporting work accidents to the Occupational Safety and Health Administration (OSHA), require time from staff members that must be accounted for when developing a time standard; a process layout or the structure of product line management may require a broader job description; automation of processes can eliminate certain aspects of the job description. Then, too, work design also affects the other areas. If the job description is not understood by employees, dissatisfaction results and productivity suffers; or enlarging a job may motivate workers and increase their satisfaction. Finally, the above four components of work design affect each other. For example, the range of job tasks determines the amount of time needed to do the job and is often directly related to compensation.

The previous discussion examines decisions about work design from a systems perspective. However, health care managers must be careful not to make the decisions in isolation. They must realize the importance of the system-wide consequences of their decisions and carefully undertake analysis to consider alternative solutions.

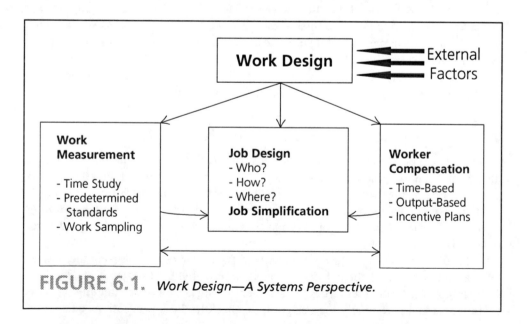

FIGURE 6.1.   *Work Design—A Systems Perspective.*

Job Design. Who is responsible for what tasks? How are they supposed to do their job? Where will they do their job and under what conditions? These are the important questions to answer when designing a job. The primary goal is to create a work system that promotes productivity, efficiency, and effectiveness while balancing costs and benefits for both the individual worker and the organization as a whole.

To be successful, job design must be consistent with the health care organizations' goals and must be in written form; it should be understood by both management and employees. The job of work design should be undertaken by experienced personnel who realize the intricacies involved. One of the most important sources of information when developing a job description and its responsibilities, for new jobs but particularly for job revisions, is the employee. Managers and coworkers also should be included in the design process.

Over time, the management principles guiding the design of jobs have changed considerably. A century ago, the management techniques concentrated on improving the productivity of an organization by standardizing labor practices. Frederick Winslow Taylor's scientific management approach (1911) relied on time studies. Taylor claimed that conflicts between management and labor arose because management did not realize how long jobs actually took. He stressed the need to collect reliable data on work times to improve productivity and efficiency. There is little doubt that his analytical, efficiency-oriented approach was very much a reaction against the wastefulness and expense of turn-of-the-century labor practices.

The work of Taylor was expanded by others, including Frank and Lillian Gilbreth with their emphasis on motion studies. Work measurement and simplification were then introduced and practiced by many manufacturers. Work was divided, labor was specialized, and parts were standardized. The result was a boom in United States productivity, particularly in manufacturing and agriculture. The goal of the scientific management or efficiency school was ultimately to collect reliable data on the work performed and use the data to design more efficient work methods and systems. The approach worked best with routine, predictable, repetitive, and separable tasks.

Does the scientific management approach have health care applications? After all, the delivery of patient care is by no means routine, predictable, or standard. In fact, however, the principles have been applied to certain areas in health care. Of course, in any organization, there are routine and predictable activities, particularly among lower-level administrative duties. Even the development of the various levels of health care professionals—medical doctors (MDs), nurse practitioners (NPs), registered nurses (RNs), licensed practical nurses (LPNs), and nursing assistants (NAs)—is an example of the division of labor. Forms and paperwork have been standardized; information systems allow the automation of routine and predictable tasks; robots have been used in radiology and laboratory departments to perform nonjudgment tasks. Nonetheless, many responsibilities of health care personnel do not lend themselves straight-forwardly to scientific management principles, being unpredictable and requiring the exercise of judgment. Moreover, they often involve interacting with the patient who is not an object.

Aspects of scientific management that are particularly useful in health care, however, are work sampling and time measurement to identify, understand, and standardize the predictable parts of a job. The uses of those tools are discussed in the next section.

The behavioral management school, also called the human relations school, developed as an alternative to the systematic and logical emphasis of the efficiency school. Behavioral management focuses on satisfying the needs and wants of the employee. Its supporters reject a focus on technical efficiency as the overriding consideration in designing work systems. Rather, motivation of the workers, particularly intrinsic motivation, is viewed as the best way to improve productivity and worker satisfaction. Specialization, meaning a narrow scope of duties is claimed to create monotonous jobs that instill a sense of worthlessness in workers, resulting in low morale and high absenteeism. In health care, those dangers apply primarily to support, not professional, personnel.

The behavioral school believes that jobs can be improved through job enlargement, rotating jobs, and job enrichment. Job enlargement means giving the worker a larger proportion of the total task as horizontal loading, adding work at the same level of skill and responsibility. For instance, a nurse might be made responsible for patients in several departments. Job rotation, though important in industries (for instance, amusement park workers) is less applicable in health care, where licensing and professional requirements aim to protect the patient. Job enrichment has employees add the responsibility of planning and coordinating their tasks: vertical loading by increasing the worker's responsibilities. Job enrichment is especially common in health care. For instance, nurses are often given the responsibility of leading a continuous quality improvement program or sitting on marketing and strategic planning committees. Job enrichment aims to motivate employees by increasing their responsibilities and—importantly—their autonomy. As Herzberg (1959) puts it, increasing satisfiers (motivators) and holding dissatisfying factors (hygiene factors) constant should lead to more content workers and thus to greater productivity.

The behavioral approach to job design has serious drawbacks. First, studies have shown only a weak direct link between satisfaction and productivity. Dissatisfaction does tend to reduce productivity but only indirectly by increasing absenteeism and turnover, both of which are very costly for the organization: not only in monetary costs (for example, the necessity to hire an agency nurse at a premium wage) but also by hurting staff morale, interrupting the continuity of care, and in short, harming the quality of care. However, an organization focused primarily on improving worker satisfaction may actually find productivity decreasing while costs continue to increase. In that case an organization cannot compete successfully in a health care market that, because of factors such as managed care, emphasizes mostly profit margins; and that because of increased competition, stresses efficiency. Finally, the behavioral model fails to consider the technological aspects of the organization.

What is needed is a blending of the efficiency and behavioral schools in a socio-technical approach (see Figure 6.2). The socio-technical approach seeks both technological and sociological benefits, recognizing the choice of technology and technological changes: layout redesign, automation, and implementation of new techniques influence the social

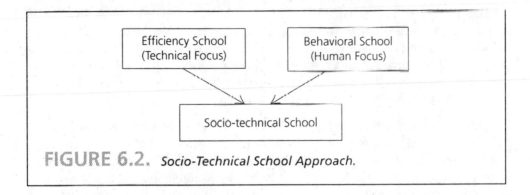

FIGURE 6.2. *Socio-Technical School Approach.*

structure of the organization and thus ultimately worker satisfaction and productivity. Job design must be consistent with both technological efficiency and the organization's social structure. As for job enrichment, task variety, skill variety, task autonomy, and feedback are all very important. However, the socio-technical approach goes one step further: it gives workers a say about what work is done and how it is done. A potential problem, however, can be managers who are reluctant to entrust any of their authority to their workers.

Another important aspect of work design is attention to working conditions. The physical environment can significantly affect worker performance, the quality of health care, and workplace accidents. Aspects of the working environment that should be considered include safety, temperature (60–70 degrees preferred), humidity, ventilation (particularly important in the operating room), colors (could you work in a hospital with red walls?), and noise, as well as pattern of work breaks. Of course, workplace regulations must be met.

Work Measurement Using Time Standards

Now that we know how the job is done, it is important to know how much time it takes to complete the job. Do you know what all the nursing personnel in your organization are doing and where they spend their time? Does a particular physician take three times as long to do his paperwork as the others in his group practice? Time standards are important in establishing productivity standards, determining staffing levels and schedules, estimating labor costs, budgeting, and designing incentive systems.

A time standard is the length of time it should take a qualified worker to complete a specified task, working at a sustainable rate, using given methods, tools, equipment, and raw materials, and facing similar workplace conditions. The abilities and skills of workers will vary and so will the conditions under which they work, so adjustments must be made for those factors. The health care manager must develop a time standard for each job, to estimate the number of employees needed to do it and also to measure their productivity.

When establishing a time standard, it is essential to capture every aspect of the job and also every factor that may influence it. A change in any of those aspects and factors shown in Figure 6.1 can change the time needed. For instance, if a robot is introduced into the lab to sort and label test specimens, the time needed for lab personnel to sort and label will be reduced, giving them more time for other work. Whenever a significant change in procedures or technologies is made, the time standard should be updated with a new study. There are three common methods of work measurement based on time standards: stopwatch time studies, historical times, and predetermined data, each of which is discussed below.

Stopwatch Time Studies. A stopwatch time study bases the time standard observations of one worker taken over a number of trials (cycles). Introduced by Frederick Taylor, time studies are now the most widely used method of work measurement (Stevenson, 2002; p. 324). A time study begins by identifying the task to be studied and informing those who work on it about the study. It is essential to explain the study to those being observed, to avoid misunderstandings and suspicions. Honest explanations can eliminate workers' fears and gain their cooperation, avoiding the Hawthorne effect. The next step is to decide on the number of cycles to observe. The number should be based on: (1) the variability of the observed times, (2) the desired accuracy, and (3) the desired level of confidence for the estimate.

Determination of Number of Cycles (Sample Size). Desired accuracy may be explained by the percentage of the mean of the observed time. For instance, the goal may be to achieve an estimate within 10 percent of the actual mean. The sample size is then determined by:

$$n = \left(\frac{zs}{a\overline{x}} \right)^2 \qquad (6.1)$$

where

z = number of standard deviations to achieve desired confidence level
s = sample standard deviation
a = desired accuracy
$\overline{x}$ = sample mean
n = sample size

Sometimes desired accuracy is expressed as an amount (for example, within one-half minute of the true mean). The formula for sample size then becomes:

$$n = \left(\frac{zs}{e} \right)^2 \qquad (6.2)$$

where

e = amount of maximum acceptable error.

To make an initial estimate of sample size, one should take a small number of observations and then compute the mean and standard deviation to use in the formula for n.

EXAMPLE 6.1

A health care analyst wishes to estimate the time required to perform a certain job. A preliminary stopwatch time study yielded a mean of 6.4 minutes and a standard deviation of 2.1 minutes. The desired confidence level is 95 percent. How many observations will be needed (including those already taken) if the desired maximum error is:

a. +/– 10 percent?

b. one-half minute?

Solution

a. Using formula (6.1) and z = 1.96 (see Appendix A), we get:

$$n = \left(\frac{1.96 \times 2.1}{0.10 \times 6.4} \right)^2 = 41.4 \text{ or } 41.$$

b. Similarly, using formula (6.2), we get:

$$n = \left(\frac{1.96 \times 2.1}{0.5} \right)^2 = 67.8 \text{ or } 68.$$

Once the cycle (sample size) is determined, observations can be made; the activity is timed and the standard time computed.

To compute a time standard, three times must be calculated—observed time, normal time, and standard time. The observed time is the average of the observed times:

$$OT = \frac{\sum x_i}{n} \tag{6.3}$$

where

OT = observed time
x_i = observed time for worker i
n = number of observations for worker i.

This average observed time must be adjusted for worker performance to yield normal time. Normal time is the observed time multiplied by a performance rating. That is done by multiplying the observed time by the performance rating that has been established for the entire job.

$$NT = OT \times PR \tag{6.4}$$

where

NT = normal time
OT = observed time
PR = performance rating

Note that this formula, (6.4), assumes that a single performance rating has been made for the entire job. A job, however, is defined as a combination of elements or tasks, and each task may have a different performance rating. For instance, if we are measuring the time it takes to obtain a clinical test result, the job is defined simply as the time it takes from test completion to charting the result. However, that job has many elements: transport of the test sample to the lab, labeling the specimen, conducting the test, recording the results, and transferring the results back to the patient's room or physician. Each element, or task, that composes this job may have a different performance rating. In this case, the normal time equals:

$$NT = \sum E_j \times PR_j \qquad (6.5)$$

where

NT = normal time
E_j = the observed time of element j
PR_j = performance rating of element j

The performance rating adjusts the observed time for the time of an average, or "normal," worker's pace. When being observed, a worker may pursue his own interests by purposely slowing the pace so that the new standard will be easier to meet. The worker being observed may be below or above the natural ability or skill level of his or her coworkers. A normal rating equals 1.0. Therefore, a performance rating above one is given to a faster-than-average worker, a rating of less than one to a worker whose pace is slower. As could be expected, because the performance ratings are subjective, they often cause conflict between the workers and their management.

Normal time represents the amount of time it takes a worker to perform the job without interruption or delay. But no one can be asked to work 100 percent of the time. Personal needs (for example, going to the bathroom and required rest breaks) and unavoidable delays (such as technological problems or waiting for a medical record) are inevitable. Thus, the normal time is adjusted by using an allowance factor, to provide a standard time:

$$ST = NT \times AF \qquad (6.6)$$

where

ST = standard time
NT = normal time
AF = allowance factor

There are two ways to compute the allowance factor. Allowances can be based on job time, where:

$$AF_{job} = 1 + A \qquad (6.7)$$

where A equals the allowance factor based on job time.

This formula is appropriate when the various jobs in a health care organization require different allowances. However, if jobs cannot be differentiated or are similar, the factor can be based on a percentage of time worked:

$$AF_{day} = 1/(1-A) \qquad (6.8)$$

where A equals the allowance factor based on a workday.

Typical allowance factors for working conditions are found in Table 6.1.

The time study method of work measurement has several limitations: the performance and allowance ratings are subjective; only those jobs that can be observed can be studied. That makes it difficult to study administrators' or managers' work, or creativity-oriented or intense mental processes. Time measurement is most

TABLE 6.1. **Typical Allowance Percentages for Varying Health Care Delivery Working Conditions.**

Allowance Level	Percent
1. Basic-low (personal, fatigue, standing)	11
2. Basic-moderate (basic-low and mental strain)	12
3. Basic-high (basic-moderate and slightly uncomfortable heat/cold or humidity	14
4. Medium-low (basic high and awkward position)	16
5. Medium-moderate (medium-low and lifting requirements up to 20 lbs.)	19
6. Medium-high (medium-moderate and loud noise)	21
7. Extensive-low (medium-high and tedious nature of work)	23
8. Extensive-medium (extensive-low and with complex mental strain)	26
9. Extensive-high (extensive-medium and lifting requirement up to 30 lbs.)	28

Source: Adapted from B. W. Niebel, 1988.

EXAMPLE 6.2

The nursing unit manager at HEALTH FINDER HOSPITAL wants to evaluate the activities in the patient care unit. The manager hired an analyst, who timed all the patient care activities for this job, which has twenty elements. The observed times (OT) and the performance ratings for six samples of a particular employee are recorded in Table 6.2. From those measurements the nursing manager wants to know the standard time for the whole job with its 20 tasks with extensive-medium level allowance. Assume that nursing tasks differ from other clinical and ancillary operations.

Solution

Table 6.3 displays the calculations summary for all 20 job elements involved in nursing care. Column (4) is the average of the six observations from column (3). Column (5) uses the normalizing formula (6.5):

NT = Sum of [(Avg. time for element j) × (Performance rating for element j)]

To calculate the standard time, an allowance factor should be determined using Table 6.1, in this case 26 percent.

The allowance factor for this job:

$AF_{job} = 1 + A = 1 + 0.26 = 1.26$.

Finally, the standard time for the nursing activities:

$ST = NT \times AF = 243.49 \times 1.26 = 306.80$ minutes or 5.1 hours.

effective for short, repetitive tasks. Time studies are prohibitively expensive for irregular or infrequently occurring tasks, they disrupt worker routine, and workers may resent them.

Standard Elemental Times and Predetermined Standards. Standard elemental times (historical times) are developed from the organization's historical time data. Over time, health care organizations can accumulate elemental times for certain tasks that are common to many jobs. These elemental times can then be combined to develop job times. Use of standard elemental times costs less and doesn't disrupt work. However, times taken from the files may be biased or inaccurate, or the files may not have all the elemental times needed for entire jobs. The applicability of elemental times to the complex job designs in health care is limited.

TABLE 6.2. Observed Times and Performance Ratings for Nursing Unit Activities.

Nursing Unit Activities	Performance Rating	Observed Time in Minutes					
		1	2	3	4	5	6
1. Patient assessment	1.08	12	11	12	9	13	12
2. Care planning	0.95	9	7	6	8	7	9
3. Treatments	1.12	8	8	7	9	10	11
4. Medication	1.05	4	3	4	5	6	4
5. Collecting blood/lab specimens	1.10	8	7	6	9	10	7
6. Passing/collecting trays, snacks, feeding patients	1.20	18	21	18	19	21	20
7. Shift report	0.97	5	6	5	7	8	6
8. Charting/documentation	0.98	8	5	6	8	9	10
9. Responding to patients' call lights	1.15	4	3	3	5	6	5
10. Staff scheduling phone calls	0.95	5	4	4	5	6	7
11. Phone calls to/from other departments	0.96	6	5	5	4	6	7
12. Transporting patients, specimens, etc.	1.05	9	11	12	11	9	10
13. Patient acuity classification	1.11	5	6	5	6	7	4
14. Attending educational in-services	1.00	75	75	75	75	75	75
15. Order transcription and processing	0.94	5	6	4	6	7	6
16. Ordering/stocking supplies and lines	0.98	6	4	5	6	7	4
17. Equipment maintenance and cleaning	0.95	9	11	8	9	11	10
18. General cleaning/room work (garbage, making beds)	1.15	12	9	12	10	9	11
19. Assisting with the admission process	1.06	11	9	10	9	8	9
20. Breaks/personal time (not including lunch)	1.00	15	15	15	15	15	15

TABLE 6.3. **Observed and Normal Time Calculations for Nursing Unit Activities.**

(1) Nursing Unit Activities	(2) Performance Rating (PR)	(3) Sample Observed Times in Minutes						(4) Observed Time (OT)	(5) Normal Time (NT) OT * PR
		1	2	3	4	5	6		
1. Patient assessment	1.08	12	11	12	9	13	12	11.50	12.42
2. Care planning	0.95	9	7	6	8	7	9	7.67	7.28
3. Treatments	1.12	8	8	7	9	10	11	8.83	9.89
4. Medication	1.05	4	3	4	5	6	4	4.33	4.55
5. Collecting blood/lab specimens	1.10	8	7	6	9	10	7	7.83	8.62
6. Passing/collecting trays, snacks, feeding patients	1.20	18	21	18	19	21	20	19.50	23.40
7. Shift report	0.97	5	6	5	7	8	6	6.17	5.98
8. Charting/documentation	0.98	8	5	6	8	9	10	7.67	7.51
9. Responding to patients' call lights	1.15	4	3	3	5	6	5	4.33	4.98
10. Staff scheduling phone calls	0.95	5	4	4	5	6	7	5.17	4.91
11. Phone calls to/from other departments	0.96	6	5	5	4	6	7	5.50	5.28
12. Transporting patients, specimens etc.	1.05	9	11	12	11	9	10	10.33	10.85
13. Patient acuity classification	1.11	5	6	5	6	7	4	5.50	6.11
14. Attending educational in-services	1.00	75	75	75	75	75	75	75.00	75.00
15. Order transcription and processing	0.94	5	6	4	6	7	6	5.67	5.33
16. Ordering/stocking supplies and lines	0.98	6	4	5	6	7	4	5.33	5.23
17. Equipment maintenance and cleaning	0.95	9	11	8	9	11	10	9.67	9.18
18. General cleaning/room work (garbage, making beds etc.)	1.15	12	9	12	10	9	11	10.50	12.08
19. Assisting with the admission process	1.06	11	9	10	9	8	9	9.33	9.89
20. Breaks/personal time (not including lunch)	1.00	15	15	15	15	15	15	15.00	15.00
								234.83	243.49
								Job—OT	Job—NT

Predetermined standards, which are obtained from published data, have these advantages: (A) standards are based on repeated observations of a large number of employees in an industry; (B) no performance rating or allowance factor has to be obtained and operations are not interrupted; and (C) standards can be established before the job is even performed (Stevenson, 2002; p. 329).

The best-known standards are those of the MTM (Methods-Time Measurement) Association. A more detailed discussion on sources and uses of predetermined standards is found in Chapter Nine, on productivity.

Work Measurement Using Work Sampling

Work sampling is a technique for estimating the proportion of time that a worker or machine spends on various activities. Work sampling does not require direct timing of an activity. Rather, observers make brief observations of a worker or machine at random intervals over a period of time and simply record the nature of the activity (Stevenson, 2002; p. 331). The resulting data are simply counts of the number of times that each category of activity or nonactivity was observed. Table 6.5 is an example of a tallying sheet for a work sampling study in a nursing unit. Work sampling has two purposes: to estimate the percentage of unproductive or idle time for repetitive jobs, and to estimate the percentage of time spent on the various tasks in nonrepetitive jobs — for example, estimating the time an RN spends on direct, on indirect, and on professional or nonprofessional tasks of patient care.

Work sampling has several advantages over time study. The observations are spread over a period of time, so results are less susceptible to short-term fluctuations. There also is little or no work disruption, and workers are less resentful. Work sampling studies are less costly and less time-consuming, and many studies can be conducted simultaneously. Observers do not need extensive skills, as long as they are trained properly to conduct the observation.

Despite the advantages, there are certain shortcomings of work sampling studies. First of all, they provide less detail on the elements and tasks of a job and often no record of the worker's method. Sometimes workers alter work patterns, which invalidates the results. If observers do not adhere to the random observation schedule, that further taints results. Work sampling studies should not be used for short, repetitive tasks.

The results obtained from a work sampling study of patient care tasks might enable a health care manager to usefully restructure the work in the nursing units. For example, if observations show that RNs are performing a high percentage of nonprofessional or indirect job activities (for example, changing sheets on an empty bed or emptying a bed pan), these activities could be assigned to employees with lower skill levels, since the tasks do not involve judgments about patient care. Thus costs would be lowered, and perhaps quality of care might be improved: non-RN employees earn less; and by directing RNs from nonprofessional, indirect tasks to direct and professional tasks, perhaps patients would receive more professional attention. Table 6.4 shows a small portion of the patient care tasks that are classified as professional, nonprofessional, direct or indirect care.

TABLE 6.4.   Abridged Patient Care Tasks in a Nursing Unit.

Patient Care Tasks	Professional	Nonprofessional	Direct	Indirect
1. Ace bandage application	*		*	
2. Admit — patient orientation	*		*	
3. Assist to/from bed, chair	*		*	
4. Bed bath	*			
5. Bed change — empty		*		*
6. Bed change — occupied	*		*	
7. Bed pan		*		*
8. Blood pressure	*		*	
9. Catheterization of bladder	*		*	
10. Census count		*		*
11. Charting	*		*	
12. Bowel control training	*		*	

To conduct a work sampling study, a health care manager or analyst must first clearly identify the work situation and its work force or the equipment that is to be observed. Once the target area of study is identified, then the number of times the work or equipment should be observed must be decided. The number of observations must statistically represent what actually takes place even when observations are not being made.

The methodological difference between a work sampling study and time study can be compared to thus: taking still pictures of a work situation and then observing different still pictures from different time frames versus videotaping the work situation, hence making continuous observations. However, it is possible, by taking enough still pictures, to reach conclusions that are statistically representative of that work situation. Because time studies require more resources than work sampling studies do, a work sampling study with a statistically representative sample could help health care managers capture necessary information quickly and more cheaply, as well as with less resentment from the staff. Table 6.5 is an example of a form collecting work

TABLE 6.5. Work Sampling Data Collection Form for Nursing Unit.

Unit: 4W   Observer: CL   Date: 11/02/05

Shift: A.M.   Time: 10:04

Observed Staff Name & Title	Prof. Direct	Nonprof. Direct	Prof. Indirect	Non-Prof. Indirect	In Communication with			On Break
					Patient	Staff	Physician	
G. Smith, RN	✓							
V. Black, RN	✓				✓	✓		
E. Masor, RN			✓					
Z. Sardee, RN		✓						
P. Bills, RN	✓						✓	

sampling data to estimate the proportions of direct, indirect, professional, and nonprofessional care in a nursing unit.

In order to collect data appropriately, the observers who collect the data must be trained to assess the nature of the work using a list of items from Table 6.4. (The complete list contains over 120 items.) An observer going into a nursing unit should be able to identify the patient care tasks done by nurses as either professional or nonprofessional, and either direct or indirect patient care.

Training Observers The selection of the observers and their training are important parts of work sampling. A balance between the costs and the expertise of the observers must be considered. For many activities, clerical workers, secretaries, and even local university students can be used. However, some observations require appropriate skill levels. For instance, a student would not produce valid and reliable results if he were to record specific direct care procedures for which an RN would have the skill to collect the data. A reliance on nurses for data collection is also warranted for observations in areas that may present a hazard to nonhealth personnel, for instance, the ICU or certain psychiatric settings.

A comprehensive training program of three steps should be standardized for all data collectors. Data collectors should be first educated as to the study's goals, protocol, collection procedures, and data submission procedures, and the guidelines for their behavior. Then, the observers should be trained in data collection. Training may include sessions using videotaped activities for practice in identifying and recording actual nursing services. In the third phase, observers participate with a project member in explaining the nature of the project to those who will be observed in the observation setting. In many studies, a standardized and comprehensive training program has produced intra-rater reliability of 90 percent or greater and inter-rater reliability of about 80 percent.

It is also possible to have workers self-report their activities. Self-reported logs are less expensive but reduce the reliability and validity of the data collected. Even with a reminder device, people may not record their activities promptly, and some may not be honest in their reports. Furthermore, self-reporting uses people's time, and it creates frustration or resentment and a lack of cooperation. Nevertheless, there are certain activities for which self-reported logging may be appropriate: those that are complex, with many variables and exceptions; activities requiring thought; activities with a long cycle; or activities performed by relatively few people doing many processes.

Determination of Sample Size. Work sampling is based on probability theory. The sampled activities are viewed as representing the total population of activities; therefore, to obtain valid and reliable results, sample size must be carefully chosen.

Inherent in any work sampling study is a degree of error. Work sampling estimates can be interpreted only as approximations of the actual time spent performing a particular activity. A goal of work sampling is to minimize the degree of error and obtain a desirable confidence interval in which the actual percentage falls. For instance, the hospital administrator may want an estimate of MRI idle time that provides a 95.5 ($z = 2.00$)

percent confidence of being within 4 percent of the actual percentage. Once the error level and confidence level are decided, the sample size can be determined using the following formulas:

$$CI = \hat{p} \pm e \tag{6.9}$$

$$e = z\sqrt{\frac{\hat{p}(1 - \hat{p})}{n}} \tag{6.10}$$

$$n = (z / e)^2 \hat{p}(1 - \hat{p}) \tag{6.11}$$

where

CI = confidence interval
e = error
z = number of standard deviations needed to achieve desired confidence
$\hat{p}$ = sample proportion (number of occurrences divided by sample size)
n = sample size

If a preliminary estimate of $\hat{p}$ is not available, use 0.5; after twenty to thirty observations, recalculate the sample size based on the new estimate. Furthermore, if the resulting sample size is not an integer, it should be rounded up to the nearest integer.

EXAMPLE 6.3

A hospital administrator wants an estimate of X-ray idle time that has a 95.5 percent confidence of being within 4 percent of the actual percentage. What sample size should be used?

Solution:

Given: e = 0.04; z = 2.00 (see Appendix A); $\hat{p}$ = 0.5 (preliminary).

Where $\hat{p}$ = 0.5: n = (2.00/0.04)² × .50 × (1 − .50) = 625 observations.

If for 20 observations, it is observed that the x-ray was breaking down on average one time, the revised estimate is then $\hat{p}$ = 1/20 = 0.05. The revised estimate of sample size is:

$\hat{p}$ = 0.05, n = (2.00/0.04)² × .50 × (1 − .50) = 118.75 or 119 observations

Once the sample size is determined, the next step is to develop the random observation schedule. That means deciding on the duration of the study (for instance, how many days over which the observations will be made). If observations are grouped too closely, the behaviors observed may not truly represent typical performance. For deciding on observation times, a random number table is a useful tool (see Table 6.6). Adjustments may have to be made to the randomly determined times. For instance, the amount of direct nursing care required on a unit may vary by week versus weekend, time of day, and seasonality. The impacts of such variations should be accounted for in the work study methodology. Before any observations are made, workers and their supervisors must be informed about the purpose of the study and how it will occur to avoid arousing suspicions that will hinder the study (Hawthorne effect). Finally, proceed with observations. Recompute the required sample size several times during the study if initial estimates are not reliable.

Development of a Random Observation Schedule. A random number table is essential to determine the observation times for a work sampling study. A random number table contains a list of unordered sequences of numbers (see Table 6.6). Numbers that are obtained from this table can be translated into particular observation times. For each observation, three numbers should be obtained: the first represents the day, the second the hour, and the third the minute when the observation will be made. The number of digits needed for each number is determined by the number of days in the study, the number of hours per day, and the minutes per hour. When using a random number table, it is important to vary the starting point from one study to another to avoid taking observations at the same times.

One method of choosing a starting point is to use the serial number on a dollar bill. Let the first number of the serial number represent the row to begin with, and the second number the column. For example, a serial number starting with 43 points to the fourth row and third column in Table 6.6, and the eight digit number there is 59830829. Appropriate selection of days, hours, and minutes takes these eight-digit numbers one after the other to develop the random observation schedule. For example, if the study covers between ten and ninety-nine days, a two-digit number is needed; if the activity is performed for eight hours daily, a one-digit hour number is needed; a two-digit number is needed for minutes, since there are sixty minutes per hour.

EXAMPLE 6.4

A nursing manager wants to observe the time a nurse spends in direct and in indirect care over a five-day period, on a unit where the shift is 8 hours.

Solution

A one-digit number will be needed for the day, one digit for the hour, and two digits for the minute. Using Table 6.6, starting from row 4, column 3, we obtain

TABLE 6.6.   Random Numbers.

	1	2	3	4	5	6	7	8	9	10
1	35491937	20651090	30546738	27696713	91854858	26470901	29600381	43662404	55790910	53368767
2	90089321	75138197	18262296	53506988	53664329	58683691	44072656	72123301	28627532	72233733
3	74264444	20553216	88880910	32182848	99227273	42091243	00185415	8357505	41837616	31852225
4	6975941	19701236	59830829	79995795	34330400	63391396	97866058	36093751	13890129	32572320
5	85104515	28079011	30791869	49069307	25601053	20059512	59547584	82327514	25940454	28633012
6	49445830	31791906	92435664	55449680	36293078	76826714	89141197	12205275	33570010	27259183
7	97984536	60317365	21508928	98014497	61529058	44276591	14715726	69340554	66688546	10818201
8	50991720	74038271	96451777	08764415	56072460	46404128	38033324	01926168	11279991	95600259
9	64349299	37831506	63182639	04789945	77658452	04272124	48648380	41902751	02079296	17430093
10	34894237	13116155	43110883	70982790	83397806	76383491	01380231	72811348	13242203	92667968
11	90761790	74867084	76963011	32548196	41697527	51249421	45324317	73925689	24228978	39762050
12	49467328	98679191	80203395	22956834	97271339	11381340	51175058	25051425	76621924	94995977
13	32794406	31342191	02913167	57792667	39337813	59751552	37057187	42319104	03677954	56886523
14	78152505	9638226	07737349	68260524	75852472	36834815	00551441	02859120	70489943	27486952
15	50075996	31935541	70044884	89925239	35183489	71073623	13252209	79970687	52414096	69996058
16	45030940	76909062	89925239	75233560	08589156	95913497	69644209	02601417	06504579	98654452
17	77637463	25848336	76968202	33535876	71755667	69560190	32893639	80542894	60040669	41588322
18	83262443	46142158	11416363	85122725	64419508	22965410	22075332	43671820	84851088	52801519
19	55924210	17405029	23887208	06435470	91190846	07104170	01882290	61773826	51088549	46474896
20	15306521	71387249	39155916	93179719	66965894	49643197	06692649	45665977	11202987	88350481

Note: Random number generator formula: =RAND( ) * 1000 (generated using Excel).

the random number 59830829. The first number is 5. Thus, we determine the day (in this case, the fifth day of the week, Friday). We move to the next number, 9, for the hour; but since activity is performed 8 hours daily, we discard that number, and move to the next one, 8. If we assume that the shift starts at 7:00 A.M., the number 8 represents 2:00 P.M. (assign 1 = 7:00 A.M., 2 = 8:00 A.M.,…, 8 = 2:00 P.M.). The minutes are derived from the next two digits, 30. Put together, the first observation is made on the fifth day, 30 minutes into the eight hours of work, or at 2:30 P.M. This procedure is repeated for each observation to be taken. Then the observations should be sorted chronologically by day, hour, and minute.

EXAMPLE 6.5

The chief of the hospital maintenance technicians wants to estimate the proportion of time that technicians spend in a part of the maintenance process. The maintenance office is open 9 hours, starting at 8:00 A.M., every day of the week. Twenty observations will be taken during a month-long investigation. Determine the random observation times and develop an observation schedule, assuming that the serial number of a dollar bill starts with 25.

Solution

Since we know the starting point in Table 6.6 is the second row and fifth column, the random number is 53664329. Next we need to choose the reading direction of the succeeding random numbers: either by moving to the right on the same row, and when the row is finished, going down one row and moving from left to right; or by going down on the same column, and when the column is finished moving to the next column right and reading from bottom to top. For this case, we choose to read in the same column, going down. For days, read two digits from left to right—select two-digit number, if higher than 31, then move to the next digit to make a two-digit day observation, and so on. Within eight digit numbers, if there are not enough digits to identify day, hour, and minutes for the observation, discard that random number and select the next one. For hours, read single digit numbers from left to right, discard 0 and assign 1 = 8:00 A.M., 2 = 9:00 P.M., and so on. For minutes, read two-digit numbers and discard numbers 60 or over. Prepare a chronological list of the observation time results by day, hour, and minute, to be given to the data collection team. If a health care facility is open ten hours for business, then single digits from 0 through 9 can be used to make assignment for hours (0 = 8:00 A.M., 1 = 9:00 A.M.,…., 9 = 5 P.M.).

Table 6.7 shows the development of a work sampling schedule. Twelve random numbers have been discarded because one cannot draw the valid numbers for day, hour, or minutes from the same string of eight digits. Table 6.8 shows the final schedule, with valid observations times sorted according to chronological order by day, hour, and minute.

TABLE 6.7. Development of the Schedule for a Work Sampling Study.

Observation	Random Number	Day	Hour	Minute	Notes
	53664329				Discarded
1	99227273	22	7 = 2 P.M.	27	
2	34330400	30	4 = 11 A.M.	00	
3	25601053	25	6 = 1 P.M.	01	
4	36293078	29	3 = 10 A.M.	07	
5	61529058	15	2 = 9 A.M.	05	
6	56072460	07	2 = 9 A.M.	46	
	77658452				Discarded
	83397806				Discarded
7	41697527	16	9 = 4 P.M.	52	
8	97271339	27	1 = 8 A.M.	33	
	39337813				Discarded
	75852472				Discarded
9	35183489	18	3 - 10 A.M.	48	
10	08589156	08	5 = 12 P.M.	15	
11	71755667	17	5 = 12 P.M.	56	
12	64419508	19	5 = 12 P.M.	08	

(continued)

TABLE 6.7. *(continued)*

Observation	Random Number	Day	Hour	Minute	Notes
13	91190846	11	9 = 4 P.M.	08	
	66965894				Discarded
	49643197				Discarded
14	07104170	07	1 = 8 A.M.	04	
	96913497				Discarded
15	71073623	10	7 = 2 P.M.	36	
	36834815				Discarded
	59761552				Discarded
16	11381340	11	3 = 10 A.M.	13	
17	51249421	12	4 = 11 A.M.	42	
	76383491				Discarded
18	04272124	04	2 = 9 A.M.	21	
19	46404128	04	1 = 8 A.M.	28	
20	44276591	27	6 = 1 A.M.	59	

TABLE 6.8. Final Work Sampling Schedule.

Observation	Day	Time
19	04	8:28 A.M.
18	04	9:21 A.M.
14	07	8:04 A.M.
6	07	9:46 A.M.
10	08	12:15 P.M.

15	10	2:36 P.M.
16	11	10:13 A.M.
13	11	4:08 P.M.
17	12	11:42 A.M.
5	15	9:05 A.M.
7	16	4:52 P.M.
11	17	12:56 P.M.
9	18	10:48 A.M.
12	19	12:08 P.M.
1	22	2:27 P.M.
3	25	1:01 P.M.
11	26	2:14 P.M.
8	27	8:33 A.M.
20	27	1:59 P.M
4	29	10:07 A.M.

Random Observation Schedule Using Excel. Excel is very instrumental to generate random observation schedule. Although this requires a few steps, however, it is more convenient than using the random number table explained earlier. User needs to determine the sample size and the start and finish dates on observations. Once these dates are determined, the following formula can be used to extract random dates and times as follows:

$$\text{Formula} = \text{RAND()} * (\text{End Date} - \text{Begin Date}) + \text{Begin Date} \quad (6.12)$$

The formula requires three columns:

1) Beginning date
2) End date
3) Formula as shown in (6.12)

In addition, hours of collection and whether observations on weekends are permissible must be delineated. User, after placing the appropriate dates and times in three columns identified above, would copy the formula to rows below based on the number of observations needed. However, if observations cannot be taken during off hours and weekends, many of the Excel generated random observations that fall in these times will be discarded. So, it is advised to generate a large number of rows of observations.

Excel has dynamic random generation method, this means once the random observations are generated, they need to be preserved by copying to another column for final processing (for example, discarding off hours/weekend observations; developing a final schedule in a chronological order). Otherwise, any entry to spreadsheet will change the random observation schedule. Example 6.6 illustrates an Excel based random observation schedule.

In order to preserve these dates (in column C), they need to be placed into another column, column E, using copy and paste special with "values" option. As soon as this operation is done, the values in column C will be changed due to the dynamic random scheme of Excel. However, this is not a concern anymore since the remaining discarding process for unwanted observations (off hours and weekends) will be conducted on column E which has the stabilized (unchanging) random observations. Figure 6.4 displays results in column E as stabilized dates and times; the reader can observe that the original values generated are now in column E and values in column C are changed.

EXAMPLE 6.6

Manager of Transesophageal Echocardiogram laboratory would like to improve efficiency of the processes in this department. To observe the proportion of time spent in various processes, a pilot work sampling study with an initial 20 observations will be taken during March 2009. Laboratory is open 8:00 A.M. to 5:00 P.M. during the week days only. Determine the random observation schedule using Excel.

Solution

Using the steps described earlier, beginning date and time of the observation schedule is placed in column A as a date function "=DATE(2009,3,1)+TIME(8,0, 0)." First parenthesis indicates year, month and day to begin observations, and the second parenthesis show 8:00 A.M. as the start time. Similarly, column B includes the last permissible observation date/time using "=DATE(2009,3,31)+ TIME(17,0,0)." Finally, the formula (6.10) is entered in column C as "=RAND()*(B3-A3)+A3." The next step would be copying these three columns to the following rows. Figure 6.3 displays the resulting random selections.

FIGURE 6.3. *Random Observation Schedule.*

The next step is to discard observations that fall off hours and weekends. It is easier to discard off hours observations (outside to working hours) shown in Figure 6.5, than making sure that the observation does not fall into the weekend. Those valid observations are identified in column F, and a numerical sequence is assigned in column G. To finalize the random schedule, the user may sort the observations in columns E through G using column G in descending sort order. Figure 6.5 displays valid dates and times after the sort. To obtain the final schedule in chronological order, valid observations in column E need to be sorted in ascending order. The result of this sort order provides the final observation schedule which is shown in Figure 6.6.

Work Simplification

An important part of work design is using common sense to find easier and better ways of performing the work. Work simplification is not just speeding up the job time

	A	B	C	D	E	F
1	From Date	To Date	Random Selection			
2			Formula = RAND()*(End Date-Begin date)+Begin Date			
3	3/1/09 8:00 AM	3/31/09 5:00 PM	3/4/09 9:08 PM		3/30/09 1:53 PM	
4	3/1/09 8:00 AM	3/31/09 5:00 PM	3/29/09 12:07 AM		3/12/09 1:16 AM	
5	3/1/09 8:00 AM	3/31/09 5:00 PM	3/21/09 11:47 AM		3/11/09 8:27 PM	
6	3/1/09 8:00 AM	3/31/09 5:00 PM	3/1/09 8:29 PM		3/13/09 2:12 AM	
7	3/1/09 8:00 AM	3/31/09 5:00 PM	3/21/09 12:25 AM		3/8/09 6:35 PM	
8	3/1/09 8:00 AM	3/31/09 5:00 PM	3/5/09 11:39 PM		3/24/09 10:13 AM	
9	3/1/09 8:00 AM	3/31/09 5:00 PM	3/19/09 2:14 AM		3/22/09 12:24 PM	
10	3/1/09 8:00 AM	3/31/09 5:00 PM	3/2/09 9:52 PM		3/10/09 5:29 PM	
11	3/1/09 8:00 AM	3/31/09 5:00 PM	3/20/09 1:54 AM		3/20/09 2:25 PM	
12	3/1/09 8:00 AM	3/31/09 5:00 PM	3/6/09 9:37 PM		3/27/09 11:06 PM	
13	3/1/09 8:00 AM	3/31/09 5:00 PM	3/14/09 9:47 AM		3/20/09 2:46 AM	
14	3/1/09 8:00 AM	3/31/09 5:00 PM	3/24/09 1:53 PM		3/15/09 11:57 PM	
15	3/1/09 8:00 AM	3/31/09 5:00 PM	3/23/09 2:58 PM		3/29/09 11:15 PM	
16	3/1/09 8:00 AM	3/31/09 5:00 PM	3/22/09 7:42 AM		3/18/09 7:09 AM	
17	3/1/09 8:00 AM	3/31/09 5:00 PM	3/17/09 4:21 PM		3/9/09 4:51 AM	
18	3/1/09 8:00 AM	3/31/09 5:00 PM	3/28/09 7:40 PM		3/22/09 9:13 PM	
19	3/1/09 8:00 AM	3/31/09 5:00 PM	3/15/09 5:21 AM		3/21/09 12:25 PM	
20	3/1/09 8:00 AM	3/31/09 5:00 PM	3/14/09 11:33 PM		3/9/09 10:37 PM	
21	3/1/09 8:00 AM	3/31/09 5:00 PM	3/17/09 10:35 AM		3/4/09 12:32 AM	
22	3/1/09 8:00 AM	3/31/09 5:00 PM	3/19/09 7:34 PM		3/1/09 4:32 PM	
23	3/1/09 8:00 AM	3/31/09 5:00 PM	3/19/09 6:32 PM		3/31/09 11:41 AM	
24	3/1/09 8:00 AM	3/31/09 5:00 PM	3/5/09 4:45 PM		3/12/09 5:54 PM	
25	3/1/09 8:00 AM	3/31/09 5:00 PM	3/11/09 10:28 AM		3/28/09 9:33 AM	
26	3/1/09 8:00 AM	3/31/09 5:00 PM	3/16/09 5:29 PM		3/29/09 9:32 AM	
27	3/1/09 8:00 AM	3/31/09 5:00 PM	3/18/09 8:23 AM		3/21/09 12:42 AM	
28	3/1/09 8:00 AM	3/31/09 5:00 PM	3/6/09 7:38 AM		3/9/09 2:28 AM	
29	3/1/09 8:00 AM	3/31/09 5:00 PM	3/17/09 10:22 PM		3/14/09 1:45 PM	
30	3/1/09 8:00 AM	3/31/09 5:00 PM	3/21/09 10:13 AM		3/29/09 7:06 PM	
31	3/1/09 8:00 AM	3/31/09 5:00 PM	3/23/09 7:34 AM		3/4/09 1:52 AM	
32	3/1/09 8:00 AM	3/31/09 5:00 PM	3/4/09 5:46 PM		3/6/09 6:37 PM	
33	3/1/09 8:00 AM	3/31/09 5:00 PM	3/16/09 4:32 AM		3/31/09 1:48 PM	

FIGURE 6.4. *Stabilized Dates and Times.*

or finding a new way of working harder or faster. Rather, work simplification seeks a way to do a job with less effort, less cost, and less time, more safely, and without hurrying. Changing work methods, not the job itself, is the aim. Work simplification can be achieved through eliminating unnecessary parts of the work, combining and rearranging other parts of the work, and simplifying the necessary parts of the work.

The three main tools used to map the work process and identify means to simplify it are work distribution charts, flow process charts, and flow charts. Layout analysis also can be used (see Chapter Five).

Work Distribution Chart. A work distribution chart defines the functions of a particular department in terms of its major activities and pinpoints each employee's contribution

FIGURE 6.5.   *Valid Dates and Times.*

to them. Table 6.9 is a partial work distribution chart for a nursing unit, such as generally prepared by an employee or supervisor. The key to an effective work distribution chart is being highly specific about the tasks. For instance, instead of saying that a nurse was doing paperwork, a more specific response is that the nurse was filling out an order for a laboratory test. The unit of analysis for analyzing the work distribution chart may be the department as a whole, an independent activity, or an individual person(s). Trouble can be identified by asking:

FIGURE 6.6. *Final Observation Schedule.*

Which activities consume the most time?

■   Are the tasks evenly and fairly distributed?

■   Is there over- or under-specialization?

■   Are employees assigned too many unrelated tasks?

■   Are talents used efficiently?

■   Is the time spent on each activity justifiable?

TABLE 6.9. Partial Work Distribution Chart for Nursing Unit.

Activity	Hours	Nurse Manager	Hours	Nurse I	Hours	Nurse II	Hours
Patient admissions	12	Coordination with Admissions Dept.	8		2		2
Communications	16	Physicians and patient family	8	Patient family	4	Patient family	4
Direct patient care	48		8	Medication administration	20		20
Indirect patient care	16	Monitor charts	4	Meals	6	Update Charts	6
Discharge planning	14		2		6		6
Scheduling & Adm	4		4				
Miscellaneous	10	Supervisory meeting Sessions with trainees	42	Emergency coverage	2		2
TOTAL	120		40		40		40

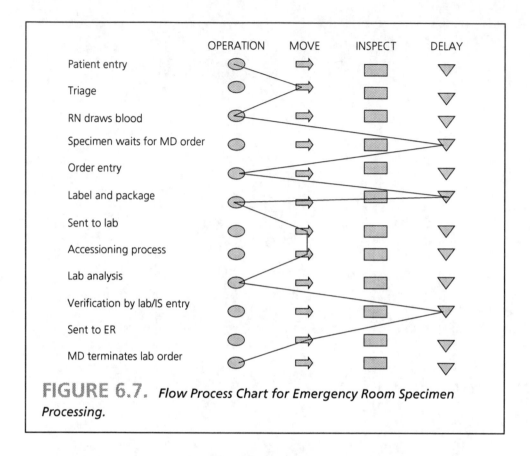

FIGURE 6.7. *Flow Process Chart for Emergency Room Specimen Processing.*

Flow Process Chart. A flow process chart records a procedure as a graphic chart, using shorthand to simplify and unify the record (see Figure 6.7). It is used to examine the overall sequence of an operation in an attempt to identify nonproductive tasks, and highlights inconsistencies and redundancies. Any task beyond the operation itself (the circles in Figure 6.7) represents a potential delay that should be evaluated and perhaps eliminated. Important questions to ask include why a task is being done, what it contributes, where it is being done, when it is being done, who is doing it, and how? Steps that can be taken by examining a flow process chart include eliminating nonproductive tasks; combining certain job elements; changing the sequence, place or person associated with the task; and improving overall operations.

Figure 6.7 depicts a flow process chart for the emergency room, where efficient total turn-around time for lab processing is essential. This emergency department has inefficient turn-around times for stat laboratory tests, with delays from three tasks. From the flow chart, one can suggest: packaging, labeling, and information system (IS) entry should be combined into one task. In addition, the task "MD terminates lab order" can be eliminated. These steps would eliminate delays and reduce unnecessary operations.

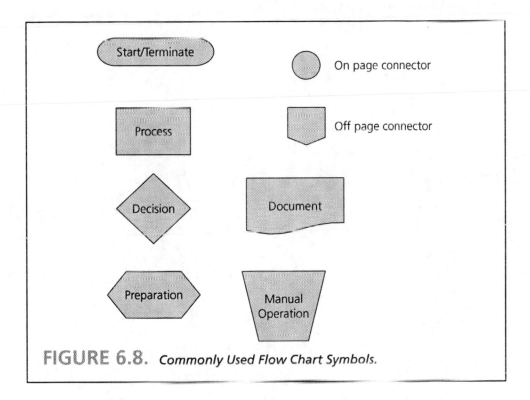

FIGURE 6.8. *Commonly Used Flow Chart Symbols.*

Flow Chart. Flow charts depict the chronological flow of work in a logical manner to help the health care manager analyze, plan, and control the work flow. Figure 6.8 depicts commonly used flow chart symbols. One can draw detailed flow charts of operations by using computer programs like Visio. Figure 6.9 depicts a flow chart for the initial process and the improvement after reengineering for the emergency department's specimen and lab work described above.

Worker Compensation

Compensation is an important matter to both the employee and the employer, though of course from divergent points of view. Without an adequate compensation package, employers may have difficulty attracting high-quality, competent employees, or may face workers with no extrinsic motivation to perform productively. On the other hand, higher wages and benefits erode the organization's profit. Because labor costs comprise approximately 40 percent or more of a health care organization's budget, establishing an appropriate wage schedule is essential to its survival in the long run.

There are two basic systems for compensating employees—time-based or output-based (incentive) systems. Time-based systems, the most common in health care, compensate employees for the time they work during a pay period. When quality is just as, or more important than, quantity, a time-based system is preferable.

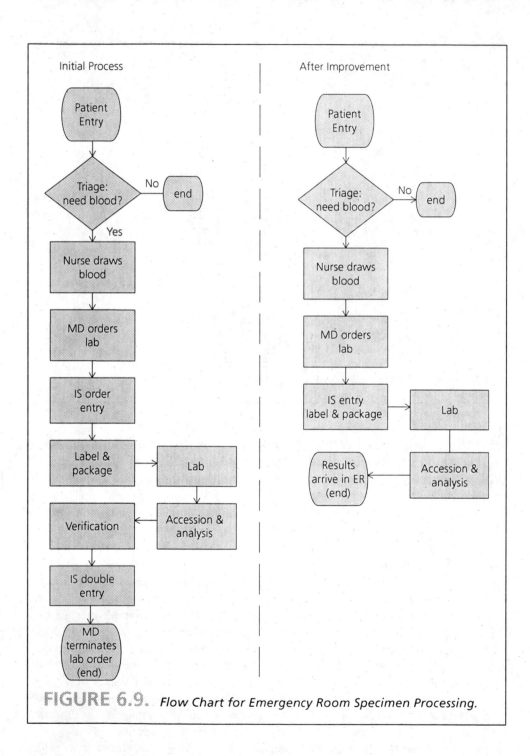

FIGURE 6.9. *Flow Chart for Emergency Room Specimen Processing.*

Output-based systems compensate employees according to how much output they produce during a pay period.

In health care, incentive-based plans are on the rise. Originally developed by hospital systems, managed care organizations, and health management companies, the incentive plans, both individual and group, are now being used more by individual hospitals, as well. Indeed, high-performing hospitals use incentive compensation. Incentive plans are designed to motivate employees to achieve certain goals of the organization: higher profits, lower costs, better quality of care, or greater productivity. Incentive programs can take one of two forms, profit sharing or gain sharing. Under profit sharing plans, employees receive a percentage of the organization's profits, under a prearranged formula. Under gain sharing plans, employees share a percentage of the cost savings achieved by increasing productivity.

SUMMARY

Reengineering is a methodology intended to overcome the difficulty in realizing TQM and CQI performance over a long duration, as well as the myopic conduct of organizational change, restructuring and downsizing approaches. To reengineer the system, health care managers must be able to understand work-design, jobs, job measurement, process activities, and reward systems—all well known concepts of industrial engineering. With that knowledge, they can recognize the bottlenecks in the old system, identify unnecessary and repetitive tasks, and eliminate them in the reengineered system of care. Time standards are important in establishing productivity standards, determining staffing levels and schedules, estimating labor costs, budgeting, and designing incentive systems. In this chapter, measurement of time standards, work sampling, and work simplification techniques were given in-depth consideration.

KEY TERMS

Work Design
Job Design
Socio-Technical School

Time Standards
Work Sampling
Work Simplification

EXERCISES

6.1 In a routine clinical process, observed times in minutes were 84, 76, 80, 84, and 76. One observed employee was working 25 percent faster than the average worker. Allowance factors for this job, based on the workday, add to 20 percent. What are the normal and the standard times?

6.2 Pre- and post-examination processing of patients in an outpatient clinic involves various tasks performed by clerks and nurses. A time study conducted by the decision support department is shown in Table EX 6.2.

a. Determine the observed time for the pre-post exam process.

b. Determine the normal time for the pre-post exam process.

c. Determine the standard time for the pre-post exam process, using the basic-moderate allowance for the job.

d. Calculate the standard time for the exam process. Do you think the time spent in the outpatient clinic, without including the exam time, is reasonable? If not, what improvements would you recommend?

TABLE EX 6.2

Activity	Performance Rating	Observations (in Minutes)										
		1	2	3	4	5	6	7	8	9	10	11
Registration	1.15	3	6	4	8	4	5	4	6	4	6	4
Copayment	0.95	7	9	11	8	12	9	6	11	9	12	10
Wait for nurse	1.00	17	15	17	12	11	17	12	19	12	20	18
Vital signs	0.96	9	8	11	12	9	8	10	12	8	12	11
Wait for exam room	1.00	12	15	12	14	21	18	11	16	9	14	18
Placement to exam room	0.98	3	5	4	6	3	5	3	6	5	4	7
Wait for physician	1.00	10	17	21	11	13	15	14	12	19	15	9
Examination	1.00	18	15	19	22	18	12	19	21	16	21	17
Test order entry	1.02	4	7	3	5	4	11	9	12	11	14	9
Referral requests	1.11	11	10	16	9	8	9	7	7	9	7	6
Follow-up appointment scheduling	1.08	3	5	3	4	3	4	4	5	3	3	5

6.3 The emergency department in a major medical center has delays in the stat laboratory tests turn-around time (TAT). According to standards, the stat lab results should be reported within 30 minutes. The analyst conducted a time study to measure the reporting times for fourteen different lab tests over fifteen observations. The performance ratings of the personnel handling the test are also recorded in Table EX 6.3.

TABLE FX 6.3

Lab Test	Performance Rating	1	2	3	4	5	6	7	8	9	10	11	12	13	14	15
		\multicolumn{15}{c}{Observations (in Minutes)}														
Hem 8	0.95	28	34	29	33	21	18	26	23	30	24	23	24	20	27	28
Hem 18	1.03	29	38	24	39	27	26	20	23	27	26	28	28	34	37	29
Apter	1.11	27	36	35	35	36	27	29	33	29	33	34	40	36	32	28
AMY	0.97	28	37	29	27	28	29	27	26	25	24	25	28	22	31	22
Ca	1.09	38	44	33	34	21	23	20	28	23	27	22	27	27	29	25
Glucose	0.98	52	54	49	43	51	56	60	37	39	40	29	43	44	50	43
Chem 7	1.01	28	37	27	35	33	30	31	27	25	33	32	34	29	25	25
K	1.04	12	25	18	11	19	27	11	19	14	15	14	15	18	16	12
HCG	0.98	18	29	16	20	23	15	15	14	16	18	19	22	18	18	21
ALP	0.97	29	39	30	32	32	34	32	34	32	34	34	38	36	33	33
ALT	0.94	29	39	30	32	29	36	23	25	28	28	31	29	33	32	33
B	1.03	29	38	36	23	25	28	32	34	32	29	38	36	23	25	28
AST	1.05	29	39	28	31	29	33	28	32	34	32	34	32	33	29	32
BBSP	0.94	26	32	18	26	39	28	31	29	26	28	31	29	19	28	32

a. Using the basic-low allowance, calculate the standard time for each lab test.

b. What is the overall standard time for stat orders?

c. Are the overall stat time and individual test times within expectations? If not, what would you recommend?

6.4 The Nursing Units Manager at HEALTH FINDER HOSPITAL wants to evaluate activities in the patient care unit. The manager hired an analyst who timed all the patient care activities, which include seventeen elements. The observed times (OT) and performance ratings for six observations are shown in the Table EX 6.4.

TABLE EX 6.4

Patient Care Unit Activities	Performance Rating	1	2	3	4	5	6
		\multicolumn{6}{c}{Observations (in Minutes)}					
1. Patient assessment	1.10	9	11	11	9	13	11
2. Care planning	0.96	10	9	7	8	7	10
3. Treatments	1.14	8	9	8	9	10	10

(Continued)

TABLE EX 6.4 *(continued)*

Patient Care Unit Activities	Performance Rating	Observations (in Minutes)					
		1	2	3	4	5	6
4. Medication	1.07	4	3	4	4	5	3
5. Collecting blood/lab specimens	1.15	8	7	6	9	10	7
6. Passing/Collecting trays, giving out snacks, feeding patients	1.12	18	21	20	21	21	20
7. Shift report	0.97	7	6	5	7	9	7
8. Charting/Documentation	0.95	8	7	8	8	9	11
9. Responding to patients' call lights	1.10	4	5	4	7	6	8
10. Phone calls to/from other departments	0.95	6	7	5	4	9	8
11. Transporting patients, specimens etc.	1.06	11	11	12	12	9	10
12. Patient acuity classification	1.10	7	6	7	6	7	6
13. Order transcription and processing	0.95	5	7	4	6	7	6
14. Ordering/stocking supplies and lines	0.97	6	7	5	6	7	6
15. Equipment maintenance and cleaning	0.96	12	11	8	10	11	9
16. General cleaning/room work (garbage, making beds)	1.14	12	10	12	10	10	12
17. Assisting with the admission process	1.05	11	9	10	9	9	10

a. Determine the average observed time for each element.

b. Find the normal time for each element.

c. Utilize Table 6.1 to develop an allowance percentage for a job element that requires a medium-low allowance.

d. Determine the standard time for the whole job (for all seventeen elements).

6.5 An initial work sampling survey to estimate the percentage of time that MRI equipment is idle between 8:00 A.M. and 8:00 P.M., found that the MRI was idle in 9 of the 120 observations.

a. Determine the percentage of idle time.

b. From the initial results, approximately how many observations would it require to estimate the actual percentage of idle time to within 4 percent, with confidence of 95 percent?

6.6 The decision support system analyst has been asked to prepare an estimate of the percentage of his time that a lab technician spends on microscopic examination of blood cultures, with a 95.5 percent confidence level. Past experience indicates that the proportion will be 25 percent.

    a. What sample size would be appropriate to have an error of no more than 64 percent?

    b. If a sample of 300 is used, what would be the potential error for the estimate?

6.7 The chief of the hospital maintenance technicians wants to estimate the percentage of their time that technicians spend in a certain part of the maintenance process. The maintenance office is open 8 hours on weekdays. Twenty observations will be taken during the month of March. Determine the random observation times, using Table 6.6 and assuming that the first two digits of a serial number from a dollar bill are 32. Prepare a list of the observation time results chronologically by day, hour, and minute, to be given to the data collection team. Assume the month is March of the current year, and the workday starts at 8:00 A.M.

6.8 The director of radiology wants to estimate the percentage of their time that radiology technicians spend readjusting the machines for various images. The radiology department is open 10 hours on weekdays (8:00 A.M. to 6:00 P.M.). Twenty-five observations will be taken during a two-week period. Determine the random observation times using Table 6.6 and assuming that the first two digits of a serial number from a dollar bill are 43. Prepare a list of the observation time results chronologically by day, hour, and minute, to be given to the data collection team.

6.9 Prepare a flow chart for a patient visit to an outpatient orthopedic clinic to show the flow for handling minor fractures requiring casts.

6.10 Prepare a flow chart for a colonoscopy exam (from scheduling to discharge).

6.11 Phlebotomy is an invasive procedure for collecting a blood sample. Prepare a flow process chart for the phlebotomy process in an outpatient setting.

6.12 Prepare a work distribution chart for the office management staff of a group practice. Assume a supervisor manager and three clerks.

CHAPTER

STAFFING

LEARNING OBJECTIVES

- Describe workload management systems: the relationship between staffing and scheduling with respect to human resource capacity planning.
- Evaluate patient acuity systems and their relation to staffing and scheduling.
- Describe the various scheduling options and relationship to human resource operations in various health care organizations.
- Develop levels of utilization and coverage factor for core level staffing in health care facilities.

The efficient and effective allocation of resources is perhaps the greatest challenge facing the health care manager today. Human capital resources represent the largest portion of the budget for most health care organizations, and therefore are of particular concern. In manufacturing, deciding on the proper staffing levels and skill mix is relatively simple. Demand for the manufactured product is predictable within certain limits, and unanticipated demand can be met with inventory surplus. Health care managers, however, face considerable uncertainty—that is, patient census and acuity levels can vary dramatically daily or even hourly. Health care managers struggle with chronic staffing shortages or surpluses, over-budget labor costs, and dissatisfied patients and staff. Balancing the quality of care with patient, physician, and nurse satisfaction is another significant challenge.

So how is the health care manager to cope with such problems created by uncertainty? One solution is to staff for peak levels at all times; however, common sense tells us that would soon become prohibitively expensive. Yet, staffing only for the minimal census and acuity levels would lead to overworked staff, patient dissatisfaction at best, and at worst, poor outcomes of care. Minimal staffing levels could be increased with part-time labor in times of high demand; but paying part-time or temporary staff at a premium rapidly raises costs. A solution is using flexible staffing methodologies. In flexible staffing, a core level of staff is established based on a long-term assessment of staff needs; that is augmented by short-term (daily) adjustments using various methods to match staffing levels to patient needs.

This chapter examines vital staffing and scheduling issues that the health care manager must handle. How many nurses and lab technicians are needed? What if patient demand suddenly rises, or several nurses are sick? Is turnover high because the demand on the nurses' workload is too high? After deciding on staffing levels, the manager must develop a successful work schedule. Should we use a four-day, ten-hour shift or a five-day, eight-hour shift? Or is a twelve-hour shift preferable? How satisfied are the nurses with the scheduling process, and how is their level of satisfaction affecting patient care? These questions, among others, are addressed here and in Chapter Eight.

WORKLOAD MANAGEMENT OVERVIEW

Workload management is a general term that refers to staffing and scheduling operations by an organization's manager. The three duties of workload management—staffing, scheduling, and reallocation—are not mutually exclusive, as illustrated in Figure 7.1. Figure 7.1 also shows the direct link among staffing, scheduling, and productivity variables.

First of all, let us define those three components of workload management. Staffing procedures decide on the appropriate number of full-time employees (FTEs) to be hired in each skill class (RN, LPN, aides). Staffing decisions are generally made annually, taking seasonal variations into account; thus, staffing decisions are tactical.

Scheduling establishes when each staff (nurse) will be on or off duty and on which shifts they will work. Weekends, work stretches, vacation requests, and potential sick days are all important considerations in scheduling decisions, which are generally considered to be operational.

The third component is the reallocation of human resources, which fine-tunes the previous two decisions. Reallocation is a daily, if not a shift-by-shift decision. The number of float nurses needed on each unit is determined daily according to unforeseen changes in need as classified by a patient acuity system. We will discuss reallocation later in the section "Reallocation Through Daily Adjustments."

Although staffing, scheduling, and reallocation are the core responsibilities of workload management, other tasks, other dimensions too, are important. The development of workload standards, for instance, is a prerequisite for effective workload management. Both workload management and workload standards development significantly affect productivity and productivity-related variables: staffing costs,

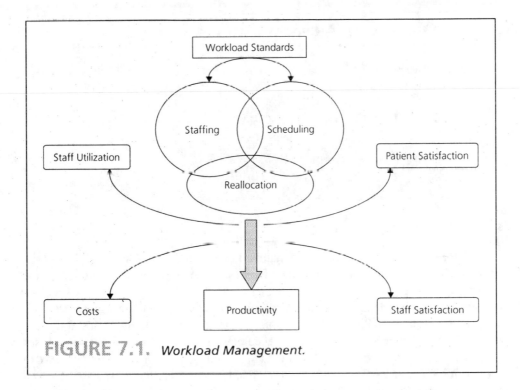

FIGURE 7.1. *Workload Management.*

job-satisfaction levels, and staff utilization. The following sections examine each of these aspects of workload management more closely.

Establishment of Workload Standards and Their Influence on Staffing Levels

Recall that staffing refers to deciding on the number of full-time equivalents to be hired for a particular unit. Because labor costs can represent 40 percent or more of a hospital or other health care organization's budget, it is vital to hire only the necessary staff. Equally important, however, is to maintain high quality patient care. Patient and staff satisfaction are also considerations, as is the premium paid to temporary staff needed on short notice.

To assist in staffing decisions, the health care manager must develop standards. A work standard is defined as the predetermined allocation of time available for a unit of service to maintain an appropriate level of quality (Kirk, 1986). The unit of service varies with the department. Nursing units, for instance, use the patient day as the unit of service. Because patient days are usually adjusted for acuity, the work standard is referred to as an acuity-adjusted standard. When the unit of service is a procedure, such as a laboratory test or X-ray, the standard is a procedural one. Examples of work standards often used today are found in Table 7.1.

TABLE 7.1. **Examples of Work Standards.**

Description of Work	Standard
Nursing care hours per patient day (medical-surgical unit)	4.5
Nursing care hours per patient day (coronary ICU)	12.0
Physical therapist hours per patient treatment	0.5
Indirect nursing hours per ER visit	0.7
Technician hours per CT scan	0.4

Historically, standards were based mainly on the average census levels of the entire organization. Queuing analysis or other forecasting techniques were applied to the patient census data to base staffing levels on previous admissions and expected lengths of stay. Although these methods did estimate overall hospital census variation with relative accuracy, their application to individual hospital units was limited. Hospital occupancy could be predicted with relative accuracy in the aggregate; however, census variations at the departmental level fluctuated widely, limiting the effectiveness of forecasting techniques. The success of the various forecasting methods also depended on the accuracy of the length-of-stay estimate. In the past such estimates often came from the physicians and could be inaccurate (Walker, 1990). Today, however, precise estimates of length of stay can be obtained from hospital information systems.

We will focus on three major areas to assist in staffing decisions: (1) patient acuity and classification systems and their usefulness for creating work standards; (2) the methods for developing work standards internally, with examples of how the standards can be translated into FTEs; and (3) some of the controversies about the development of professional and industry work standards.

Patient Acuity Systems

According to Warner (1976), there are three important components of any staffing decision. (1) A reliable patient classification and acuity system must be used to determine the need for services based upon such patient specific characteristics as age, diagnosis, acuity, and so on. (2) Time standards should be established that reflect the time necessary to care for each patient within each unit, using the patient classification system. (3) A method must be adopted to convert the total number of minutes of coverage needed into the appropriate number of full-time equivalents and FTE skill mix. The conversion method must adjust for factors such as expected sick days, vacations, and substitution among nursing skill levels. This sub-section discusses focus on Warner's first requirement—development of a patient classification system. The second and third requirements will be discussed in detail.

The modern hospital relies greatly on the departmental acuity-adjusted census, rather than on an aggregate census estimate, to establish work standards. Shukla (1991) notes that fewer subsequent adjustments to staffing levels are needed when an admissions monitoring system is based on the unit's patient care requirements rather than on unit census. Indeed, the use of an acuity standard is intuitively appealing. For example, the time and supervision per day required to care for an elderly gentleman in the intensive care unit is surely more than that required for a patient recovering from a minor surgical procedure. When such differences are not reflected in the nursing workload standards, the number of FTEs would be based solely on the fact that two patients were in the hospital at a particular time (patient census), regardless of the time needed to treat each. The result would be an inappropriate staffing pattern.

There is another reason for adopting acuity-adjusted standards. Today the population entering the hospital is sicker than it was a decade ago, and that trend is likely to continue. Coupled with this greater acuity is a decline in reimbursement and growing emphasis on cost control. The use of acuity-adjusted work standards can help to ensure that staffing is adjusted to meet the needs of a sicker population, thus maintaining a high quality of care.

In order to adopt acuity-adjusted standards, the health care organization must first implement a patient acuity system, which is a workload measurement system that measures the amount of care required by any given patient (Piper, 1989). Patient acuity systems, often called patient classification systems, are used routinely in nursing, since a Joint Commission standard requires nursing departments to "define, implement, and maintain a system for determining patient requirements for nursing care on the basis of demonstrated patient needs, appropriate nursing intervention, and priority for care" (Piper, 1989; p. 43). However, it is important to understand that acuity level is not synonymous with severity of illness. An extremely ill individual, for example someone with chronic obstructive pulmonary disease (COPD), may require only basic, palliative care. On the other hand, a less severe condition can nevertheless require large time commitments from the staff.

According to Piper (1989; p. 46), acuity systems fall into two categories—prototype and factor-analysis systems. Prototype systems classify patients according to the type of care needed. Patients are usually grouped into one of three to ten levels based upon expected nursing time commitments, diagnosis, mobility, medications, and education needed for either the patient or the family. Prototype systems are relatively simple to set up and use, but they are highly subjective.

A factor analysis system establishes classifications by summing the relative values assigned to individual tasks or indicators of patient need. For instance, on a scale of activities of daily living (ADL), a patient needing no assistance may receive a 10, a patient needing minimal assistance in one or two ADLs may receive a score of 20, and a patient needing total care in five or six areas will receive a 50. Factor analysis techniques provide a highly developed set of workload data. The health care manager can identify the reasons for fluctuations in patient acuity, which can assist in deciding on the staff skill mix needed for the unit. However, developing a factor analysis method is both time consuming and difficult.

An example of a factor-analysis system is the GRASP system. This workload management system was designed to help resolve inefficiencies that arose from fluctuating workloads. The program's goal was to replace state and national average standards with internally developed standards, to prevent over- and under-staffing. The approach of the system was simply to match patient care needs with the available nursing care.

GRASP System. The GRASP system was developed as a management information tool that could help reduce errors and inefficiencies arising from uncontrolled and fluctuating nursing work loads. The goal, as stated before, was to provide local-level data, rather than national averages, for use in staffing budget determination. The system essentially matches nursing care available to patient care needs.

The amount of nursing care available is easy to measure. GRASP defines one hour of nursing care as a single nursing care unit (NCU). Thus, one nurse who works 10 hours equals 10 NCUs. On the contrary, patient care needs are much more difficult. Strict reliance on census figures, or simply the number of beds available, is inadequate. Instead, the care needs of each individual patient must be collected—GRASP is designed to accomplish this task. GRASP considers all patient-related variables in its determination of the amount of care each patient should receive daily. One hour of required patient care is defined as one patient care unit (PCU); the care needs of each patient in terms of PCUs are assessed upon admission and reassessed daily for the patient's length of stay.

The total amount of care needed for each patient is determined by giving a point value to each of the following areas: direct physical care, indirect care, and teaching time. Delay and fatigue factors are also added. Physical care activities include diet, toilet, cleanliness, vital signs, turning and assisted activities, medications, suctioning, and respiratory aids. Time standards for each were developed (which must be modified for each hospital using the system).

Within each nursing unit, a wall chart lists these activities and assigns a point value to each (each point is equal to 6.5 minutes). Daily assessment of needs is made by circling the number of points that corresponds to the level of care required of the patient based on physician orders. The points are then totaled for each patient. The total points represent 85 percent of total physical care. The remaining 15 percent includes unmeasured care activities and is assigned on a predetermined basis.

Indirect care is relatively constant for all patients and therefore is not assessed on an individual basis. A standard time for teaching and emotional support is also added. Finally, all time standards are increased by 12 percent, an industrial engineering standard to account for interruptions, delays, and fatigue. The number of points is then converted to the number of PCUs required (Meyer, 1978).

Another similar system was developed by the Medicus Systems Corporation and is called the Nursing Productivity and Quality System (NPAQ).

NPAQ System. This system was designed to assist in the area of nursing resource management. The development of the system's methodology by Medicus Systems

Corporation cost several million dollars of research and development spread over more than ten years.

The Medicus patient classification system uses factor evaluation techniques that objectively categorize patients based on thirty-seven key indicators (forty for psychiatry). Five categories are created based on the number of care hours the staff should provide over a given twenty-four-hour period. The classification process is usually done using a preprinted classification tool. Each day, nurses on each unit mark the indicators appropriate for each patient, a process that generally takes fewer than ten minutes per unit (fifteen to thirty patients). The scoring of the forms is automated and each indicator is weighted during the scoring process.

The classification process produces two parameters that describe the nursing workload requirements for the unit—a workload index and average acuity index. Together, these indexes provide a basis for the objective determination of nursing workload per unit. This workload value can be converted into staffing and skill mix requirements using a separate module of the Medicus system—the Staff Planning and Allocation Module (Medicus Systems Corporation, 1989).

Patient acuity systems are necessary to accurately calculate the core staffing level necessary to meet patient requirements. Tables 7.2 and 7.3 illustrate how patient acuity systems operate. Table 7.2 lists the number of patients in a medical or surgical unit on each day of January in a given year. The census hours have been collected retrospectively from a hospital information system. Also recorded are the numbers of patients in each of the acuity levels, with level one patients requiring the least amount of care and level four the most.

Remember that historically, staffing levels were based mostly on total census, which as we noted could lead to staffing inefficiencies. Compare, for instance, January 5 (census = 9) and January 7 (census = 12). If the staffing requirements were based solely on census, a greater number of FTEs would be used on January 7. However, when we look at the acuity levels of the patients, we observe that nearly 80 percent of the patients on January 5 are in category three, compared to only 17 percent of the patients in this category on January 7. The greater acuity is reflected in the required hours per patient day (HPPD). Notice that the HPPD value for January 5 is 4.8, and for January 7, 3.6 hours. Multiplying the census times by the required HPPD, we see that the acuity-adjusted census is the same for both days: 43.2 hours of care are required. Viewed in this way, the staffing requirements for both days are the same, although the skill mix may differ.

Similarly, even when census levels are the same for two days, the number of nurses required for each day may not be equal if patient needs differ. On January 21 and January 23, for instance, the patient censuses are equivalent (census = 13.0 patients). However, on January 23, the required hours of direct care is 1.6 hours more. The reason for this difference is seen in the distribution of patients across the various acuity levels; on January 21, a higher percentage of patients is in the low acuity categories. Again, despite similar census patterns, more staff members are needed on January 23.

TABLE 7.2. Daily Census, Required Labor Hours, and Acuity Level Statistics for a Medical or Surgical Floor.

Date	Day of Week	Census				Based on Patient Classification—Required Hours per Patient Day				Number of Patients in Acuity Level			
		A.M.	P.M.	Night	Total	A.M.	P.M.	Night	Total	1	2	3	4
01/02/yy	SUN	12	13	12	12.3	2.3	1.4	0.8	4.5		6	7	
01/03/yy	MON	13	12	12	12.3	1.9	1.6	0.9	4.4		6	7	
01/04/yy	TUE	22	22	10	18.0	2.1	1.7	1.0	4.7	1	5	16	
01/05/yy	WED	9	9	9	9.0	2.1	1.7	1.0	4.8		2	7	
01/06/yy	THU	11	11	9	10.3	1.8	1.4	0.9	4.1	3	3	5	
01/07/yy	FRI	12	12	12	12.0	1.6	1.3	0.7	3.6	6	4	2	
01/08/yy	SAT	12	12	11	11.7	2.0	1.6	0.9	4.6	3	3	4	2
01/09/yy	SUN	14	14	14	14.0	1.7	1.4	0.8	3.9	4	3	5	
01/10/yy	MON	14	13	13	13.3	2.0	1.6	1.0	4.6	2	4	7	
01/11/yy	TUE	12	12	10	11.3	1.3	1.1	0.6	3.0	7	5		
01/12/yy	WED	18	20	13	17.0	2.1	1.7	1.0	4.8		4	14	
01/13/yy	THU	13	13	13	13.0	1.9	1.5	0.9	4.3	2	4	6	
01/14/yy	FRI	13	13	13	13.0	2.0	1.5	0.9	4.4	2	2	9	
01/15/yy	SAT	13	12	10	11.7	1.9	1.5	0.9	4.2	2	4	7	
01/16/yy	SUN	11	12	11	11.3	1.7	1.3	0.8	3.7	3	4	3	
01/17/yy	MON	11	10	10	10.3	1.9	1.5	0.9	4.2		6	5	
01/18/yy	TUE	9	10	8	9.0	2.0	1.5	0.9	4.5		3	6	
01/19/yy	WED	9	9	9	9.0	1.9	1.4	0.9	4.2	1	3	4	
01/20/yy	THU	10	11	10	10.3	1.6	1.3	0.8	3.7	1	7	1	
01/21/yy	FRI	13	13	13	13.0	1.8	1.5	0.9	4.1	2	4	5	
01/22/yy	SAT	12	12	12	12.0	1.8	1.5	0.9	4.2	2	6	3	1
01/23/yy	SUN	13	13	13	13.0	2.5	2.0	1.2	5.7		1	4	2
01/24/yy	MON	12	10	6	9.3	1.9	1.6	1.0	4.5	1	7	2	2
01/25/yy	TUE	8	8	8	8.0	1.3	1.1	0.6	2.9	4	2		
01/26/yy	WED	6	5	5	5.3	1.9	1.6	0.9	4.4	1	2	3	
01/27/yy	THU	7	5	5	5.7	1.4	1.1	0.6	3.1	3	4		
01/28/yy	FRI	6	6	6	6.0	2.0	1.4	0.8	4.2	1	1	4	
01/29/yy	SAT	7	7	7	7.0	1.8	1.3	0.8	3.9	2	1	3	
01/30/yy	SUN	9	9	9	9.0	1.8	1.3	0.7	3.8	2	2	3	
01/31/yy	MON	9	9	9	9.0	1.9	1.6	0.9	4.4	1	3	5	
Statistics													
Mean		11.3	11.2	10.1	10.9	1.9	1.5	0.9	4.2	18.9	*32.7*	45.9	2.5
Minimum		0.0	0.0	0.0	0.0	0.0	0.0	0.0	0.0	0.0	0.0	0.0	0.0
Maximum		22.0	22.0	14.0	18.0	2.5	2.0	1.2	5.7	7.0	7.0	16.0	2.0
Std. deviation		3.8	4.4	3.1	3.5	0.5	0.3	0.2	0.9	1.5	1.9	3.5	0.7

TABLE 7.3. ~monthly~ **Average Census, Required Labor Hours, and Acuity Level Statistics for a Medical or Surgical Floor**

Year	Month	Average Census				Based on Patient Classification—Avg. Required Hours per Patient Day				Percent of Patients in Acuity Level			
		A.M.	P.M.	Night	Total	A.M.	P.M.	Night	Total	1	2	3	4
1	January	14.1	13.8	13.8	13.9	1.8	1.5	0.9	4.1	26.3	26.9	45.0	1.7
	February	14.9	14.3	14.1	14.4	1.8	1.5	0.9	4.1	26.2	31.8	38.6	3.3
	March	15.3	14.9	14.6	14.9	1.9	1.5	0.9	4.3	19.7	27.5	48.8	3.5
	April	18.7	18.4	18.2	18.4	1.8	1.4	0.8	4.1	27.3	26.4	44.3	2.0
	May	19.8	19.5	19.3	19.5	2.0	1.6	0.9	4.4	21.7	21.0	52.7	4.3
	June	19.2	18.5	18.3	18.7	1.8	1.5	0.9	4.2	23.8	24.9	50.2	1.1
	July	18.4	17.5	17.0	17.6	2.0	1.6	0.9	4.5	15.9	24.8	53.7	4.9
	August	22.8	22.2	21.9	22.3	1.8	1.5	0.9	4.2	26.5	29.2	38.6	5.2
	September	19.9	19.4	18.7	19.3	1.7	1.4	0.8	3.9	35.3	28.4	33.4	2.9
	October	22.1	20.9	20.6	21.2	1.6	1.3	0.8	3.7	38.0	29.2	31.4	1.4
	November	17.1	16.5	15.7	16.4	1.8	1.5	0.8	4.1	29.2	26.3	40.0	4.2
	December	10.2	9.6	9.2	9.7	1.7	1.4	0.8	4.0	28.1	26.8	43.8	1.3
2	January	20.9	19.8	19.3	20.0	1.8	1.4	0.8	4.1	27.7	27.7	42.3	2.3
	February	19.1	18.7	18.1	18.6	1.9	1.5	0.9	4.2	22.4	31.6	42.2	3.7
	March	16.6	16.0	15.6	16.1	1.8	1.4	0.8	4.1	25.1	30.2	41.6	3.1
	April	4.5	4.4	4.1	4.3	1.9	1.5	0.9	4.3	12.2	39.1	43.7	5.0
	May	9.7	9.5	8.9	9.4	1.9	1.5	0.9	4.2	14.1	36.8	47.1	2.0
	June	8.3	8.5	7.8	8.2	1.9	1.5	0.9	4.2	15.0	33.3	50.4	1.2
	July	8.7	8.2	7.5	8.1	1.7	1.4	0.8	4.0	18.0	43.4	38.1	0.6
	August	8.0	7.5	6.7	7.4	1.6	1.4	0.8	3.7	23.1	44.8	32.1	
	September	7.4	6.9	6.5	6.9	1.8	1.4	0.8	4.0	15.4	44.6	38.2	1.7
	October	6.4	6.1	5.3	5.9	1.8	1.5	0.9	4.1	13.0	39.7	47.3	
	November	13.5	13.2	12.7	13.1	1.8	1.4	0.8	4.1	28.7	30.4	38.3	2.6
	December	13.3	12.6	11.2	12.4	1.6	1.3	0.7	3.7	30.3	43.6	25.7	0.4
3	January	11.3	11.2	10.1	10.9	1.9	1.5	0.9	4.2	18.9	32.7	45.9	2.5
Statistics													
Mean		14.4	13.9	13.4	**14.0**	1.8	1.5	0.8	**4.1**	23.3	32.0	42.1	2.4
Minimum		4.5	4.4	4.1	4.3	1.6	1.3	0.7	3.7	12.2	21.0	25.7	0.0
Maximum		22.8	22.2	21.9	22.3	2.0	1.6	0.9	4.5	38.0	44.8	53.7	5.2
Std. deviation		5.3	5.1	5.2	5.2	0.1	0.1	0.0	0.2	6.7	6.7	6.8	1.5

summary of table 7.2

As seen in the previous example, the patient acuity system translates the acuity levels of the patients into a time estimate for the direct care hours required of the FTEs. This direct time estimate can then be translated into the standard from which the number of FTEs needed can be determined. The ability to develop required care hours from automated patient classification systems can save significant time and money. The methods used to first assign the time levels associated with each census and acuity level, and the methods used to convert these standards into the number of FTEs needed, are discussed in the next section.

The Development of Internal Workload Standards

Workload standards can be either adopted from external agencies or developed internally. Although externally developed standards have the advantage of lower cost, internally developed standards often result in more accurate staffing decisions. The desired balance between costs and accuracy is a decision that rests with each institution and should not be generalized. An important component of the decision, however, should be a retrospective analysis of past staffing problems and their costs to the institution.

Before staffing can begin, workload standards must be adopted; as noted, developing them internally often results in more adequate staffing. The first step in the internal development of these standards is careful identification and documentation of the activities in the department or unit being examined. All activities performed should be carefully identified and documented, to reduce the possibility of misinterpreting the data, and also to improve the usefulness of the data in future evaluations (Page and McDougall, 1989; p. 71). Flow and process charts can document activities adequately.

It is also helpful to classify all the activities recorded as either variable or fixed. Fixed activities are those that do not vary with the volume of services. Examples include routine janitorial work, inventory checks, and team meetings. Variable activities do fluctuate with the services rendered and include X-rays, recording of medical records, and billing. Activities also can be classified as either direct or indirect. Direct care activities occur as care of the patient; indirect activities are support services, for instance, documenting medical records, scheduling, X-ray transport, and code cart checks.

After identifying the activities of the department, the times to perform them must be estimated. It is not feasible, however, in terms of costs and time to examine all activities within a department, and it also would seem fruitless to develop time standards for activities that occur only rarely or that require little time. But whatever activities are chosen must be representative of the workload of the entire department. Some departments use an 80/20 rule, choosing indicators from the 20 percent of activities that make up 80 percent of the volume; data on service volume can often be obtained from the hospital's billing system. However, some departments naturally require more specific and detailed time estimates than others. Remember that the more detailed the desired estimates, the greater the financial and time commitments for data collection and analysis, and therefore the better the case for using external standards.

Departments that offer a wide variety of procedures without similar service times should examine each activity separately. For example, orthopedic surgeon A, who lives in a small town and faces a relatively constant service mix, could develop standards based on the average time to set a broken leg. However, orthopedic surgeon B, who does a number of knee replacements and hip surgeries, would find that surgeon A's method would severely underestimate the time required for his work. Therefore, surgeon B should develop categories of services (broken legs and arms, knee and hip replacements, back surgeries, and like).

Many methods are available to measure the time necessary to perform the activities detailed in step one of the staffing process. These methods include estimation, historical averaging, predetermined time systems, work sampling, engineered time study, stopwatch methods, continuous work sampling, and micro motion study. More specifically:

- Estimation is low in cost and takes minimal time, is biased by the estimator, and does not always consider current internal and external conditions.

- Historical averaging is easiest and least expensive, and therefore widely accepted; it can be imprecise and perpetuate inefficiencies. Example: a unit worked 10,000 hours to treat 2,000 patient days. Thus, 5,000 nursing care hours per patient day are needed.

- Logging is a low-cost data collection method where staff members log their activities and the times needed to complete them. It can be used to identify time values for patient classification system categories and can be used to determine total time involvement by classification, by nursing plan, by diagnosis, or by standards of care; this method is often time-consuming and prone to recording errors or bias.

- Time studies and work sampling are random observations that measure time spent doing certain activities (see Chapter Six for detailed discussions); these are often done by an outside source, for example a consultant or industrial engineer (Kirk, 1986; p. 5).

After the estimate of the total hours necessary for the given activity is made, it is divided by total volume to determine the workload standard. For example, if personnel in the radiology department work 1,500 hours to perform 3,000 X-rays, the workload standard would be 30 minutes per X-ray performed (1,500 hours/3,000 X-rays). Again, a standard such as this could be obtained from industry or from professional publications, which provide ratios that should then be adjusted for the unique characteristics of the individual institution. Whatever the source of a standard, it is used to compute the required number of FTEs.

Utilization of FTEs. Another important issue for staffing levels is the expected utilization of employees—that is, setting the performance expectations for the unit or department (Page and McDougall, 1989; pp. 75–76). In actuality, many operational factors prevent 100 percent utilization. Such factors may be controllable or uncontrollable. Controllable factors are staff scheduling, avoidable delays, scheduling of vacations, and reducing downtime by letting unnecessary employees go when the workload permits. Uncontrollable factors affecting utilization include substantial work fluctuations due to changes in census, physicians' ordering patterns, sick leave, and market constraints limiting the availability of part-time staff. The factors influencing the desired utilization of any specific department must be established by the health care manager.

Page and McDougall (1989), although noting that utilization targets are difficult to determine, suggest three possible estimation methods: (1) Review the historical levels of utilization among administration, management engineering, and department management to negotiate an acceptable target. (2) Quantify delays and downtime, decide what delays are unavoidable, and determine utilization based upon those delays, allowing for acceptable levels of downtime. (3) Calculate an "overall weighted average utilization based upon the distribution of work load by shift and the accepted utilization levels by shift." An example of this third method, for a hospital laboratory, is presented in Table 7.4.

As mentioned above, the standard can be either based on acuity or procedurally based. There are subtle differences in how each method is used, so we present an example of each. Example 7.1 establishes the required staff for a laboratory. Example 7.2 uses an acuity-based standard to establish the staffing for a medical or surgical unit.

TABLE 7.4. **Weighted Average Utilization for a Laboratory Based on Workload Fluctuations by Shift.**

Shift	Percent of Work Load (A)	Expected Utilization (Percent) (B)	Weighted Utilization (A x B)
Morning	45	95	.428
Afternoon	35	85	.298
Evening	7	90	.063
Night	13	85	.111
Total	100		0.900

Weighted Average Utilization Target = 90%.

Source: Adapted from Page and McDougal, 1989.

EXAMPLE 7.1

A teaching hospital's laboratory routinely performs nine microscopic procedures. Average monthly volume of each procedure has been determined from the historical data. An earlier time study also revealed the workload standard for each procedure, as shown in Table 7.5.

Solution

The first step in setting staff levels for a procedure is to discover the number of procedures to be performed (Step 1). By multiplying the volume for each procedure by the workload standard, a time estimate for each activity is made. The sum of the standard hours represents the total time needed to perform the procedures (Step 2). Because this total represents only the direct procedure hours of the technicians, it must be augmented by the indirect (support) hours, which in this example are estimated at 0.21 hour per procedure (Step 3). Table 7.6 depicts these calculations.

TABLE 7.5. **Workload Standards for Microscopic Procedures in Laboratory.**

Variable Activities	Volume (# of Procedures per 30-day Period)	X	Workload Standard (Hours per Procedure)	=	Standard Hours for 30-day Period
Procedure 1	350		.12		42.00
Procedure 2	222		.30		66.60
Procedure 3	185		.45		83.25
Procedure 4	462		.26		120.12
Procedure 5	33		.84		27.72
Procedure 6	12		.88		10.56
Procedure 7	96		.362		34.75
Procedure 8	892		.46		410.32
Procedure 9	26		1.9		49.4
TOTALS	2,278				844.72

Source: Adapted from Page and McDougall, 1989.

TABLE 7.6. **Calculation of Staffing Requirements for Microscopic Procedures.**

Step	Description	Results
1	Total volume of activities (tests)	2,278
2	Total direct procedure hours	844.72
3	Indirect support hours [.21 × (1)] (assume 0.21 hours per procedure) 2278×0.21	478.38
4	Subtotal variable hours required [(2) + (3)] $844.72 + 478.38 = 1,323.10$	1,323.10
5	Department utilization target [from Table 7.3]	90.0%
6	Total variable hours required (normalized) [(4) ÷ (5)]	1,470.11
7	Constant hours (30 days at 12.28 hours per calendar day)	368.40
8	Total target worked hours required [(6) + (7)]	1,838.51
9	Total target FTEs required [(8) ÷ 173.33] [40 hrs./wk. x 52 wks. ÷ 12 months = 173.33]	10.65
10	Vacation/holiday/sick FTE allowance [(9) x 9.8%] (percentage varies by hospital department)	1.04
11	Total Required Paid FTEs [(9) + (10)]	11.65

Source: Adapted from Page and McDougall, 1989.

The sum of the direct and indirect hours (Step 4) gives us the variable hours required for all procedures. This sum must be adjusted for the utilization level that was determined in Table 7.4. After the adjustment—made by dividing the value found in Step 4 by utilization level in Step 5—we get a normalized total variable hour estimate (Step 6), meaning that it is based upon a utilization target of 100 percent "for purposes of being able to compare staff requirements of one department with those of other departments" (Page and McDougall, 1989; p. 79).

Next, the number of constant hours must be determined (Step 7). Constant hours represent the time spent in fixed activities (meetings, inventories, etc.). By adding values in Step 6 to Step 7, we determine the target for worked hours required (Step 8). The total targeted work hours are divided by 173.33 (hours per FTE worked per month) to compute the total target FTEs required (Step 9). However, quantity (9) must be adjusted for vacation, sick days, and holidays. It is estimated that the adjustment factor is 9.8 percent, giving a leave of absence allowance of 1.04 FTE. By adding this allowance (Step 10) to the total target FTEs (Step 9), we determine the total number of FTEs required in the laboratory, 11.65 FTEs.

Determination of FTEs for Nurse Staffing. Determination of the FTEs required to staff a nursing unit requires several steps. First, the minutes of required care are determined using the following formula:

$$
\begin{aligned}
\textit{Minutes of Care Required} &= \textit{(Average Census)} \\
&\times \textit{(Average Required Minutes per Patient)}.
\end{aligned}
\tag{7.1}
$$

This equation then should be divided by the number of minutes available to work per nurse per day (equals 8 hours/day × 60 minutes/hour, or 480 minutes available) to determine the number of unadjusted FTEs. Thus, in the second step, unadjusted FTEs are calculated using the next formula:

$$
\textit{Unadjusted FTEs} = \frac{\text{Total Minutes of Care Required}}{\text{Minutes Available to Work per Nurse per Day}}.
\tag{7.2}
$$

However, this method of calculation assumes 100 percent utilization of the staff, an assumption that is clearly unrealistic for the reasons mentioned earlier. Suppose that the administration has established a utilization standard of 0.75; that is, 25 percent of each employee's time will be spent in unproductive activities, or activities unrelated to direct patient care. The number of minutes available to work per nurse per day (example, 480 minutes) must be adjusted by the utilization standard; hence in the third step, core level FTEs are determined with this formula:

$$
\textit{Core Level FTEs} = \frac{\textit{(Average Required Minutes per Patient)} \times \textit{(Average Census)}}{\textit{(Utilization Standard)} \times \textit{(Available Work Minutes)}}.
\tag{7.3}
$$

Example 7.2 below illustrates the calculations.

EXAMPLE 7.2

The nursing manager would like to determine the number of nursing staff needed for the medical or surgical unit. Table 7.2 and Table 7.3 provide census and acuity information for a medical or surgical floor.

Solution

Table 7.2 provides information on the daily census for January 2005. Table 7.3 aggregates the monthly data to provide the average census over a 25-month period. Notice that the mean values presented in Table 7.3 are the same as those found in the year 3 January row in Table 7.3. It is important to realize that the core staffing levels in this example are found through a retrospective analysis of average monthly census and required hours per patient day.

When determining a core staffing level, there are two particular calculations of interest: average census and average required hours per patient day for the 25-month period. Examining those numbers, we see that the medical or surgical unit should staff for an average of fourteen patients daily, requiring 4.1 hours of direct care, on average.

The first step of the staffing calculation is to find the total number of minutes of care required, using formula (7.1):

$$\textit{Minutes of Care Required} = \textit{(Average Census)}$$
$$\times \textit{(Average Required Minutes per Patient).}$$
$$\textit{Minutes of Care Required} = (14 \times 4.1) \times 60 \textit{ minutes} = 3{,}444 \textit{ minutes.}$$

The second step uses formula (7.2) to divide the number of minutes available to work per nurse per day (480 minutes) to determine the number of unadjusted FTEs required.

$$\textit{Unadjusted FTEs} = \frac{3444}{480} = 7.0 \text{ , which in this case is 7 nurses.}$$

The third step determines the core level FTEs, using formula (7.3).

$$\textit{Core Level FTEs} = \frac{3444}{0.75 \times 480} = 9.6 \text{ nurses.}$$

In this example, the core level of FTEs, assuming a 0.75 utilization standard, equals 9.6 FTEs.

Coverage Factor. One other adjustment must be made to make sure that the core staffing levels are as accurate as possible. The above calculation assumes that employees will be available to work 365 days per year, without vacations, sick days, or holidays. To adjust for these factors, we must calculate a coverage factor. An example of the coverage factor adjustment is found in Table 7.7. The first step in its determination is subtracting weekend days per year and benefit days from the required coverage days per year (365 in most any health care organization), to arrive at a total of available days per FTE (line 5). By dividing the total number of required days per year by the total available days, we obtain a coverage factor. This coverage factor is then multiplied by the unit FTE requirements to calculate the total unit FTE requirements.

$$\text{Final Core Level FTEs} = \text{Core Level FETs} \times \text{Coverage Factor.} \quad (7.4)$$

For instance, under 5/40 plan, final unit requirements would be:

Final Core Level FTEs = 9.6 × 1.55 = 14.9 or 15 nurses.

This example illustrates how the coverage factor is affected by scheduling and institutional policies. When ten-hour shifts are used (the 4/40 plan), the coverage factor is elevated due to the greater number of weekend days per employee.

TABLE 7.7. **The Effect of Shift Alternatives on Staffing—The Coverage Factor.**

Assumptions	5/40 or 2/12 & 2/8 Plans	4/40 or 4/36 Plans
(1) Required coverage days per year	365	365
(2) Weekend days per year (days off)	104	156 — *more days off/wk, 3 days off/wk*
(3) Benefit days	~~10,771~~ (25)	~~10,771~~ (25)
* Vacation	10	6
* Sick days	7	7
* Holidays	7	7
* Other	1	1
(4) Total allowance days of FTE (2) + (3)	129	181
(5) Total available days of FTE (1) − (4)	236	184
(6) Coverage Factor (1) ÷ (5)	1.55	1.98

Shift Alternatives	Unit FTE Requirement	× Coverage Factor =	Total Unit FTE Requirements
5/40	9.6	1.55	15 *14.88*
4/40	9.6	1.98	19 *19.008*
4/36	9.6	1.98	19
2/12 & 2/8	9.6	1.55	15

Under the 4/40 plan, final unit requirements would be:

$$Final\ Core\ Level\ FTEs = 9.6 \times 1.98 = 19\ nurses.$$

The consequence is a higher total unit FTE requirement and consequently higher costs. (Further discussion on this subject is found in the section on scheduling.) The coverage factor is further affected by institutional policies on holidays, vacation, sick leave, training and continuing education, and by vacancies and employee turnover.

Reallocation Through Daily Adjustments. Once the final core level of FTEs is established, it must be adjusted on a daily, shift-by-shift basis to make sure that proper staffing levels are available to meet patients' requirements. Figure 7.2 illustrates an elasticity zone in which the core level staff is expected to handle patient needs. As

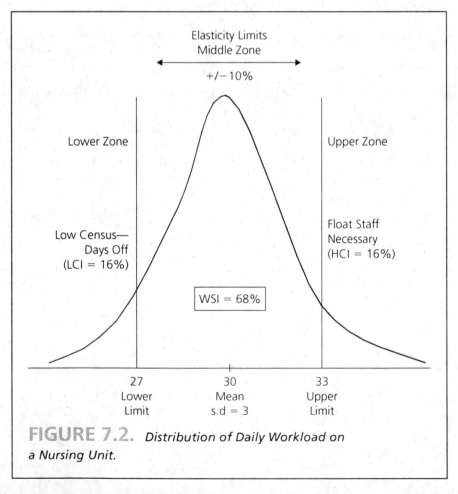

FIGURE 7.2. *Distribution of Daily Workload on a Nursing Unit.*

Source: Adopted from Shukla, R. K. *Theories and Strategies of Health care: Technology-Strategy-Performance,* Chapter Four, unpublished manuscript, 1991.

long as the workload stays within this zone, no additional staff is necessary. However, when workloads are greater than 10 percent of the standard, float staff must be hired, often at a premium. Similarly, on low census days, employees can be given time off or encouraged to catch up with in-service continuing education. The workload stability index (WSI) is a measure of how often workload stays within the limits where no additional staff or time-offs are necessary (Shukla, 1991).

If development of internal standards is prohibitively expensive for your organization, it is possible to adopt externally developed standards.

External Work Standards and Their Adjustments

External standards can be either of two types, industry based or professionally based. Industry standards can be adapted to a particular institution if adjusted carefully for factors such as case mix. Industry standards have the advantage of being available at much lower cost than the development of institutional standards. They are extremely credible in most cases, having been evaluated by industry experts (Kirk, 1986).

One of the first professional standards was published in 1979 by the Oncology Nursing Society (ONS) with the collaboration of the American Nurses Association, in a manual entitled *Outcome Standards for Cancer Nursing Practice*. Updated in 1987, this publication aimed to provide nurses with the tools to determine the degree of nursing care a patient should receive (Lamkin and Sleven, 1991; p. 1,242). Other groups that have developed professional standards are the Nurses Association of the American College of Obstetrics and Gynecology (*Guidelines of Perinatal Care* [1988]; *Standards for Obstetric, Gynecological, and Neonatal Nursing* [1986]; *Considerations for Professional Nurse Staffing in Perinatal Units* [1988]) and the American Association of Critical-Care Nurses (AACN) (*Standards for Nursing Care of the Critically Ill* [1989]). Many of these professionally published manuals make relatively specific recommendations— for example, the AACN publication's statement: "utilization of at least 50 percent RN staff on each shift . . . [and a] nurse patient ratio [reflecting] the patient's acuity and required nursing care. Staffing patterns should be reviewed regularly by the Critical Care Committee to ensure the delivery of safe care." (Lamkin and Sleven, 1991; p. 1,242).

To avoid the possibility of inaccuracies when using industry standards or professionally determined staffing standards and the costs that inappropriate staffing level may incur, such external standards must be evaluated and adjusted for the unique characteristics of a particular organization. A partial list of factors referred by the ONS is as follows:

- Size and design of facility

- Average length of stay

- Non-nursing responsibilities

- Nursing responsibilities

- Intensity/acuity levels of patients

- Reliability of patient classification system

- Clinical expertise of available staff

- Organized system of patient education

- Staff mix

- Research and data management responsibilities

- Patient transport responsibilities

- Physician practice patterns

- Facility census patterns

Regardless of the standard developed, whether internal or external, it is important for the manager to thoroughly understand a department and its operations before applying standards. What work is currently done and by whom? Where are the potential bottlenecks? How satisfied is the staff with the current system? One of the best ways to answer these questions is through direct interviews or surveys with the department or unit employees. Not only can direct observation and employee contact improve the development of a new staffing or scheduling plan; it also helps the employees accept any changes that occur if they have participated in planning them. Again, a careful look at the factors suggested above can greatly benefit the development and application of work standards.

It is important to recognize that no standard is absolute. Some room must be left for flexibility in staffing. Figure 7.3 demonstrates how statistical analysis can reveal whether the staff is meeting the standards. The number of hours to provide a service n times over a particular period of time in a specific unit serving clients of similar acuity levels should be plotted. When the times used lie outside the upper and lower tolerance limits, it is the manager's responsibility to determine the reason. It certainly should not be assumed that the problem lies with the staff; it is possible that the standard is unfair or outdated and should be reevaluated.

FIGURE 7.3. *Workload Standard Tolerance Ranges.*

Work standards, once adopted, can be used to evaluate the productivity of the organization, a department, or even an individual employee. Without the development of such standards, the success of workload management programs aimed at improving organizational productivity cannot be assessed.

Productivity and Workload Management

Productivity is traditionally measured as the ratio of outputs to inputs (see Chapter Nine). The outputs generally consist of an organization's performance expectations (profit, quality of care, services provided, and so on); inputs include labor hours, materials, and others. Productivity measurement is important for staffing decisions, and staffing decisions can affect not only the organization's productivity, but the quality of care rendered, as well.

Departmental productivity is often measured as the ratio of the required, or standard, hours (for example, those found in Table 7.3, which are developed using the patient acuity system) to the number of hours actually worked. Thus, departmental productivity is a measure of the effective utilization of the unit's staff. Two very important staffing considerations that profoundly influence employee utilization are the appropriateness of employee skills and the matching of these skills to the appropriate job description (Page and McDougall, 1989; p. 61). For instance, registered nurses would not be used effectively if they were to change all patients' bedding or spend the majority of their time filling out medical records. Such jobs would be more efficiently handled by less expensive nurse's aides or licensed practical nurses, thereby freeing time for an RN to perform more complicated medical duties for which an aide or LPN may not be trained. Therefore, when staffing a department, the health care manager must take not only numbers of employees into account, but also skill levels.

Other factors that affect productivity are worker satisfaction and work organization. Job satisfaction or the lack of it can significantly affect organizational costs: hiring, firing, training, and low productivity arising from dissatisfaction can elevate costs dramatically. Job satisfaction can be evaluated by examining three areas: retention, recruitment, and transfers. It is generally assessed through a survey that includes a staff profile at both the professional and the personal level, satisfaction with current scheduling, preferences in terms of shifts or units, perceived flexibility, and attitude toward benefits. The important point is that the health care manager should aim to keep the staff as happy as possible, and that carefully made staffing and scheduling decisions support that goal.

Work can also be organized so as to improve effectiveness. Work simplification procedures can identify unproductive activities and eliminate them. Changes in facility layout can reduce travel time and improve traffic flow. Enhanced environmental conditions such as lighting and temperature can enhance productivity and staff satisfaction, and patient satisfaction as well.

When attempting to improve productivity through workload management, the health care manager must be aware of potential problems. Problems related to staffing and scheduling operations include workload volume fluctuations, workload scheduling, skill mix, and staffing patterns (Page and McDougall, 1989; p. 61).

Workload volume fluctuates daily and seasonally with significant effect on productivity calculations. Page and McDougall (1989) cite an instance in which a hospital's operating room was affected by three surgeons who were avid hunters. Every year, all three surgeons were absent for the first week of hunting season, significantly reducing the productivity of the operating room staff; yet staffing patterns had not been adjusted for what should have been a predictable volume change.

Appropriate workload scheduling can help a department become more productive. Leveling the workload, that is, reducing the peaks and valleys so common in any service industry with random service and arrival pattern, can often be accomplished with sophisticated workload scheduling software. Techniques used to schedule the hospital employees are discussed in the next chapter.

SUMMARY

Staffing patterns must involve matching the human resources available to the fluctuating demand for their services. When an efficient match is maintained, productivity is enhanced. Alternative staffing patterns can improve flexibility, reduce costs, maintain continuity of patient care, and increase worker and patient satisfaction. Options for changing current staffing patterns are presented under Scheduling in Chapter Eight. In sum, workload management operations can significantly affect organizational productivity.

KEY TERMS

Workload Management
Patient Acuity System
Full Time Equivalent (FTE)

Staff Utilization
Work Load
Coverage Factor

EXERCISES

7.1) A mammography center performs ten different procedures. The volume of each procedure during an eight-month period and the standard hours per procedure are shown in Table EX 7.1.

TABLE EX 7.1

Procedure Description	Volume	Standard Hours
SC BX Breast IM Guide	220	.20
SC PLC CLIP Breast	195	.25
SC PLC Wire Breast	121	.50
SC PLC Wire Breast Add	24	.60

Procedure Description	Volume	Standard Hours
Mammo Spec Board	103	.75
Mammogm DIAG UNI	1,494	.25
Mammogm DIAG BI	1,505	.33
Mammogm SCR BI	8,924	.33
XR NDL/WIRE Breast LOC	136	.45
XR Surgical Specimen	318	.75
XR STERO Breast BIOP	226	.75

The target utilization rate for the center is 85 percent. Indirect support time is 0.20 hour per procedure, and total administrative hours by all staff average ten hours per day. The fringe benefits comprising vacation/holiday/sick compensation amount to 10 percent of required FTEs.

    a. Calculate the standard hours per month.

    b. Determine the indirect support hours per month.

    c. Determine the variable hours per month.

    d. Normalize the variable hours per month.

    e. Determine the total required hours.

    f. Determine the target FTE level.

    g. Determine the required FTEs with fringe benefits.

7.2 Utilize the information from exercise 6.2, where pre- and post-examination processing of patients in an outpatient clinic involves various tasks performed by clerks and nurses.

    a. Excluding the wait times by patients, recalculate the standard time.

    b. If there were an average of 1,800 patient visits to the outpatient clinic, what would be the standard hours per month?

    c. If the target utilization rate of the facility is 80 percent; the indirect support time per visit is 0.10 hour; and the total administrative time by all staff in a given day is five hours, what is the target FTE level for the clinic?

    d. If fringe benefits account for 9 percent of the target FTEs, what are the required FTEs?

7.3 Utilize the information from Exercise 6.3, where the standard turn-around-times (TAT) for handling stat laboratory tests were estimated. The automated machine times for these tests and the monthly volumes are given in Table EX 7.3.

TABLE EX 7.3

Lab test	Machine Time	Monthly Volume
Hem 8	15	2,200
Hem 18	18	2,200
Apter	25	1,800
AMY	20	3,200
Ca	19	2,400
Glucose	25	2,400
Chem 7	22	2,200
K	10	2,000
HCG	12	1,800
ALP	25	1,000
ALT	24	1,500
B	20	1,000
AST	25	800
BBSP	16	900

a. Recalculate the standard time for each test by subtracting the machine time.

b. Determine the standard hours per month for staff handling these tests.

c. If the target utilization rate of the facility is 90 percent, the indirect support time per test is 0.05 hours, and the total administrative time by all staff in a given day is seven hours, what is the target FTE level for this part of the laboratory?

d. If fringe benefits account for 9.5 percent of the target FTEs, what will be the required FTEs?

7.4 In a staff model HMO, the requirement for MDs' time is estimated to be 11,000 minutes per day. The utilization target for MDs is 90 percent. Human resources' benefit plan for them includes eleven holidays, ten sick days, and twenty-one paid vacation days per year. Determine the core level of MD FTEs for the HMO.

7.5 In the emergency department of a medical center, the requirement for staff MDs' time is estimated to be 20,000 minutes per day. The utilization target for MDs is 95 percent. The medical center's benefit plan for staff MDs includes ten holidays, ten sick days, and twenty-one paid vacation days per year.

a. Determine the core level of MD FTEs for the emergency department.

b. Determine the final core level of MD FTEs if all staff are scheduled for eight-hour shifts, using a 5/40 scheduling plan.

c. Determine the final core level of FTEs if MDs work on a 4/40 scheduling plan.

7.6 Table EX 7.6 depicts the average RN minutes needed on a daily basis in various units.

TABLE EX 7.6

ICU	CCU	SURG	MED	PED	OB/GYN
7,000	8,000	8,500	9,000	7,500	6,500

a. Assuming an 85 percent utilization level and that everything else is constant, how many RN FTEs should be hired to satisfy the patient care demand in each unit?

b. The FTEs hired for SURG, MED, PED, and OB/GYN are scheduled for eight-hour shifts on a 5/40 plan, and they will get ten holidays, six sick days, and fifteen paid vacation days per year. How does this information affect your FTEs?

c. The FTEs hired for the ICU and CCU are to be scheduled for ten-hour shifts on a 4/40 plan, and ICU and CCU nurses get the same benefits as do other unit nurses. How does this information affect your FTEs?

7.7 For Famous Health care System (FHS), consultants from O&A determined the average daily patient demand for various nursing professionals. Table EX 7.7 depicts the average number of minutes for Registered Nurses (RNs), Licensed Practical Nurses (LPNs), and Nursing Aides (NAs) needed daily in various patient care departments of FHS.

TABLE EX 7.7

Departments	RN Minutes	LPN Minutes	NA Minutes
ICU	7,000	3,500	1,500
CCU	8,000	4,750	2,500
Surgical	10,500	6,500	4,000
Medical	12,500	7,500	4,500
Pediatric	9,500	3,500	2,500
OB/GYN	10,500	7,500	4,000

FHS decided that utilization targets for RNs, LPNs and NAs should be 85 percent, 80 percent, and 80 percent, respectively. FHSs' human resources benefit plan for RNs has seven holidays, five sick days, and eighteen paid vacation days per year. The benefit package for LPNs has seven holidays, five sick days, and fourteen paid vacation days per year. The NA benefit package has seven holidays, five sick days, and ten paid vacation days per year. FHS wants to reevaluate staffing levels according to the patient demand measurements provided by O&A, as follows:

   a.   Determine the core level of FTEs for each department.

   b.   Determine the final core levels of FTEs for the Surgical, Medical, Pediatric, and OB/GYN departments if all staff are scheduled for eight-hour shifts using a 5/40 scheduling plan.

   c.   Determine the final core levels of FTEs for the ICU and CCU departments if RNs and LPNs work on a 4/40 and NAs work on a 5/40 scheduling plan.

CHAPTER

8

SCHEDULING

LEARNING OBJECTIVES

- Describe the various shift patterns and cyclical and flexible scheduling alternatives.
- Review concepts that are important for computerized scheduling.
- Evaluate scheduling alternatives for operating rooms.
- Describe factors that affect efficient utilization of operating rooms.

Scheduling for staff and resources are recurring and time-consuming tasks for health care managers. If not done skillfully, scheduling of either can waste resources and reduce the revenue of the health care organization. In this chapter, we discuss staff scheduling, mostly pertaining to nursing staff, and resource scheduling, mainly for surgical suites (operating rooms). While both of these are, respectively, the major resource consumption areas, the latter is one of the major revenue-generating centers of the hospitals.

STAFF SCHEDULING

Staff scheduling allocates the budgeted FTEs to the proper patients in the proper units at the proper times. There is controversy about the most effective and efficient scheduling pattern, centering on shift length: Is the eight-, ten-, or twelve-hour shift preferable? The choice can affect turnover, absenteeism, and overall job satisfaction. Moreover, scheduling relates directly to the quality of patient care by affecting coverage and continuity of care, as well as staff morale.

The five factors to consider when scheduling are: coverage, schedule quality, stability, flexibility, and cost. Coverage refers to how well patients' needs are met: does the schedule meet patients' needs, maintain continuity of care, and provide even coverage for all patients? Schedule quality refers to how well the staff likes the plan. That is influenced by factors such as equalization of rotation, weekends, days off, and work stretch. A third element is the stability of the schedule. Can the nurses count on predictable schedules? Or, are their schedules always changing? On the other hand, flexibility of the schedule is also an important concern. Can the schedule adapt to environmental changes, for example, nurses changing among shifts, orientation and continuing education programs, and understaffing. Finally, given the revenue constraints facing many organizations, costs are an important concern. Are resources being consumed wisely? Would an alternative schedule produce better care at lower cost?

As noted, one important issue is shift length, which should be decided in light of the criteria presented above. A 5/40 shift refers to a five-day, forty-hour week; thus, the employee works eight hours per day. Similarly, a 4/40 shift refers to a four-day workweek of forty hours, or ten hours daily.

Traditionally, the eight-hour, five-day workweek (5/40) has predominated. However, with recognition that employee satisfaction, schedule flexibility, and high quality of care must be sought, innovative approaches have turned toward the option of a compressed workweek. The change would be made either in days (such as from a 5/40 to a 4/40 plan), in hours worked (from a 4/40 to 4/36 plan), or in both days and hours (from a 5/40 to a 3/36 plan). Many organizations have chosen to change the number of days worked in a week but to keep the total hours the same. For changes in shift hours, the most popular alternatives to the traditional eight-hour shift are the ten- and twelve-hour shifts.

In general, ten-hour shifts, compared to eight-hour shifts, provide several consecutive days off, more weekend days off, opportunity to work with other shift workers, more staff during busy periods, increased continuity of care, and provide time for meetings and in-service education. However, this shift pattern requires more staff and may increase staff fatigue. Moreover, twelve-hour shifts similarly provide several consecutive days off, more weekend days off, and increased continuity of care. In addition, this shift pattern requires one less shift report and is attractive for hiring new staff. Nevertheless, it may require more staff and promote fatigue. Although considerable research on the use of different shift lengths has been reported by experienced health care professionals, there is considerable disagreement among them (Newstrom and Pierce, 1979).

The four-day, forty-hour workweek gained popularity in the early 1970s, although it was first tried in the 1940s, by both the Gulf and Mobil Oil companies (Newstrom and Pierce, 1979). Today, many nursing units are seeking the advantages of the ten-hour shift. For instance, it creates a shift overlap, which allows hospitals to cope with daily peak demand periods, thereby avoiding extensive reallocation of staff and staff overtime. The overlap in the ten-hour shift system can be designed to occur during the periods of greatest patient need. The improved communication between shifts should

FIGURE 8.1. *Comparison of Eight- and Ten-Hour Shifts.*

enhance the continuity of care. Since having a three-day weekend is perceived as a benefit to the nursing staff, morale and productivity may also improve. However, the increased number of days off per year and the overlap of shifts mean that more employees must be hired to staff a ten-hour rotation. Recall the staffing coverage factor from Chapter Seven. The resulting increase in labor costs can be a major drawback of the system. Figure 8.1 compares the eight-hour and the ten-hour schedules.

A modification of the traditional 4/40, in which the worker works four days and then has three days off, is the "eight-day week." Under this system, employees work four ten-hour days, after which they have a four-day break before beginning the cycle again. Thus, two shifts of employees can alternate between being on and off of the 4/40 work cycle throughout the year.

The twelve-hour shift provides the most days off weekly, which can help in recruiting and retaining staff. It also reduces the number of shifts that administrators must prepare and gives the staff more open days for continuing education. However, working the long hours of the twelve-hour shift has the potential for employee burn-out. Some organizations may allow workers to alternate eight- and twelve-hour shifts, in an attempt to realize the benefits of each. An example of this alternating pattern is seen in Figure 8.2.

The following section provides some examples of programs that have been tried to improve nurses' recruitment, satisfaction, and retention, as well as aspects of patient care, by altering scheduling and shift patterns.

The Eight-, Ten-, and Twelve-Hour Shifts—Studies of Shift Patterns. Many health care organizations have experimented with changing shift lengths to address a variety of concerns. Some organizations may want to reduce staffing levels; others may want

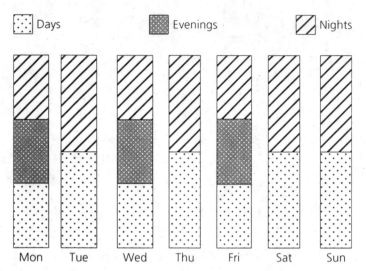

FIGURE 8.2.   *Pattern of Alternating Eight- and Twelve-Hour Shifts.*

to reduce costs. Supporting staff recruitment and retention when medical personnel are in short supply is another aim. Other aims might be to improve nurses' productivity or their job satisfaction, which would mean less necessity to hire part-time nursing personnel from outside agencies. Improving the continuity of care, and thus patient satisfaction, is also cited as benefit.

An Ohio hospital, recognizing the need for greater flexibility in scheduling and also the importance of more time off for nurses who work under highly intense conditions, adopted a ten-hour shift (Velianoff, 1991). Rather than relying on the traditional 7 A.M., 3 P.M., 11 P.M. starting times for shifts, with two hours of overlap, they created six different shifts. Depending on the workload, either five or six daily shifts are used. As a result of the change, the organization reported reduced overtime, and greater productivity. Moreover, nurses were less distracted from patient care by their job satisfaction issues. Ninety percent of the hospital's nurses preferred the ten-hour shift over previous systems.

The advantages of the ten-hour shift are not recognized by all health care managers, however. The director of a nursing unit in New York, for example, claims that ten-hour shifts are not cost-effective and that such advantages as do exist do not outweigh the extra costs of hiring additional staff (the coverage factor). In the 1990s, she argued, "We need to promote nurse satisfaction in addition to continuous, cost-effective, quality care." (Corsi, 1991). In response, the editor of *Nursing Management* recognized that ten-hour shifts are not the most cost-effective. However, she noted that if they reduce turnover and absenteeism, the expenses are justified. It is apparent that the perceived merits of the ten-hour shift depend largely on the goals or guidelines of the individual institution.

A comparison of nurses' work patterns in the eight- and twelve-hour shifts was completed at a 132-bed, not-for-profit community hospital in Southern California. Overall, the study found that shift length did not significantly influence job performance in the sample. Of particular interest are the similar absenteeism rates for both shifts. Contrary to the literature, which often predicts higher absenteeism for the eight-hour shift schedule, the number of shifts missed was the same for both the eight- and the twelve-hour work patterns. Noting that the primary reason for absences was personal illness, the author suggests that a health promotion program may be more effective than a change in the schedule system in lowering the absenteeism rate. Notice also that the hours spent in continuing education did not differ significantly and were in fact higher for the eight-hour shift. Though, a commonly cited advantage of the twelve-hour shift is that it leaves more time open for nurse education.

Palmer (1991) further claims that twelve-hour shifts are preferable in areas where the nurse-to-patient ratios are low, such as in intensive care and the emergency room. In these units, a nurse can care for up to four patients at a time for the twelve-hour period. When the nurse is not overburdened and continuity of patient care is enhanced, a twelve-hour shift can have substantial advantages. In other areas of the hospital, the possibility of burnout may prohibit the use of the twelve-hour shift. For instance, Palmer has found that twelve-hour shift nurses who float to medical units often request an eight-hour shift to avoid unacceptable levels of fatigue. Concluding her study, she notes that although twelve-hour shifts may give the hospital a competitive advantage in recruitment and retention, its personnel policies and compensation packages must be carefully examined to maintain productivity.

In sum, the success of a change in shift length varies greatly from organization to organization. Each facility must evaluate where it wants to head and what aspects of its operations it wants to improve. No one system suits every health care organization, and the choice depends on the particular institution's goals.

The implementation process can also significantly affect the success of a program to change shift lengths. Involving the nursing staff in the planning and incorporating their views in the final decisions will greatly improve the possibilities for a successful program. To address some of the flaws with straight eight-, ten-, and twelve-hour work shifts, many organizations are turning to flexible working schedules.

Cyclical Scheduling. Work schedules can be classified as either permanent (cyclical) or flexible (discretionary). Under a cyclical work schedule, employees do not rotate shifts. The schedule is usually planned for a four- to six-week period, and is repeated period after period. Exhibit 8.1 illustrates the cyclical staffing schedule concept for both a four- and a five-week scheduling period. The "0" in the illustration indicates a day off. The system allows the employees to select the shift that best fits their schedule. However, having chosen it, the nurses are locked into that shift. This can create difficulties in hiring new nurses to replace those who leave, because they must be willing to take the schedule of the departing nurse.

EXHIBIT 8.1 Cyclical Staffing Schedules for Four and Five Weeks.

The Four Week Schedule

Weeks → 1 … 2 … 3 … 4 … 5

Employee	S	M	T	W	T	F	S	S	M	T	W	T	F	S	S	M	T	W	T	F	S	S	M	T	W	T	F	S	S	M	T	W	T	F	S
A	O	O								O	O								O	O		O						O	O	O					
B			O	O								O	O		O						O	O	O								O	O			
C					O	O		O						O	O	O								O	O								O	O	
D	O						O	O	O								O	O								O	O		O						O
# of Staff Scheduled	2	3	3	3	3	3	3	2	3	3	3	3	3	3	2	3	3	3	3	3	3	2	3	3	3	3	3	3	2	3	3	3	3	3	3

The Five Week Schedule

Weeks → 1 … 2 … 3 … 4 … 5

Employee	S	M	T	W	T	F	S	S	M	T	W	T	F	S	S	M	T	W	T	F	S	S	M	T	W	T	F	S	S	M	T	W	T	F	S
A	O	O								O	O								O	O		O						O						O	O
B			O	O								O	O		O						O						O	O	O	O					
C					O	O		O						O						O	O	O	O								O	O			
D						O	O						O	O	O	O								O	O								O	O	
E						O	O	O	O								O	O								O	O		O						O
# of Staff Scheduled	3	4	4	4	4	3	3	3	4	4	4	4	3	3	3	4	4	4	4	3	3	3	4	4	4	4	3	3	3	4	4	4	4	3	3

The cyclical schedule, although it does promote even coverage, high stability, and lower scheduling costs, is inflexible to environmental changes such as nurses who ask to change from full- to part-time, or rotating nurses between departments according to patient census and acuity. Therefore, cyclical schedules are best used in a stable environment where nurses (or allied health professionals) do not rotate between shifts and where the supply of employees is sufficient to ensure that a new one can easily be hired into an open cyclical slot.

Flexible Scheduling. As you well know, today's health care environment is highly unstable, and personnel shortages, particularly of nurses, make recruitment difficult. Consequently, hospitals have turned to discretionary work systems. Discretionary work systems fall into two categories—staggered and flexible schedules. The staggered start system, while not changing the number of hours worked per week, allows employees to decide when to start their work day. A variation on the staggered start is the staggered week, or flex week. Under this system, employees maintain eight-hour days and average forty hours per week. However, they alternate, for instance, between a 4/32 and 6/48 plan.

Because coverage is essential and managing a staggered start system to ensure it is expensive, the flexible working hour system is much more common in health care. Under a flexible system, the health care manager can cope with fluctuations in demand. A core level of staff is established, based on a long-term assessment of staff needs (see Chapter Seven for detailed discussion), and is augmented by daily adjustments (reallocation) using various methods to ensure that staffing levels meet patient needs. Nurses must be willing to change shifts to meet fluctuations in patient demand. Besides that, a pool of full- and part-time nurses is formed for use during periods of high patient demand (either through census or acuity), and scheduling procedures must be adapted for their use. The organization must also be flexible in responding to its employees' needs, in order to reduce turnover.

With flexible scheduling, the nurses select the schedule pattern that best meets their needs, given the scheduling system adopted by the administrator of the unit. Some form of part-time shift is usually necessary to meet a unit's staffing needs. Often, the part-time shift positions are filled by a pool of float nurses hired directly by the hospital. Another source of temporary or part-time nurses is staff relief agencies, also known as supplemental nursing services, external temporary agencies, and registries (Rasmussen, 1982). The health care organization pays the agency, which in turn pays its employees. Nurses from these agencies can be let go when not needed and otherwise relieve an overburdened hospital staff. However, they are often viewed as outsiders by the regular nursing staff, especially since they usually paid more per hour than the hospital pays its nurses.

Flexible scheduling is common because of the increasing uncertainty and costs facing health care facilities. In 1990, the American Nurses Association adopted a statement on flexible scheduling and part-time work, to ensure that nurses would be allowed opportunities for part-time work. The Association argues that nurses need options if they are to "manage multiple personal and professional roles" (Kinney, 1990).

Findlay (1994) provides a comprehensive review of the literature on flexible work systems in nursing and gives an account of the flexible working system he developed for the thirty-bed continuing care psychiatric unit where he worked. His system was based on a 37.5-hour workweek; nurses worked five days on and two days off, with no more than eight hours of work per day, Monday through Friday, and no more than 9.5 hours per day on weekends. Overlaps between all shifts ensured the continuity of care, and duty rosters were assigned in six-week cycles. Nurses could choose their shift preferences on a first-come-first-served basis. Daily, ten-minute overview meetings dispersed essential patient information, and a weekly, thirty-minute meeting handled issues unrelated to the patients.

An evaluation of this system after six months showed that flexible schedules used nursing resources more effectively. Patients benefited from improved continuity of care, and staff no longer had to be routed from other units. By not having to hire staff agency nurses or pay overtime, the unit reduced its expenditures by 15 percent in the six months after implementation. With nurses freed from a rigid schedule, innovations in patient care were developed and implemented. Surveys of the nurses indicated that they too believed that care continuity had improved. Additional benefits identified by the nurses included: more time for patient-related activities, boosted morale, higher job satisfaction, greater unity on the ward, less tiring workload, and more flexibility in annual leave and public holidays.

When flexible scheduling results in different nurses being with the same patient over his or her hospital stay, clinical information must be transferred from shift to shift. All nurses caring for a particular patient must be aware of all the factors affecting the patient's care. Only when nurses are aware of the history of the patient can they together provide continuous care of high quality.

In sum, flexible staffing programs can help the health care organization meet the five scheduling criteria presented at the beginning of this section. Coverage can be maintained by adjusting staffing patterns when necessary while ensuring continuity of care and comprehensive knowledge of patients' histories. From the literature, flexible scheduling appears to promote schedule quality in terms of job satisfaction. Although flexible staffing does not always allow a stable schedule for nurses, it also must be remembered that often they are working when they wish to. In that sense, changes in scheduling patterns are assumed to meet the needs of the staff. The very term "flexible staffing" tells us that the fourth criteria, flexibility, is being met. Finally, flexible staffing usually cuts costs by reducing the need for overtime and hiring temporary nursing personnel at a premium. Nonetheless, without proper implementation even the most thought-out flexible staffing program can fail. Computerized scheduling technology has made flexible scheduling more feasible and it is discussed next.

Computerized Scheduling Systems. In 1976, Warner estimated that less than 1 percent of all hospitals used a computerized scheduling system. Today many more do, as they recognize the value of such systems. Computerized acuity systems, such as the Medicus NPAQ system discussed in Chapter Seven, can translate workload estimates into the appropriate required staffing and skill mix levels. Computerized scheduling can ensure that staffing levels are high enough to meet patient needs, while producing schedules that promote satisfaction among the staff. Computerized scheduling systems can easily take both employee preferences and institutional policies into account. Furthermore, they tend to cost less in terms of money and time than traditional, "by hand" scheduling methods do. The advantages of computerized systems are most pronounced when the nursing environment encounters unexpected change, and therefore should be of particular use today.

Implementation of a New Work System. After spending several months evaluating the current staffing patterns, reviewing the literature, analyzing systems in other institutions or nursing units of a hospital that use a different scheduling pattern, and finally developing a pattern for the nursing unit, it is important not to rush its implementation. Unless the implementation is handled well, all the previous months' efforts will have been in vain.

Employees naturally resist change. Those barriers to change must be dissolved before any system can be effective. The process must begin during the initial planning: From the outset, employees should be persuaded that their views about the current staffing patterns are being sought in order to develop a pattern that will suit them better. The nursing staff should participate at all levels of the planning process, and their input should be understood to be important.

A written proposal outlining the change should be developed and circulated to all nursing staff on the unit. Its advantages and disadvantages and the effectiveness of similar scheduling patterns at other institutions and as described in the literature should be documented. Questions and concerns should be openly addressed, and then strategies to minimize the disadvantages should be developed. Careful attention must be paid to issues such as lengths of breaks, especially for ten- and twelve-hour shifts; vacation and sick-day policies; pay, especially shift differentials and overtime; and times for staff education.

Only after the staff has considered the changes, their advantages and disadvantages, and their roles in the process, should implementation begin. During implementation, head nurses and the administrator must assess the effectiveness and efficiency of the new patterns. The administrator should be routinely available to address questions and concerns, identify problems, and make adjustments as seen necessary. After implementation, it is important to evaluate the program through surveys, productivity and utilization data, and evaluation of the financial results.

Newstrom and Pierce (1979) identify several considerations of importance during planning and then implementation. The first such consideration is workforce values; they can be ascertained through surveys and personal interviews with the staff. Any policy that goes to counter those values will be difficult if not impossible to apply without serious consequences. A second consideration is the evaluation of alternative forms. A careful review of the literature can help the health care manager to identify potential alternatives and their attributes, as well as pitfalls to avoid. Often, systems used at other institutions would have to be adapted to meet the values, goals, and concerns of your institution. Even after a plan is developed, it may need adjustments to work well. Another concern is employee acceptance. The literature shows that without this acceptance, success will be in jeopardy. Involving employees in planning, implementation, and evaluation should increase acceptance. Another recommendation is the use of a pilot test; instead of applying the new work system to several units at once, or even to the entire unit, it should be applied to a small, representative sample. A pilot test should help to iron out the bugs in the system, producing a model to which the remainder of the unit or other units can adhere.

After implementation, the system must be evaluated. Are the employees more satisfied than before? Is their productivity increasing? Have patient complaints diminished? Are continuity of care objectives being met? Are costs being saved. If not, why? Is the new system flexible? These questions are just a few of many that must be answered during evaluation. However, if problems do exist, that does not mean the new system is a complete failure and should be abandoned. Rather, steps should be taken to recognize inadequacies and make adjustments. A goal of evaluation, after all, is to ensure that the quality of both the staffs' and the patients' care and lives is enhanced under the new system.

Surgical Suite Resource Scheduling

The surgical suite is a major source of revenue for the modern hospital, so careful scheduling is critical to its profitability. The surgical suite also offers a major area for cost containment, because (1) surgical suites have high costs and traditionally low facility and personnel utilization rates, and (2) surgical patients constitute a significant portion of the demand served by other hospital departments (Magerlein and Martin, 1978; Dexter and Traub, 2002). Surgical suite patient scheduling assigns patients, staff (surgeon[s], anesthesiologists, nurses, and so on), equipment, and instruments to specific rooms within the surgical department. Efficient scheduling can both raise revenues and reduce costs, thereby increasing profits.

Inefficient scheduling leads to idle time between cases, significant overtime costs, increased patient anxiety due to delays, and quite possibly, dissatisfied surgeons. Surgeon satisfaction may be among the more important factors to consider in scheduling because they are in essence the "customers" of the operating room (OR). Their satisfaction can be attained by ensuring high probability for surgical start times and creating a schedule they perceive as fair. In addition, the OR scheduling must be carefully coordinated with other areas of the organization, particularly the post-anesthesia care unit (PACU), beds, and surgical and floor nurse schedules.

The goals of surgical suite scheduling mentioned most often in the literature include:

- Effective use of the surgical suite by reducing delays and turnover time
- Satisfaction of surgeons

■ Safety and satisfaction of patients

■ Satisfaction of the operating room staff

■ Simplicity and ease of scheduling

■ Effective use of the PACU

■ Achieving a low case-cancellation rate

When assessing the use of the OR, these alternative measures have been used, including:

■ Total minutes the OR is in use

■ Total utilized time divided by total available time

■ Idle time of nurses as percent of total available OR time

■ Turnover time

■ Idle time of anesthesiologists as a percent of total available OR time

■ Hours utilized within the block time divided by available block hours (Williams, 1971; Gordon and others, 1988; Breslawski and Hamilton, 1991; Dexter and others, 2003)

The OR scheduling systems in hospitals use the various methods briefly described below.

First Come/First Served (FC/FS). One of the two most common methods for scheduling surgical suites, the FC/FS scheduling method allocates surgery times to the first surgeon requesting them. A limit on the number of times allocated to that surgeon, or to the estimated surgical time, may be imposed; though not in all hospitals. The problems with FC/FS scheduling are:

■ A high cancellation rate due to overbooking

■ Different levels of OR use among surgical specialties, possibly causing frustration on the part of surgeons who perceive that as unfair

■ Simultaneous overtime and idle time: canceled cases lead to idle time, and surgical complications create overtime (Hackey, Casey, and Narasimhan, 1984; Dexter and Traub, 2002)

The major advantages of this approach are the ease of scheduling and greater flexibility.

Block Scheduling. With block scheduling, the second most popular system, a block of OR time is allocated to each surgeon or group of surgeons. Blocks are usually one-half to a full day in length. The block is reserved for the surgeon's or group's exclusive use until a cutoff date, usually a day or two before surgery, at which time unused time is made available to other surgeons (Magerlein and Martin, 1978; Dexter and others, 1999).

The big advantage of the block system is that it increases utilization through better afternoon use of the surgical suite usage. The system also allows surgeons to know surgical start times well in advance, and "guarantees" them. Any afternoon overruns are attributable to the surgeon's performance, thereby giving him or her nowhere to shift responsibility for the delay. Finally, block scheduling reduces surgeons' competition over surgical scheduling and may reduce administrative work, cancellations, and the overall surgery waiting list.

The major drawback of the system is that unused block time is often held by surgeons up until the cutoff day, even when they may have no need for it. This leads inevitably to costly idle time. In addition, blocked OR time may delay urgent surgery cases until the patient's surgeon has a block scheduled. An example of a block schedule is shown in Exhibit 8.2.

Dynamic Block Scheduling. This method is a variation of block scheduling in which individual surgeons' or surgery groups' use of block time is regularly reviewed (quarterly or semi-annually). The assigned amount of block time is adjusted based on the basis of the analysis.

Longest Case First (LCF). LCF scheduling allocates the longest procedures to the earliest slots available. This system inherently allows certain specialists (such as thoracic surgeons) to always get early morning slots, which can frustrate other specialists. The system assumes that the longer the surgery, the higher the variability in surgical time. Therefore, as the day goes on, later cases can be shifted in the schedule to complete the surgical workload on time, or as closely as possible to that.

Shortest Case First (SCF). SCF is used to maintain an even load in the PACU; the shortest procedures are done in the morning. An LCF system generally causes under-utilization and idle time in the PACU in the early morning hours.

Top Down/Bottom Up. This method is also a modified block scheduling system, in which the day is divided into two blocks. Long cases are scheduled FC/FS during the morning block, and short cases are scheduled FC/FS at the end of the day. If idle time develops in the long block, the next patient who arrives for a short procedure is assigned in the gap. If time in the long block runs out, then a long case can be scheduled at the beginning of the short case block. Surgeons with multiple surgeries are scheduled in the same room to reduce idle time between surgeries.

Multiple Room System. Surgeons are usually assigned to a room; however, under a multiple room system, surgeons are scheduled to rotate from room to room. The system attempts to eliminate surgeon waiting time between cases during cleanup, room

EXHIBIT 8.2 An Example of OR Block Schedule: Surgical Suite Scheduling Method.

RM	MONDAY	TUESDAY	WEDNESDAY	THURSDAY	FRIDAY
CYSTO	0730 Urology Surgeon #1	0730 ENT Surgeon #1	0730 Urology Associates	0730 General Surgeon #1	0730 Oral Surgery / 1400 Associates (CYSTO, ORAL)
2	1330 General Surgeon #2	0730 General Surgeon #2	0730–1200 Oral / 0730–1130 Surgery Associates	0730/0815 ENT Surgeon #1 (ENT)	0730 ENT Surgeon #3 (ENT)
3	0730 ENT Surgeon #2	0730 General Surgeon #2			
4	0730 ENT Surgeon #3	0730 ENT Surgeon #2	0730 General Surgeon #2	0730/0815 ENT Surgeon #4	0730 ENT Surgeon #1 (ENT)
5	0730 Ortho Assoc. #1	0730 Ortho Assoc. #2	0730 Ortho Assoc. #1	0730/0815 Ortho Assoc. #2	0730 Ortho Assoc. #4 (ORTHO)
6	0730 Ortho Assoc. #4	0730 Ortho Assoc. #3	0730 Ortho Assoc. #2	0730/0815 Ortho Assoc. #1	0730 Ortho Surgeon #1 / 1130 Ortho Surgeon #2 (ORTHO)

Times (per block column): 0730, 1130/1330, 1530, 1730; 0930, 1330

(Continued)

EXHIBIT 8.2 (Continued)

RM	MONDAY	TUESDAY	WEDNESDAY	THURSDAY	FRIDAY
7	0730 Neuro Associates / 1530 / 1730	0730 Neuro Associates / 1530 / 1730	0730 Neuro Associates / 1500 / 1530 / 1730	0730/0815 Neuro Surgeon #1 / 1530 / 1730	0730 General Surgeon #2 / 1130 / 1300 General Surgeon #3 / 1530 — NEURO
8	0730 Neuro Associates / 1530	0730 Neuro Associates / 1530	0730 Neuro Associates / 1530	0730/0815 Neuro Surgeon #2 / 1530	0730 / OPEN / 1530 — NEURO
9	1730 / 0730 / OPEN / 1300 / 1530 / 1730	0730 General Surgeon #1 / 1330 Ortho Surgeon #3 / 1530 / 1730	0730 Surgical Assoc. #3 / 1330 / 1530 / 1730	0730/0815 / 0930 General Surgeon #6 / 1530 / 1730	0730 General Surgeon #4 / 1130 General Surgeon #5 / 1530 / 1730 — GEN
10	0730 Gen. Surgeon #2 / 1330 / 1530 / 1730 / 0730	0730 Surgical Assoc. #1 / 1530 / 1730 / 0730	0730 Surgical Assoc. #2 / 1530 / 1730 / 0730	0730/0815 Gen. Surgeon #6 / 1130/1215 Gen. Surgeon #5 / 1530 / 1730	0730 General Surgeon #1 / 1500 / 1530 / 1730 — GEN
11	OPEN / 1530 / 1730	0730 Plastic Surgeon #1 / 1130 Gen. Surgeon #3 / 1530 / 1730	1130 Gen. Surgeon #5 / 1530 / 1730	0730/0815 Plastic Surgery Associates / 1530 / 1730	0730 Surgical Assoc. #1 / 1200 / 1530 / 1730 — PLAS

setup, and anesthesia preparation. Because the time between cases has been estimated at between 20 and 45 minutes, the multiple room system can save considerable costs for surgeon and lower staff overtime.

Assessment of Scheduling Alternatives

According to a simulation test of FC/FS, SCF, and LCF, longest-time-first scheduling provided the highest use (measured as the ratio or the number of minutes utilized to the number of minutes in the work day) and the lowest overtime. Shortest-time-first was the poorest of the three systems according to the simulation (Breslawski and Hamilton, 1991; Dexter and Traub, 2002). However, each scheduling system meets certain objectives of the organization better than others. For instance, if the only goal is to reduce staff overtime, it is easy to select a system—either the top down/bottom up block or the longest-time-first. Unfortunately, the decision is not usually so easy; in most cases the organization has a series of decision criteria.

The OR manager must assess the stated mission of the OR to establish the decision criteria, rank the criteria by importance, and eliminate alternatives that do not satisfy the most important criteria. This step must be repeated, applying each scheduling method to the criteria in most important to least important order. That process, can produce a satisfactory decision.

Estimation of Procedure Times

Several of the previous systems schedule procedures according to their length. But how are we to know which procedure will constitute a long and which a short procedure? Moreover, the scheduling intervals' significant consequences for the utilization and effectiveness of the surgical suite must be considered. For instance, if time estimates are consistently low, the OR will be overloaded, with consequent cancellations, overtime, and frustrated surgeons, staff, and patients. On the other hand, excessive time estimates lead to costly idle time. Accurate estimates are needed to reduce daily variability in the OR scheduled load.

Magerlein and Martin (1978) identify the three methods for estimating procedure times: surgeon's estimates, OR scheduler's estimates, and historical averages. Most hospitals use either surgeons' or OR scheduler estimates. Although surgeons' estimates are often used, only a few attempts have been made to validate them (Denbor and Kubic, 1963; Phillips, 1975; Goldman, Knappenberger, and Sharon, 1970; Bendix, 1976), and those attempts have significant limitations and ambiguous findings. In general, the shorter the expected procedure is, the more accurate is the surgeon's estimate. Neither OR scheduler estimates nor historical averages have been validated (Rose and Davies, 1984; Kelley, Easham, and Bowling, 1985).

With computerized surgical suite scheduling systems, the use of databases to predict case block length is now more common. Databases can adjust historical averages for case complexity. Shukla, Ketcham, and Ozcan (1990) compared four data-based models for predicting case block length on the basis of: (a) procedure, (b) procedure and surgeon, (c) procedure and case complexity, and (d) procedure, case complexity, and surgeon. Their research demonstrated that hospitals can improve OR block scheduling systems by developing predetermined block time by considering the differences among surgeons and among case complexities. The study showed that surgeons tend to overestimate a surgery's required time, possibly to avoid any delays extending beyond their time blocks. Database systems facilitate reliable and equitable scheduling, reducing the surgeons' motivation to overestimate their time blocks. Health care managers must convince the surgeons that improving OR efficiency benefits not only the hospital, but also the surgeons themselves, since they would then have more time available to operate.

SUMMARY

In this chapter, we discussed staff scheduling mostly pertaining to nursing staff and patient scheduling mainly for the surgical suite. Staff scheduling allocates the budgeted FTEs to the proper patients in the proper units at the proper times. The scheduling choice can affect turnover, absenteeism, and overall job satisfaction. Moreover, scheduling relates directly to the quality of patient care by affecting coverage and continuity of care, as well as staff morale. If not done skillfully, scheduling of either can waste resources and reduce the revenue of the health care organization.

The surgical suite is a major revenue-generating and cost center of the hospitals, and thus must be managed carefully. Surgeons are confronted daily with delays and turnover times, but they may not understand their consequences for costs and the surgical suite's perishable capacity. It is the health care manager's duty to analyze ongoing inefficiencies and their root causes and then educate the surgical staff, including surgeons, anesthetists, nurses, and others, about methods that would work effectively for the surgical suite. Measures that are paramount for achieving efficiency include periodic examining of block utilization, turnover rates, delays and delay reasons, and updating surgery estimation times. Health care managers should give them constant attention.

KEY TERMS

Coverage
Schedule Quality
Schedule Stability
Eight-, Ten-, and Twelve-Hour Shifts
Flexible Scheduling

Cyclical Scheduling
Surgical Suite Resource Scheduling
Block Scheduling
Dynamic Block Scheduling.

EXERCISES

8.1 Use the information from Exercise 7.7; first determine the final core-level FTEs for the ICU and CCU departments, where RNs and LPNs work on a 4/40 and NAs on a 5/40 scheduling plan; then re-evaluate the final core-level staffing requirements if all staff work on either a 5/40 or a $(2 \times 8 + 2 \times 12)/40$ scheduling plan, and make recommendations.

8.2 Prepare a cyclical work schedule for a behavioral care practice with three staff members.

8.3 Prepare a cyclical work schedule for a small group practice with nine staff members.

(Hint: Use three-week or four- and five-week combinations.)

CHAPTER

9

PRODUCTIVITY

LEARNING OBJECTIVES

- Describe the meaning of productivity in health care organizations.
- Develop measures of productivity in various health care operations.
- Describe commonly used productivity ratios.
- Describe the concept of multi-factor productivity.
- Review adjustment methods for inputs and outputs of the productivity ratios.
- Compare productivity within and across the health care organizations.
- Describe the relationships between productivity and quality in health care.

Health care professionals must learn to manage constraints. Cost containment strategies such as the Medicare Prospective Payment System (PPS), private insurers' reimbursement ceilings, and managed care contracting place tremendous pressures on institutions—whether hospitals, nursing homes, mental health facilities, or home health agencies—to produce good quality care using the most efficient and effective combinations of human and capital resources. Under those pressures, the health care manager has to find efficient methods of using the resources at his or her disposal to produce high-quality outcomes.

This chapter examines the concept of productivity as applied to health care. The recent decades' changes in reimbursement strategies aimed to end waste and promote

205

innovative and cost-efficient delivery systems. To what degree have these strategies been successful? What trends are apparent in health care output and labor productivity? How is productivity measured, and how has its measurement changed over time? What are new directions and trends in productivity analysis and improvement? This chapter will answer these questions, among others.

TRENDS IN HEALTH CARE PRODUCTIVITY: CONSEQUENCES OF PPS

An underlying goal of the Medicare PPS system was to encourage organizations to use their resources more productively. With a capitated payment, organizations that could not improve productivity would either decline financially or be forced to reduce their quality of care, both potentially negative effects of PPS.

Unfortunately, productivity gains from PPS have not materialized to the extent predicted. Inpatient stays have been shortened, with many replaced by more cost-effective outpatient procedures; that shift increased productivity. However, the positive productivity trend did not last more than a couple of years. Hospitals now employ more people to treat fewer patients, and the increase is not accounted for by the greater severity of patient illness in the late 1980s and 1990s. Even strategies adopted by managed care have been only mildly successful. Although employers, insurers, and the public are spending less on inpatient care, the rising use of outpatient procedures has simply increased costs in that area, which counters the savings (Altman, Goldberger, and Crane, 1990).

The constraints that force health care institutions into the role of cost centers, coupled with shifting patterns of inpatient acuity, tight health care labor markets, and society's expectations of high quality of care are leading organizations to a "productivity wall." When the wall is reached, it is quality of care that inevitably is sacrificed for the sake of productivity and profit (Kirk, 1990). It must be recognized that there are limits to ratcheting up productivity. It is not always possible to do more with less. The reversal of the productivity improvements realized in the first two years after the introduction of PPS suggests that managers may have reached the limits of the savings to be realized through shorter admissions and improved scheduling and staffing (Altman, Goldberger, and Crane, 1990). In the next section, we examine definitions of productivity, and why the do-more-with-less philosophy is often unrealistic.

Productivity Definitions and Measurements

Productivity is one measure of the effective use of resources within an organization, industry, or nation. The classical productivity definition measures outputs relative to the inputs needed to produce them. That is, productivity is defined as the number of output units per unit of input:

$$Productivity = \frac{Output}{Input}$$

(9.1)

This ratio can be calculated for a single operation (productivity of a heart sur-geon), department (productivity of the nursing staff), or organization. Naturally, a higher value for that equation is preferable; at least no other considerations are applied.

Sometimes, an inverse calculation is used that measures inputs per unit of output. Care must be taken to interpret this inverse calculation appropriately; the greater the number of units of input per unit of output, the lower the productivity. For example, traditionally productivity in hospital nursing units has been measured by hours per patient day (HPPD). That requires an inversion of the typical calculations, meaning total hours are divided by total patient days.

$$HPPD = \frac{Total\ Hours}{Patient\ Days}$$

EXAMPLE 9.1

Nurses in Unit A worked collectively a total of twenty-five hours to treat a patient who stayed five days, and nurses in Unit B worked a total of sixteen hours to treat a patient who stayed four days. Calculate which of the two simi-lar hospital nursing units is more productive.

Solution

First, define the inputs and the outputs for the analysis. Is the proper measure of inputs the number of nurses or of hours worked? In this case the definition of the input would be total nursing hours. When the total number of nursing hours worked per nurse is used as the input measure, then the productivity measures for the two units are:

$$HPPD_A = \frac{Total\ Hours}{Patient\ Days} = \frac{25}{5} = 5$$

$$HPPD_B = \frac{Total\ Hours}{Patient\ Days} = \frac{16}{4} = 4$$

Now the question is: Which unit is more productive? If the productivity ratio is expressed as output over inputs, then a higher value indicates better productivity. However, if the productivity ratio is expressed as input over output, as in this case, then a lower value indicates better productivity. Since HPPD is an input-over-output ratio, Unit B in this example provides better productivity than Unit A does.

Productivity Benchmarking. Productivity must be considered as a relative measure; the calculated ratio should be either compared to a similar unit or compared to the productivity ratio of the same unit in previous years. Such comparisons characterize benchmarking. Many organizations use benchmarking to help set the direction for change. Historical benchmarking is monitoring an operational unit's own productivity or performance over the last few years. Another way of benchmarking is to identify the best practices (best productivity ratios of similar units) across health organizations and incorporate them in one's own. We will examine how benchmarking is done in practice later in the chapter.

Multi-factor Productivity. Example 9.1 demonstrated a measure of labor productivity. Because it looks at only one input, nursing hours, it is an example of a partial productivity measure. Looking only at labor productivity may not yield an accurate picture. It is increasingly realized that the workers are not the sole determinant of productivity. Low labor productivity does not necessarily mean that people doing the tasks are performing poorly; it may be the management system that is deficient. There may not be high quality evaluation tools, technical support, adequate pay and incentives, or a climate that motivates employees. Therefore, newer productivity measures tend to include not only labor inputs, but the other operating costs for the product or service as well. When we have more than one input, yet not all, the measure is referred to as multi-factor productivity.

$$Multi\text{-}factor\ Productivity\ = \frac{Service\ Item\ \times Price}{Labor\ +\ Material\ +Overhead} \quad (9.2)$$

Total productivity measures include all inputs, thereby being the most complete and precise. Total productivity measures, however, are difficult to operationalize. Example 9.2 illustrates a case for multi-factor productivity calculation and also demonstrates historical benchmarking.

EXAMPLE 9.2

A specialty laboratory performs lab tests for the area hospitals. During its first two years of operation the following measurements were gathered:

Measurement	Year 1	Year 2
Price per test ($)	50	50
Annual tests	10,000	10,700
Total labor costs($)	150,000	158,000
Material costs ($)	8,000	8,400
Overhead ($)	12,000	12,200

Determine and compare the multi-factor productivity for historical benchmarking.

Solution

Using formula (9.2), multi-factor productivity for Year 1 and Year 2 is as follows:

$$\text{Multi-factor Productivity}_{Year-1} = \frac{10,000 \times 50}{150,000 + 8,000 + 12,000} = 2.9.$$

$$\text{Multi-factor Productivity}_{Year-2} = \frac{10,700 \times 50}{158,000 + 8,400 + 12,200} = 3.0.$$

Comparison of the two years' productivity ratios finds marginal productivity improvement in the second year with respect to the first year of operations.

Example 9.2 assumes that each test represents an equal amount of output (or assumes outputs are homogeneous) and that quality is constant. Therefore the measure is only as accurate as those assumptions. Yet for the hospital industry in general and nursing services in particular, outputs and inputs are difficult to define precisely. For instance, suppose two nursing units with the same staffing levels each treat thirty patients on a given day. It would appear that both units are equally productive. An important piece of information that must be taken into account, however, is that one of the nursing units is located in intensive care and the other in routine care. With this additional information, we realize that the intensive care nursing unit is probably more productive because it handles a more complex case mix. Even if case mix were constant across both units, one unit might be providing a higher quality of care than another. In short, to define and operationalize the concept of productivity for the purpose of comparisons between systems (either internal or external), we must be sensitive to the issues of *case mix* and *quality*.

Given today's reduced reimbursement, tight financial constraints, and decreased human resources, the measure of HPPD fails to monitor the actual cost of care. As budgets are developed, more and more emphasis is placed on unit cost versus productivity. Skill mix is one way of maintaining resources and productivity while reducing the cost per unit (patient day or office visit). In hospital units, substituting the less skilled LPNs and nurse aides for the highly skilled RNs keeps the number of staff per patient the same, and cuts costs. A similar strategy can be applied in outpatient settings such as physician group practices, with general practitioners and nurse practitioners substituting for specialists as it is deemed appropriate.

With this model of staffing it is essential for roles to be clearly defined and for the tasks each person does to fit within the role definition. The remainder of this chapter defines several approaches to these issues in productivity measurement and discusses some advantages and disadvantages of each.

Commonly Used Productivity Ratios

Although economists define productivity in terms of a ratio of outputs to inputs, they tend to define outputs and inputs in aggregate terms. For instance, inputs in health care may be aggregated as FTEs or as hours worked, and outputs may be aggregated as patient days or as weighted aggregate patient days. In outpatient settings, visits or weighted aggregate visits may be used as outputs.

In contrast, the more refined approach taken from industrial engineering focuses on a micro-analysis of employee time, using either an individual employee or a nursing unit as the unit of analysis. Productivity under this approach is viewed as the ratio of time spent on productive tasks to the total time worked. Although both perspectives provide useful information to assess, compare, and improve productivity, our discussion here will concentrate on the economic perspective. (The engineering perspective is covered in Chapter Six, in the sections on work sampling and work measurement.)

The measures of labor productivity, developed from the economic perspective, hours per patient days (per discharge, or per visit) are presented below. Notice that the inputs; cost of labor, hours, and direct care hours, are standardized or adjusted for skill mix. Similarly outputs, number of patient days, discharges, and visits are adjusted for case mix.

Hours per Patient Day (or Visit). According to this measure, two units that have the same staffing levels and treat the same number of patients are equally productive. This conclusion is correct only if we can assume that both case mix and the quality of care for the two units are equal. Data for this measure are generally available from hospital information systems (inpatient), or from physician billing systems (outpatient). In inpatient settings, the output data can be obtained from the census report, and the input data from personnel payroll systems. Other sources of data are various subscription services that provide not only productivity data for the subscribing hospital, but also comparative statistics for similar size (peer) hospitals. In outpatient settings, physician billing systems not only can provide output data for visit information, but also, through Common Procedure Terminology (CPT) coding, can provide necessary input data. However, whether inpatient or outpatient, comparisons of productivity ratios must be made cautiously if variations in case mix and quality are not considered. The general formula for inpatient settings can be stated as:

$$Hours \ per \ Patient \ Day = \frac{Hours \ Worked}{Patients \ Days} \qquad (9.3a)$$

Example 9.3 illustrates use of this productivity measure for inpatient settings.

EXAMPLE 9.3

Annual statistical data for two nursing units in Memorial Hospital are as follows:

Measurements	Unit A	Unit B
Annual patient days	14,000	10,000
Annual hours worked	210,000	180,000

Calculate and compare hours per patient day for two units of this hospital.

Solution:

Using formula (9.3a), for two units we get:

$$Hours\ per\ Patient\ Day_{Unit\ A} = \frac{210,000}{14,000} = 15\ hours.$$

$$Hours\ per\ Patient\ Day_{Unit\ B} = \frac{180,000}{10,000} = 18\ hours.$$

Using this measure without any adjustments, Unit A appears to be more productive.

Applying the concept on outpatient settings, formula (9.3a) can be expressed as:

$$Hours\ per\ Patient\ Visit = \frac{Hours\ Worked}{Patient\ Visits} \qquad (9.3b)$$

Example 9.4 illustrates the application of this formula.

EXAMPLE 9.4

Performsbetter Associates—a two-site group practice, requires productivity monitoring. The following initial data are provided for both sites of the practice:

Measurements	Suburban	Downtown
Annual visits	135,000	97,000
Annual paid hours	115,000	112,000

Calculate and compare the hours per patient visit for the suburban and the downtown locations of this practice.

Solution

Using formula (9.3b) for each site, we get:

$$Hours\ per\ Patient\ Visit_{Suburb} = \frac{115,000}{135,000} = .85\ hour\ or\ 51\ minutes$$

$$Hours\ per\ Patient\ Visit_{Downtown} = \frac{112,000}{97,000} = 1.15\ hours\ or\ 69\ minutes.$$

Using this measure without any adjustments, the suburban location appears to be more productive using this measure.

Adjustments for Inputs

Ratios calculated above did not consider any standardization for its components. Here, we introduce standardization with adjustments to inputs by skill mix adjustment and adjustment to hours or standardizing the cost of labor (Shukla, 1991).

Skill Mix Adjustment. The first measure we have applied does not differentiate the skill mix of the nursing care providers. To make such distinctions, we can weigh the hours of personnel of different skill levels by their economic valuation. The economic valuation (calculation of weights) can be driven by various methods. One approach is to calculate weights based on the average wage or salary of each skill class. To do that, a given skill class wage or salary would be divided by the top class skill salary. For example, if RNs, LPNs, and aides are earning $35.00, $28.00, and $17.50 an hour, respectively, then one hour of a nurse aide's time is economically equivalent to 0.5 hour of a registered nurse's time; and one hour of a licensed practical nurse's time is equal to 0.8 hour of a registered nurse's time.

Another approach to obtain weights would be a more detailed, engineering approach (Shukla, 1991), using the percentage of tasks that the less skilled staff are permitted to perform, compared to the duties of the most skilled staff (for example, the percentage of the RN tasks that can be performed by LPNs as allowed by licensure and laws as well as professional associations). However, because this approach has aroused controversy, using wage or salary information to determine the weights should suffice.

Adjusted Hours. From the above discussion and example, the adjusted labor hours can be formulated as:

$$Adjusted\ Hours = \sum w_i X_i \tag{9.4}$$

where

w_i indicates the weight for skill level i, and

X_i represents hours worked by skill class i.

More explicitly,
Adjusted Hours = 1.0 (RN hours) + 0.8 (LPN hours) + 0.5 (Aide hours),
and adjusted hours per patient day can be expressed as:

$$Adjusted\ Hours\ per\ Patient\ day = \frac{Adjusted\ Hours}{Patients\ Days} \qquad (9.4a)$$

Similarly, in outpatient settings, if one hour of a nurse practitioner's (NP) time is economically equivalent to 0.6 hours of a specialist's (SP) time, and if one hour of a general practitioner's (GP) time is equal to 0.85 hours of a specialist's time, adjusted hours would be calculated as:

Adjusted Hours = 1.0 (SP hours) + 0.85 (GP hours) + 0.6 (NP hours), and adjusted hours per visit can be expressed as:

$$Adjusted\ Hours\ per\ Visit = \frac{Adjusted\ Hours}{Patients\ Visits} \qquad (9.4b)$$

EXAMPLE 9.5

Using data from Example 9.3, and economic equivalencies of 0.5 Aide = RN, 0.8 LPN = RN, calculate the adjusted hours per patient day for Unit A and Unit B. Unit A at Memorial Hospital employs 100 percent RNs. The current skill mix distribution of Unit B is 45 percent RNs, 30 percent LPNs, and 25 percent nursing aides (NAs). Compare unadjusted and adjusted productivity scores.

Solution

The first step is to calculate adjusted hours for each unit. For Unit A, since it employs 100 percent RNs, there is no need for adjustment. Using formula (9.4), we get

$$Adjusted\ Hours_{(Unit\ B)} = 1.0(180,000 \times .45) + 0.80(180,000 \times .30)$$
$$+ 0.50(180,000 \times .25).$$
$$Adjusted\ Hours_{(Unit\ B)} = 1.0(81,000) + 0.80(54,000) + 0.50(45,000).$$
$$Adjusted\ Hours_{(Unit\ B)} = 146,700.$$

In this way, using the economic equivalencies of the skill mix, the number of hours is standardized as 146,700 instead of 180,000. Hence, using formula (9.4a), we get

$$Adjusted\ Hours\ per\ Patient\ Day_{Unit\ A} = \frac{210,000}{14,000} = 15.0\ hours$$

$$Adjusted\ Hours\ per\ Patient\ Day_{Unit\ B} = \frac{146,700}{10,000} = 14.7\ hours$$

Using adjusted hours, Unit A, which appeared productive according to the first measure (see Example 9.3), no longer appears as productive. If unit B is more productive than A according to the adjusted measure, yet less productive according to the unadjusted measure, this must be due to unit B having a high proportion of aides or LPNs. Under the assumption that both units offer an equal quality of care to patient populations with the same case mix, Unit B would be more productive by providing the same quality of care using less equivalent labor.

Cost of Labor. This measure no longer uses labor hours as the input, but rather labor costs. The costs of nursing labor per patient day should include overtime, holidays, annual leave, and other benefits. Because differences in wage structures and in longevity of employment influence salary levels among hospitals, labor cost is more difficult to compare across systems. However, when large numbers of nurses are included in the analysis, we can assume that the longevity factor is normally distributed and that the mean lengths of employment on two large units or in two hospitals are equal.

Standardized Cost of Labor. Total labor cost comprises the payments to various professionals at varying skills. To account for differences in salary structure across hospitals or group practices, cost calculations can be standardized using a standard salary per hour for each of the skill levels (Shukla, 1991). Thus, first we need to formulate the labor cost of care, differentiating these payments. The labor cost based on hours and wages earned in each skill mix class can be formulated as:

$$Labor\ Cost = \sum c_i X_i \tag{9.5}$$

where

c_i indicates the wage for skill level i, and

X_i represents hours worked by skill class i.

More explicitly, nursing labor costs can be written as:

Labor Cost = RN wages (RN hours) + LP wages (LPN hours) + Aide wages (Aide hours).

Productivity ratios for the labor cost of care are shown in formulas (9.5a) and (9.5b), respectively as:

$$Labor\ Cost\ Patient\ Day = \frac{Labor\ Cost\ of\ Care}{Patient\ Days}. \qquad (9.5a)$$

$$Labor\ Cost\ per\ Visit = \frac{Labor\ Cost\ of\ Care}{Patient\ Visits}. \qquad (9.5b)$$

EXAMPLE 9.6

Performsbetter Associates in Example 9.4 pays $110, $85, and $45 per hour, respectively, to its SPs, GPs, and NPs in both locations. Currently, the suburban location staff comprises 50 percent SPs, 30 percent GPs, and 20 percent NPs. The downtown location, on the other hand, comprises 30 percent SPs, 50 percent GPs, and 20 percent NPs. Calculate and compare the labor cost of care and labor cost per visit for both locations.

Solution

First, use formula (9.5) to calculate Labor Cost of Care for each location.

$$Labor\ Cost = SP\ wages \times (SP\ hours) + GP\ wages$$
$$\times (GP\ hours) + NP\ wages \times (NP\ hours),$$
$$Labor\ Cost_{Suburban} = \$110(115,000 \times 0.50) + \$85(115,000 \times 0.30)$$
$$+ \$45(115,000 \times 0.20).$$
$$Labor\ Cost_{Suburban} = \$110(57,500) + \$85(34,500) + \$45(23,000).$$
$$Labor\ Cost_{Suburban} = \$10,292,500.$$
$$Labor\ Cost_{Downtown} = \$110(112,000 \times .30) + \$85(112,000 \times 0.50)$$
$$+ \$45(112,000 \times 0.20).$$
$$Labor\ Cost_{Downtown} = \$110(33,600) + \$85(56,000) + \$45(22,400).$$
$$Labor\ Cost_{Downtown} = \$9,464,000.$$

Next we use formula (9.5b) for each site, and obtain:

$$Labor\ Cost\ per\ Visit_{Suburban} = \frac{10,292,500}{135,000} = \$76.24.$$

$$Labor\ Cost\ per\ Visit_{Downtown} = \frac{9,464,000}{97,000} = \$97.57.$$

There is a marked difference between the two locations in labor cost per visit. Despite the higher utilization of GPs in the downtown location, because volume is lower there the cost per visit is 28 percent higher.

Adjustments for Outputs

None of the measures considered thus far adjusts for outputs, namely for case mix. Hence, those measures are useful primarily for comparing large numbers of patients of similar type in general community hospitals; comparisons across specialties or hospital types may not be valid. For instance, medical/surgical patients in an acute care center are likely to utilize more resources than medical/surgical patients in a general community hospital. Comparisons between such institutions must be made with caution. Especially, assumptions must be identified. Similarly, outpatient visits can be adjusted based on CPT codes that reveal the acuity level of the outpatient visit. Methods of adjusting for patient case mix are discussed below.

The assumption that all patients receive the same amount of care, that each patient represents a homogeneous output, is not realistic. Patients require varying levels of care and use varying amounts of resources. Productivity measures therefore should adjust the output, patient days, for differences in resource consumption.

Two approaches are cited in the literature by health care researchers and managers: service mix adjustment and case mix adjustment. We will consider each of these approaches in turn, and note the advantages and disadvantages of each.

Service Mix Adjustments. Service mix adjustment is a useful tool for comparison of, for instance, two community hospitals that provide different services or have significantly different distributions of patients among their services. The service mix adjusted volume is weighted by a normalized service intensity factor (Shukla, 1991). This weight factor is calculated using the following formula:

$$W_i = \frac{H_i}{\sum H_i \,/\, n} \qquad (9.6)$$

where

W_i = weight for i^{th} service,

H_i = number of hours care required per patient day in service i,

n = number of services.

To calculate the weights for each service, simply divide the number of hours of care required per patient day in a service into the average hours of care required per patient day. Volume adjustment (for instance, patient days, or discharges) can be calculated after weights are obtained, using the following formula:

$$Adjusted\ Volume = \sum W_i X_i \qquad (9.7)$$

EXAMPLE 9.7

Two hospitals, each with unadjusted volume of 10,000 patient days per month, provide only two services, S₁ and S₂, requiring respectively three and seven hours of nursing time per patient day. Hospital A has a service mix distribution of 2,000 patient days for S₁ and 8,000 patient days for S₂; hospital B has 8,000 days for S₁ and 2,000 days for S₂. Calculate adjusted patient days for both hospitals.

Solution

In this case, total unadjusted volume is simply the sum of the volume for each service in each hospital, or Unadjusted Volume = $X_1 + X_2$.

	Hospital-A	Hospital-B
Service S₁ (3 hours/patient day)	$X_1 = 2000$	$X_1 = 8000$
Service S₂ (7 hours/patient day)	$X_2 = 8000$	$X_2 = 2000$
Total unadjusted volume	10,000	10,000

Adjusted volume requires use of formula (9.7): Adjusted Volume = $W_1X_1 + W_2X_2$. The next step is to calculate weights W_1 and W_2, using formula (9.6).

$$W_i = \frac{H_1}{\sum H_i / n} = \frac{3}{(3+7)/2} = \frac{3}{10/2} = \frac{3}{5} = 0.6.$$

$$W_i = \frac{H_2}{\sum H_i / n} = \frac{7}{(3+7)/2} = \frac{7}{10/2} = \frac{7}{5} = 1.4.$$

Adjusted volume for Hospital-A = 0.6 × 2,000+1.4 × 8,000 = 12,400.
Adjusted volume for Hospital-B = 0.6 × 8,000+1.4 × 2,000 = 7,600.

The adjusted volume in patient days for hospitals A and B would thus be 12,400 and 7,600 patient days respectively, in contrast to the unadjusted volumes of 10,000 each.

Service-mix-adjusted patient days can be used as the output (the denominator) in the four economic productivity measures presented above. Note, however, that this service mix method is valid only if we can assume that the average amount of care required per patient for a service is homogeneous, or at a minimum has similar distributions in the two systems. Given that, the method is especially helpful for comparing systems over a long period. It is not useful, though, for managers monitoring productivity weekly or daily, because the assumptions of homogeneity or similarity in the distribution of nursing care requirements are not reliable for analysis of a short period.

Within any service mix, there can be significant daily variation in resource consumption. If productivity management systems are to be useful on a daily basis, they must take these variations into account. Bear in mind that, the economic perspective is a macro approach, and so cannot provide sensitive enough case mix measurements for such management purposes.

Case Mix Adjustments

Patient classification systems, discussed in Chapter Seven, categorize patients daily into several categories of acuity. Nursing departments can use these acuity categories to manage productivity and achieve the best possible care given their budgetary constraints. Patients in each category require similar amounts of nursing care over a given twenty-four-hour time period; however, across categories the care requirements differ significantly. For acuity, the focus is on patients' direct care requirements. The ratio of the hours of direct care provided to the total hours worked is another measure of productivity.

The methodology for case mix adjustment is similar to that for service mix adjustment. Although most hospitals rely on advanced acuity systems, each system is based on the weight factors for the different acuity categories. For example, in a patient classification system designed for a medical/surgical unit with five acuity categories, we can use formula (9.6) to calculate weights. Besides the weights, we must know the percentage of patients in each acuity category. Then we can calculate the case mix index as follows:

$$Case\ mix\ index_j\ =\ \sum W_i P_{ij} \tag{9.8}$$

where

W_i = weight for i^{th} category care

P_{ij} = percent of patients for acuity category i in unit j.

EXAMPLE 9.8

Unit A and Unit B (from Example 9.3), medical care units in Memorial Hospital, classify patients into four acuity categories (Type I through Type IV), with direct care requirements per patient day being respectively, 0.5, 1.5, 4.0, and 6.0 hours. Annual distributions of patients in these four acuity categories in Unit A were 0.15, 0.25, 0.35, and 0.25. Annual distributions of patients in Unit B were

0.15, 0.30, 0.40, and 0.15. Calculate the case mix for these two units, and determine which unit has been serving more severe patients.

Solution

Using formula (9.6), first calculate the weights for each of the four categories.

$$W_1 = \frac{H_1}{\sum H_i / n} = \frac{0.5}{(0.5 + 1.5 + 4.0 + 6.0) / 4} = \frac{0.5}{12 / 4} = \frac{0.5}{3} = 0.17$$

$$W_2 = \frac{H_2}{\sum H_i / n} = \frac{1.5}{(0.5 + 1.5 + 4.0 + 6.0) / 4} = \frac{1.5}{12 / 4} = \frac{1.5}{3} = 0.5$$

$$W_3 = \frac{H_3}{\sum H_i / n} = \frac{4.0}{(0.5 + 1.5 + 4.0 + 6.0) / 4} = \frac{4.0}{12 / 4} = \frac{4.0}{3} = 1.33$$

$$W_4 = \frac{H_4}{\sum H_i / n} = \frac{6.0}{(0.5 + 1.5 + 4.0 + 6.0) / 4} = \frac{6.5}{12 / 4} = \frac{6.0}{3} = 2.00$$

Then apply formula (9.8) to calculate the case mix as:

$$Case\ mix\ index_A = \sum W_i P_{iA} = (0.17 \times 0.15) + (0.5 \times 0.25) + (1.33 \times 0.35) + (2.00 \times 0.25) = 1.12.$$

$$Case\ mix\ index_B = \sum W_i P_{iB} = (0.17 \times 0.15) + (0.5 \times 0.30) + (1.33 \times 0.40) + (2.00 \times 0.15) = 1.01.$$

From the case mix calculations, we can conclude that Unit A handled more severe patients.

Once the case mix is determined, the output side of the productivity ratios can be adjusted by simply multiplying volume (patient days, discharges, visits) by case mix index as:

Adjusted Patient Days = Patient Days × Case mix index
Adjusted Discharges = Discharges × Case mix index
Adjusted Visits = Visits × Case mix index.

Productivity Measures Using Direct Care Hours

The amount and the percentage of direct hours of care are often considered proxy measures for the quality of care. However, applying those measures can help health care managers to assess not only the quality of care, but also the productivity.

Hours of Direct Care. "Hours of direct care" is an important component of productivity ratios. It serves as a building block for other ratios. To illustrate its development, let us assume that patients are categorized into acuity groupings requiring H_1, H_2, H_3,..., H_m hours of direct nursing care per patient day. Further, assume that there are N_1, N_2, N_3,..., N_m annual patient days in units 1 through m. The total amount of direct nursing care in nursing unit j would be calculated as follows:

$$\text{Hours of Direct Care}_j = \sum_{i=1}^{n}(H_i P_{ij} N_j) \tag{9.9}$$

In this way we use the hours of direct care as the output, basing our productivity measures on the hours of direct care rather than total hours.

Percentage of Hours in Direct Care. This is an additional measure that can be derived from the "Hours of Direct Care" calculation, as the ratio of direct care hours to total care hours.

$$\text{Percent of Hours in Direct Care} = \frac{\text{Hours in Direct Care}}{\text{Hours Worked}} \tag{9.10}$$

Percentage of Adjusted Hours in Direct Care. We also can determine the percentage of adjusted nursing hours as adjusted for skill-mix in direct patient care by using formulas (9.4) and (9.9) to obtain:

$$\text{Percentage of Adjusted Hours in Direct Care} = \frac{\text{Hours in Direct Care}}{\text{Adjusted Hours}}. \tag{9.11}$$

EXAMPLE 9.9

Using information from Examples 9.3 and 9.8: calculate (a) hours of direct care, (b) percentage of hours in direct care, and (c) percentage of adjusted hours in direct care for Units A and B of Memorial Hospital. Compare these results in terms of percentage of adjusted hours in direct care.

Solution

Memorial Hospital uses an acuity classification system with four categories of direct hours of care per patient day: 0.5, 1.5, 4.0, and 6.0 hours. The annual distributions of patients in these four acuity categories in Unit A were 0.15, 0.25, 0.35, and 0.25. The annual distributions of patients in Unit B were 0.15, 0.30, 0.40, and 0.15. Annual patient days for Unit A were 14,000, and for unit B 10,000. Annual hours worked were 210,000 and 180,000, respectively.

The first step is to calculate the hours of direct care for each unit, using formula (9.9.).

$$\text{Hours of Direct Care}_j = \sum_{i=1}^{n}(H_i P_{ij} N_j)$$

(handwritten annotations in right margin:)
annual patient days   14,000 | 10,000

categories of direct hours of care per patient day   A   B

	A	B
0.5	0.15	0.15
1.5	0.25	0.30
4.0	0.35	0.40
6.0	0.25	0.15

Hours of Direct Care$_A$ = (0.5 × .15 × 14,000) + (1.5 × .25 × 14,000)
     + (4.0 × .35 × 14,000) + (6.0 × .25 × 14,000)
    Hours of Direct Care$_A$ = 46,900

Hours of Direct Care$_B$ = (0.5 × .15 × 10,000) + (1.5 × .30 × 10,000)
     + (4.0 × .40 × 10,000) + (6.0 × .15221 × 10,000)
    Hours of Direct Care$_B$ = 30,250

The second step is to calculate the percentage of hours in direct care, using formula (9.10).

$$\text{Percentage of Hours in Direct Care}_A = \frac{\text{Hours in Direct Care}}{\text{Hours Worked}} = \frac{46,900}{210,000}$$
$$= 0.223 \text{ or } 22.3 \text{ percent.}$$

$$\text{Percentage of Hours in Direct Care}_B = \frac{\text{Hours in Direct Care}}{\text{Hours Worked}} = \frac{30,250}{180,000}$$
$$= 0.168 \text{ or } 16.8 \text{ percent.}$$

The last step is to calculate the percentage of adjusted hours in direct care, using formula (9.11).

$$\text{Percentage of Adjusted Hours in Direct Care}_A = \frac{\text{Hours in Direct Care}}{\text{Adjusted Hours}} = \frac{46,900}{210,000}$$
$$= 0.223 \text{ or } 22.3 \text{ percent.}$$

$$\text{Percentage of Adjusted Hours in Direct Care}_B = \frac{\text{Hours in Direct Care}}{\text{Adjusted Hours}}$$
$$= \frac{30,250}{146,700}$$
$$= 0.206 \text{ or } 20.6 \text{ percent.}$$

From the "Percentage of Hours in Direct Care," Unit A appears to be providing a higher quality of care. However, care is provided with 100 percent RN staffing, and the RNs may be doing many tasks that could be done by staff with lower skill levels. Hence, when we examine the "Percentage of Adjusted Hours in Direct Care," the advantage of Unit A in terms of productivity diminishes. One can calculate the costs of care, using formula (9.5), to see the cost differential for the 1.7 percent extra adjusted direct care for Unit A.

The measures of case mix, while more appropriate for managerial use, are only as valid as the patient classification system. Therefore that system must be objective and not rely simply on subjective staff judgments. A system of checks and balances among staff nurses, head nurses, and supervisors should be in place to avoid over-classification. Over-classification may occur in the interest of defending nurses' productivity against under-assessment.

None of the measures discussed so far explicitly control for quality. Davis (1991) points out that evidence suggests that in actuality the quality of inputs are more important than their quantity. If so, health care organizations should be working to improve quality of inputs and thus the quality of care they provide. How can quality be incorporated into productivity measurements, if indeed at all? That is the question addressed in the following section.

The Relationships Between Productivity and Quality in Hospital Settings

Though two units appear to have equal productivity, as measured using both skill and case mix adjustments, it still is not possible to say with accuracy that the units are performing equally. The reason is simply that the quality of care may differ, resulting in either better clinical outcomes or greater efficiency of care—thus requiring fewer days of hospitalization. Few would dispute that the unit that provides the highest quality of care with a constant set of inputs is more productive.

Unfortunately, this intuitive concept is difficult to operationalize. The effort is bedeviled by lack of agreement on the definition of quality and uncertainty about the relationship between quantity and quality in medical care. A theoretical approach to including quality in productivity measurements requires two assumptions: that a uniform definition of quality exists; and that the relationship between the quality and the quantity of medical care resources is known. It does seem safe to assume diminishing marginal returns to quality from simply continually increasing medical resources; and indeed that the marginal productivity in terms of a ratio of quality of outputs to medical care inputs may eventually become negative. Figure 9.1 depicts this relationship for two hospitals, A and B, which we assume provide the same quantity of output in terms of their case mix adjusted patient days. Figure 9.1 shows that Hospital A is providing better quality of care for a given set of inputs.

Although productivity as measured by hours (or $) per case mix adjusted patient day, is the same (I_1) for Hospitals A and B, the quality of care provided by Hospital A is better. Therefore, Hospital A is more cost-effective and more productive in terms of per quality points. To develop a measure of productivity that explicitly considers quality of care, the advantage in quality must be converted to an equivalent resource advantage. Drawing a line from point B to point A9, we see that Hospital B is providing quality level Q_B using resources I_1. However, Hospital A can employ I_2 to reach this same level of quality. The difference between I_1 and I_2, ΔI, represents the additional

FIGURE 9.1. *Productivity and Quality Trade Off.*

Source: Adapted from Shukla, R. K., *Theories and Strategies of Health Care: Technology-Strategy-Performance*, Chapter Four, unpublished manuscript, 1991.

resources not needed by Hospital A to provide the same quality of care as Hospital B. The advantage of Hospital A over Hospital B depends upon the value of ΔI, which is itself affected by the quality-quantity characteristics of Hospitals A and B.

How then can Hospital B improve its quality and productivity? At point A', we can consider Hospital B at the same operating characteristics as Hospital A, where it reduces its resources by ΔI without sacrificing its quality (at Q_B). Now, consider point A", Hospital B operating on Hospital A's operational characteristic curve, where Hospital B has reduced its inputs from I_1 to $I_{A"}$ (productivity improvement) while improving its quality of care from Q_B to $Q_{A"}$. Hence, theoretically, Hospital B can improve both productivity and quality simultaneously if the health care manager in Hospital B adopts the operating characteristics of Hospital A.

The technological advances and reengineered delivery systems are what define Hospital A's operating characteristics. The health care manager of Hospital B could pay for the costs of advanced technology and reengineering in a few years from the savings created on ΔI ($I_1 - I_{A"}$).

A quality-adjusted productivity measurement constructed in this manner is possible only if the two assumptions of a uniform quality definition and a known quality-quantity relationship hold true. Research is badly needed to develop accurate methodologies for including cost-quality or quantity-quality considerations in hospital care delivery systems. Many factors can influence quality as well as performance, among them organizational characteristics, management capabilities, and employee-related variables. To complicate matters further, these variables are often not exogenous of each other, but instead related and often in a stochastic and recursive manner. The relationships are often also synergistic. For instance, systems for delivery of primary nursing care (all RN staffing) and for decentralized unit dose medication distribution together may influence quality to a greater degree than does the sum total of their independent influences. To develop a reliable productivity measure that is adjusted for quality, we must understand the multi-dimensional factors affecting quality.

Summary of Productivity-Related Dilemmas in the Hospital Setting

To increase productivity within the hospital as a whole, it is necessary to better match the appropriate resources (the inputs) with the care to be provided (the output). Care must be both timely and of high quality. The health care manager must not only assure that tasks are done correctly, but also that all the necessary things are done. It is easy to pronounce that more must be done with less; however, accomplishing such a task while satisfying the staff, physicians, and payers—to say nothing of the patients—is a difficult matter.

Health care organizations are susceptible to fluctuations in demand and census levels that can make scheduling and staffing a nightmare. These variations can profoundly affect a hospital's profit, largely because of the hospital's large percentage of fixed costs. Yet, abruptly shifting workloads to make efficient use of the staff can distress patients and create dissatisfaction in the staff and physicians (Anderson, 1989).

Altman, Goldberger, and Crane (1990) argue that changes in the labor market have made it essential to improve productivity. Labor costs make up 40 percent or more of many hospital budgets. Until recently, health care employers had drawn on a large pool of female and minority workers, whom they were able to pay relatively low wages. However, demographic and cultural trends are reducing the health care labor force, which especially in the context of rising demand for health care services, have allowed those workers' wages to rise. Employers who are unable to tie rising wages and job redesign to improved productivity will face financial ruin.

The issues presented above often must be managed at the departmental level. In addition to the general difficulties outlined above, each department or unit has distinctive characteristics that may require special knowledge and skills for productivity assessment. For example, in surgical suites, key productivity issues might be case scheduling methods, turnaround time, and utilization; in radiology—staff and equipment utilization; in housekeeping—cleaning frequency, effective supplies and equipment, and communication; in supply chain—product standardization, inventory reduction, contract negotiations (Anderson, 1989).

In sum, to realize productivity gains, it is vital to match resources with workload patterns. A successful match requires adequate communication, technological advances, cooperation, timeliness, attention to patient and physician convenience, and tradeoffs. Organizations that cannot improve productivity will face exploding costs and no longer be competitive in the health care marketplace. Yet, achieving productivity is only the initial step. What is probably more difficult is to sustain productivity—through administrative commitment, flexibility, and the rethinking of traditionally held assumptions.

Dealing with the Multiple Dimensions of Productivity: New Methods of Measurement

New methods of measuring productivity, in particular, data envelopment analysis (DEA), can be used to assess the multiple dimensions of productivity and are discussed here.

It is a familiar statement: health care managers must develop efficient methods to use the resources at their disposal to produce effective and high quality medical outcomes. However, those frequently used terms, efficiency and effectiveness, are often used with only a somewhat vague sense of their meanings in the health care context. *Efficiency* generally refers to using the minimum number of inputs for a given number of outputs. Efficient care, therefore, means a health care facility produces a given level of care or quantity that meets an acceptable standard of quality, using the minimum combination of resources. Improving productivity should lead to greater efficiency, while holding constant the quality, staff skill mix, and case mix. *Effectiveness,* in contrast, more specifically evaluates the outputs of medical care. For instance, are the necessary inputs being used in order to produce the best possible outputs? A hospital can be efficient, but not effective; it can also be effective, but not efficient. The aim is to be both.

The next two sections examine some complex aspects of efficiency. Efficiency can be examined from technical and from economic perspectives.

Technical Efficiency. Technical efficiency examines the relationships between various inputs and the related output. An organization is technically efficient if it uses the minimum combination of resources to produce a given quantity or level of care. For an example, we can look at the substitution of nurse practitioners (NPs) for physicians (MDs). Assume that a particular hospital can use one of two combinations of MDs and NPs to provide care in the intensive care unit (ICU). The first combination uses 3 MDs and 2 NPs (point A in Figure 9.2); an alternative is to use 1 MD and 5 NPs (point B in Figure 9.2). Let us suppose that both combinations of inputs result in the same quality of care. We can then say that both of these points are technically efficient, because they use the minimum number of resources to provide a given level of care. Point C, on the contrary, is a relatively inefficient point: it uses 3 MDs and 3 NPs to care for the ICU patient population, but we have already stated that the hospital provides the given level of care with 3 NPs and only 2 MDs, obviously a more efficient combination of resources. Note also that diminishing marginal productivity to both MDs and NPs is exhibited in Figure 9.2. That is, as we use fewer MDs, they become relatively more valuable; therefore, we must substitute more NPs for each MD we sacrifice.

The economist would refer to the curve in Figure 9.2 as an isoquant. An *isoquant* shows all the technically efficient combinations of inputs that can be used to produce a given quantity of output (at the same quality). Its slope is equal to the negative ratio of the marginal productivities of the inputs, in this case nurse practitioners and physicians. Although all points on the isoquant are technically efficient, they are not necessarily economically efficient.

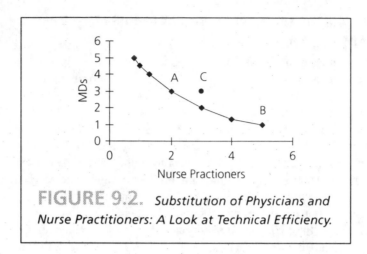

FIGURE 9.2.   *Substitution of Physicians and Nurse Practitioners: A Look at Technical Efficiency.*

Economic Efficiency. Economic efficiency adds an additional element to technical efficiency—cost. Although the isoquant shows us which combinations of inputs can be used efficiently to produce the desired output, it does not take the cost of the outputs into account. In the above example, suppose the annual compensation of an MD is $150,000, and for the NP is $80,000. The total costs of option 1 (point A) are then $610,000 ($150,000 × 3 + $80,000 × 2). Option 2 (point B) has a cost of $550,000, which clearly represents a better alternative than option 1. Point B is therefore the more economically efficient point in this example. In economics, the point of economic efficiency is found by the tangency between the isoquant and the iso-cost constraint, which is the ratio of the input prices. This point of tangency represents the point where the marginal, or additional, outputs produced from each input per dollar spent are equivalent across all inputs. Thus, the point of economic efficiency is the point where the given level of output is produced with the minimum number of resources and at the lowest possible cost, holding technology constant.

The example using nurse practitioners and physicians appears here for a particular reason. It illustrates how hospitals may be restricted as to the substitutability of their inputs. The hospital may not be able to reach point B, although that is preferable in economic terms, because legal restrictions prohibit nurse practitioners from providing certain elements of care. The prohibition arose from concerns about the effectiveness of care; the caution is that nurse practitioners, because their training is less comprehensive than that of physicians and because they are not licensed, may have fewer medical skills. If that is so, the quality of care may suffer in certain situations if nurse practitioner services are substituted for those of a medical doctor. In short, although using nurse practitioners is efficient both technically and economically, the care they provide may not be as effective.

The distinctions just clarified among technical efficiency, economic efficiency and effectiveness are essential to understand. Recent techniques for benchmarking and productivity measurement, such as data envelopment analysis, often assume an understanding of this terminology.

Data Envelopment Analysis

The assessment of productivity is often difficult, because it is a multi-dimensional construct. One measure, for example, the productivity of labor, may not give a complete picture of overall performance. Often it is necessary to look at several inputs simultaneously, along with the multiple outputs they produce. DEA uses linear programming to search for the optimal combinations of inputs and outputs as revealed in the actual performance of physicians, hospitals, or any other units of analysis, which are termed decision-making units (DMUs). The technical efficiency of each DMU is assessed relative to optimal patterns of production, which are computed from the performance of hospitals with input/output combinations that are the best of any peer DMU. Efficiency scores are then calculated for each DMU, with a score of 1 representing technical efficiency.

DEA measures relative efficiency by the ratio of total weighted output to its total weighted input and is considered to be a total factor productivity measure. DEA allows each DMU to select the weights for each input, provided that the weights are only positive and are universal.

DEA addresses the limitations of ratio analysis and regression. Additionally, DEA uses multiple outputs and multiple inputs to identify efficiencies and inefficiencies, and also to project how inefficient DMUs can become more efficient, by identifying best practices. A best-practice function can be built empirically from observed inputs and outputs. The idea of DEA is to project a frontier estimating technical efficiency for each DMU, in this case found in a peer group of teaching hospitals or physician groups. DEA calculations maximize the relative efficiency score of each DMU. The objective is to establish norms of best achieved practice, so hospitals that fall short of the frontier can aspire to reach it by modeling the practice patterns of those on the frontier. The type of orientation for the DEA model means specification of the type of strategy that must be used to enhance efficiency. Since it can be assumed that managers of hospitals or outpatient facilities are likely to have more opportunities to reduce the inputs used to produce patient outputs than to increase patient outputs (patient days, discharges, visits), an input-oriented model would be appropriate.

An input-oriented DEA model to compute efficiency scores can be expressed in the following linear programming problem as shown in Cooper, Seiford, and Tone (2000).

$$\text{Maximize } E_o = \frac{\sum_{r=1}^{s} u_r y_{ro}}{\sum_{i=1}^{s} v_i x_{io}} \qquad (9.12)$$

Subject to:

$$\frac{\sum_{r=1}^{s} u_r y_{ro}}{\sum_{i=1}^{s} v_i x_{io}} \leq 1 \qquad (9.13)$$

$$u_r \geq 0; \quad v_i \geq 0 \qquad (9.14)$$

where

E_o = efficiency score for each facility in the set of $o = 1\ldots s$ facilities,

y_{ro} = selected output "r" produced by each facility in the set "o"

x_{io} = selected input "i" used by each facility in the set "o,"

y_{rj} = selected output "r" produced by facility "j,"

x_{ij} = selected input "i" used by facility "j."

In this formulation, u_r and v_i are the weights assigned respectively to output "r" and input "i," both obtained from DEA.

Efficiently operating units, those with efficiency scores of 1, can be used to create an efficiency frontier or data envelope. Figure 9.3 depicts a simple two-input, one-output scenario. It can be seen that four physicians are using two inputs (supplies and length of stay) to produce the same output (hip replacement surgery). Each point on the graph (P1–P4) represents a physician with the same number of hip replacement surgeries, but who uses different resource combinations. P1, for instance, uses two units of both length of stay and supplies. P2 uses one unit of LOS and four units of supplies, while P3 uses three units of LOS and one unit of supplies. P4 obviously uses more of both inputs as compared to P1. The physicians using the least amount of resources (P1, P2, and P3) are the most efficient; they form the efficiency frontier, having efficiency scores of one. P4 is relatively inefficient as compared to physicians on the frontier. DEA can also be used to determine inefficiencies, that is, the reduction in resources that an inefficient provider can accomplish to become efficient. It is easy to see from the graph that if P4 uses one unit less of supplies, the physician will become efficient.

Data envelopment analysis has many uses beyond simply evaluating physician or hospital efficiency. It can also be used, for instance, to combine multiple productivity measures into one score comparable across peer groups. For example, various financial ratios may be aggregated into a single measure (Ozcan and McCue, 1996). DEA also offers a way to incorporate the measurement of quality. A quality performance ratio may be combined with a productivity measure; customer satisfaction measures can be combined with a measure of the promptness of service (Ozcan, 1998; Ozgen and Ozcan, 2002; Ozgen and Ozcan, 2004; Ozcan, Merwin, Lee, and Morrissey, 2004; Ozcan, 2008).

Inputs	Physicians			
	P1	P2	P3	P4
LOS	2	1	3	2
Supplies	1	4	1	3

FIGURE 9.3. *Example of DEA Efficiency Frontier Formulation.*

When using DEA, it is important to ascertain that outputs and inputs are homogeneous across decision making units. Also, note that efficiency scores are relative measures, and are computed as performance relative to peer DMUs' performance. Therefore the selection of peers significantly influences the computations. For example, in a study on hospital productivity, it is vital to limit comparisons to hospitals within a particular state and market size. Doing so implicitly controls for factors such as state regulation, demand structures, and area wealth (Ozcan and Lynch, 1992; Ozcan, 1998; Ozcan, Merwin, Lee, Morrissey, 2004).

Overview on Improving Health Care Productivity

Wickham Skinner (1986), in an article entitled "The Productivity Paradox," examines productivity improvement programs of United States industries that had lost their competitive edge during the late 1970s and early 1980s. In many cases, productivity programs failed to increase the market share or competitiveness of industries. Skinner believes that the focus on cost-cutting techniques and traditional productivity measures was a reason for the continued problems of industrial performance. By targeting direct costs, primarily direct labor, industry focused on short-term fixes at the expense of developing a long-range plan to improve productivity. In many cases, the industrial firms ignored the loss of quality and the flexibility costs of laying off workers. Skinner claims that the best industrial productivity strategy is to invest in capital equipment to improve product quality and responsiveness to the market. The end result should be improved customer satisfaction, a variable that should be included in the industry's arsenal of productivity measures.

Does Skinner's productivity paradox apply to health care? How can health care institutions develop productivity improvement plans that have as their objectives improved quality of care, greater market responsiveness (flexibility), and more customer satisfaction? The Ashby and Altman study discussed earlier indicates that hospitals did become more efficient during the 1980s, quite possibly because the quality of the labor force improved. In health care, the quality of inputs, not the quantity, is often the important factor (Davis, 1991). Educational programs, particularly those for the nursing staff, can be invaluable for improving productivity. Recognition of the value of a high skill level for nurses has led to legal requirements, such as Public Law 100–203 (1987), which requires use of more RN staffing and also a minimum of 75 hours of nurse's aide training.

In health care, increasing capital inputs may not be a beneficial strategy. Although technology and capital expansion have been key in improving productivity, they can ultimately mean higher costs if implemented without careful planning. Moreover, the technological advances that have improved diagnostic accuracy and allowed many conditions to be treated in outpatient facilities have consequently increased the number of services provided. That phenomenon has caused aggregate productivity of hospitals to decline, even as the efficiency of service production has increased (Ashby and Altman, 1992).

One of the capital inputs in which hospitals and other health care institutions may have underinvested, however, is computer information systems. In the early 1990s, hospitals spent, on average, 1 to 3 percent of their budgets on computer systems, as compared to the service industry average of 7 to 10 percent (Sinclair, 1991). Bedside "point-of-care" systems have resulted in better care, improved documentation, and raised productivity (Cerne,1989; Gross, 1989a). Information systems with decision support capabilities can lift the burdens of routine tasks from the nursing staff while also improving clinical decisions. Gross (1989b) estimates that lower overtime costs due to the reduction in redundant nursing tasks range from $50,000 to $375,000 in the first year after a nursing information system's implementation. Furthermore, in a particularly needed advance, information systems that document nursing assessments, diagnoses, interventions, and outcomes, make it possible to carefully monitor the quality of care by comparing actual care to quality standards.

Bar coding is becoming increasingly common in health care. Besides increasing productivity, bar-coding also improves documentation. It can be used, for example, to classify patients into an acuity category. Nurses can be given a list of criteria to apply to each patient. Next to each criterion is a bar code. Using a portable, handheld device, nurses can scan the bar codes next to the criteria that a particular patient meets. Depending upon the combination of bar codes selected, the patient is placed into one of several acuity classifications. In this use, bar-coding can save nursing time for direct care, establish an objective classification system that is accurate and flexible—as long as properly scanned—and reduce paperwork and documentation (Addams, Bracci, and Overfelt, 1991). The next generation of productivity improvements will come with nanotechnology, which for materials, will eventually outdate bar coding. Instead, the molecular structures of items will mark identity, eliminating bar coding for all materials and processes.

In addition to using the methodologies explained above, health care organizations can take several key overall steps to improve productivity. The following suggestions are drawn from Stevenson (2002, p. 36):

1. Develop productivity measures for all operations in an organization.

2. Look at the system as a whole (do not sub optimize) in deciding on which operations or procedures to focus productivity improvements.

3. Develop methods for achieving productivity improvements, and especially benchmarking by studying peer health care providers that have increased productivity; and reengineer care delivery and business processes.

4. Establish reasonable and attainable standards and improvement goals.

5. Consider incentives to reward workers for contributions and to demonstrate management's support of productivity improvements.

6. Measure and publicize improvements.

SUMMARY

Health care organizations will continue to face turbulent times and more intense competition. Health care managers must face up to promoting and improving productivity within their institutions if those are to survive. There is not a per se formula for improving productivity. Each service and procedure must be examined individually. In some areas, the organization may have to increase the inputs used to improve quality. Nevertheless, in other areas more must be done with less while holding quality constant. Determining the proper mix of inputs and outputs will always be one of the most difficult tasks of the health care manager.

KEY TERMS

Benchmarking

Input

Output

Patient Days

Visits

Multi-factor Productivity

Skill Mix

Service Mix

Productivity and Quality

Data Envelopment Analysis (DEA)

EXERCISES

9.1 The chief at the ultrasound division of the radiology department in a community hospital would like to measure the multi-factor productivity for a "complete abdomen" procedure. The last three years of data were accumulated, as shown in Table EX 9.1.

TABLE EX 9.1

Measurement	Year 1	Year 2	Year 3
Price ($)	880	883	886
Volume	5,583	6,312	6,129
Labor ($)	75,000	77,000	80,000
Materials ($)	2,750	2,900	3,100
Overhead ($)	6,500	6,700	7,000

a. What are the multi-factor productivity ratios for these years?

b. What can you conclude about the productivity trend for this procedure?

9.2 Data from the outpatient mammography operations in a health care facility were accumulated in Table EX 9.2.

TABLE EX 9.2

Measurement	Year 1	Year 2	Year 3	Year 4
Price ($)	140	145	147	150
Volume	16,387	19,336	18,555	17,557
Labor ($)	275,000	307,000	318,000	325,000
Materials ($)	6,750	7,250	7,100	7,000
Overhead ($)	24,500	26,700	28,600	28,000

c. What are the multi-factor productivity ratios for these years?

d. What can you conclude about the productivity trend for mammography operations?

9.3 The weekly output of a radiology process is shown in Table EX 9.3, together with data for labor and material (X-ray film) inputs. The standard charge value of the output is $125 per unit. Overhead is charged weekly at a rate of $1,500 plus .5 times direct labor cost. Assume a forty-hour week and an hourly wage of $16. Material cost is $10 per image. Compute the average multi-factor productivity for this process.

TABLE EX 9.3

Week	Output	# of X-ray Technicians	# of X-ray Films
1	412	6	2,840
2	364	5	2,550
3	392	5	2,720
4	408	6	2,790

9.4 Calculate the case mix index for the following hospitals, which use the same patient classification system, using the data in Table EX 9.4.

TABLE EX 9.4

Patient Classification	Direct Care Hours	Hospital 1	Hospital 2	Hospital 3	Hospital 4
Low-level care	3.0	0.50	0.35	0.30	0.20
Medium-level care	6.0	0.35	0.40	0.30	0.25
High-level care	9.0	0.10	0.15	0.22	0.30
Extreme care	12.0	0.05	0.10	0.18	0.25

9.5 Statistical Data for Nursing Unit A in HADM Memorial Hospital

Using the data provided in Table EX 9.5, calculate the following ratios and compare them to the benchmark values of a peer group shown in brackets "[ ]":

a. Case-mix index [1.20]. Does Unit A serve more severe patients?

b. Adjusted Nursing Hours per Adjusted Discharge [32.81]. What would be the reasons for the difference between Unit A and the benchmark productivity ratio?

c. Nursing Salary Expense per Adjusted Discharges [1,294.27]. What steps would you take based on this ratio?

d. Percentage of Adjusted Nursing Hours in Direct Patient Care [.64]

TABLE EX 9.5

Measurements	Unit A
Annual Hours Worked (paid)	210,000
Annual Patient Days	14,500
Average Length of Stay	4.5

Patient Classification	
Low-Level Care (3.0)*	0.35
High-Level Care (9.0)*	0.65

Skill-Mix Distribution	
RNs ($40/hr)	0.70
LPNs ($30/hr)	0.20
NAs ($15/hr)	0.10

Assume that 1 LPN = .75 RN and 1 NA = .50 RN.

*Direct nursing care hours

9.6 Statistical Data for Two Nursing Units are shown in Table EX 9.6:

TABLE EX 9.6

Measurements		Unit 1	Unit 2
Annual Hours Worked (paid)		200,000	175,000
Annual Patient Days		15,000	12,000
Average Length of Stay		5	6

Patient Classification	Direct Care Hours	Distribution of Patients	
Low-Level Care	2.0	0.20	0.25
Medium-Level Care	4.5	0.40	0.55
Medium-High-Level Care	6.0	0.30	0.15
High-Level Care	8.5	0.10	0.05

Skill-Mix Distribution			
RNs ($35/hr)		0.40	1.00
LPNs ($20/hr)		0.30	0.00
NAs ($14/hr)		0.30	0.00

Assume that 1 LPN = .80 RN and 1 AID = .60 RN

Using the data provided above, analyze and compare the productivity of the two nursing units (for each productivity ratio indicate which unit is more productive) with respect to:

a. Adjusted Nursing Hours per Adjusted Discharge

b. Nursing Salary Expense per Adjusted Discharge

c. Percentage of Adjusted Nursing Hours in Direct Patient Care

9.7 The PERFORMSBETTER MEDICAL CENTER (PMC), a three-site urology group practice, requires productivity monitoring. To create a benchmark for future years and to be able to compare performance to similar peer practices, the data in Table EX 9.7 were gathered for each of the three locations.

TABLE EX 9.7

Measurements/Sites	Location 1	Location 2	Location 3
Annual Visits	135,000	94,000	101,000
Annual Paid Hours	115,000	112,000	125,000
Patient Classification (Based on CPT Coding)			
Initial Visit (.55)*	.30	.10	.15
Low-Level Decision Making (.50)	.40	.20	.15
Medium-Level Decision Making (.75)	20	.40	.35
High-Level Decision Making (1.40)	.10	.30	.35
Skill-Mix Distribution			
Specialists ($110/hr) †	.50	.30	.70
General Practitioners ($85/hr)	.30	.50	.30
Nurse Practitioners ($45/hr)	.20	.20	.00

* Represents total hours of direct care required per patient visit within the category.

† Represents hourly compensation including fringe benefits for the skill level.

Assume that 1 general practitioner = .75 specialists, and 1 nurse practitioner = .35 specialists for economic measure of skill substitution.

Calculate:

a. Work hours/visits

b. Adjusted work hours/visits

c. Work hours/adjusted visits

d. Adjusted work hours/adjusted visits‡

e. Total salary expense/visits

f. Total salary expense/adjusted visits‡

    g.   Percent of work hours in direct patient care

    h.   Percent of adjusted work hours in direct patient care[+]

    i.   Total salary expense/hours of direct patient care[+]

[+]Use these measures for the final comparison among the three sites, and discuss potential problems at each site or overall for the company. What are your recommendations to correct them?

CHAPTER

RESOURCE
ALLOCATION

LEARNING OBJECTIVES

- Recognize the concept of resource allocation in health care organizations.
- Describe linear programming methodology and its use for allocation in health care facilities.
- Recognize the difference in applications of maximization and minimization problems.
- Recognize the use of integer linear programming in staff scheduling.

Among the frequent operational problems in health care are resource allocation, service mix, scheduling, and assignment. Linear programming (LP) is an excellent tool to apply to those problems. In practice, software for nurse scheduling and operating room scheduling, empowered by linear programming and its extensions such as integer programming, provides optimal resource allocation and scheduling. In this chapter, we will describe both linear and integer programming applications in health care.

LINEAR PROGRAMMING

Linear programming is a powerful tool that can incorporate many decision variables into a single model to attain an optimal solution. For example, a nurse scheduling problem in a medical center would involve many decision variables: various shift assignments and patterns, rotations, off days, weekend day designations, vacation requests, and holidays—all of which have to be considered simultaneously. When the requirements set up for health care management problems are translated into what is called constraints, it is possible for there to be so many that no solution to the problem appears to be feasible. However, health care managers can then reassess the requirements and relax some to seek possible solutions. To do that, one has to understand the nature of linear programming, and its structure. One must be able to observe simple problems (with few decision variables) graphically, and be able to conceptualize problems with many decision variables and constraints.

The structure of linear programming includes decision variables; an objective function; constraints; and the parameters that describe the available alternatives or resources.

The **decision variables** represent the levels of activity for an operation (for example, number of inpatient hospitalizations, number of outpatient visits); their values are determined by the solution of the problem. The variables are shown with symbols x_1, x_2, x_3, and so on in a linear equation. Decision variables cannot have negative values.

The **objective function** describes the goals the health care manager would like to attain (creating a reasonable margin for the survival or the financial health of the health care organization). Such a goal might be maximization of revenues or margins, or minimization of costs. The objective function is a linear mathematical statement of these goals (revenue, profit, costs) described in terms of decision variables (per unit of output or input). That is, the objective function is expressed as a linear combination of decision variables that will optimize the outcome (revenue, profit, costs) for the health care organization.

Constraints are the set linear equations that describe the limitations restricting the available alternatives and or resources. Especially in health care, scarce resources impede the management of facilities and the development of new health care services. The constraints to which the objective is subject arise from the health care organizations' operating environment. By factoring in constraints, a health care manager can see whether offering a new health care service would be feasible at all.

Parameters are the numerical values (values of available resources) that describe the fixed resources. Linear programming models are solved given the parameter values. This means that health care managers can emulate situations with "what if" questions by changing the values of the parameters in order to find alternative solutions. General structure of the linear programming model is as follows:

$$\text{Maximize (or minimize)} \; Z = c_1 x_1 + c_2 x_2 + c_3 x_3 + \cdots + c_n x_n \qquad (10.1)$$

Subject to:

$$a_{11} x_1 + a_{12} x_2 + a_{13} x_3 + \cdots + a_{1n} x_n (\leq, =, \geq) b_1 \qquad (10.2)$$

$$a_{21} x_1 + a_{22} x_2 + a_{23} x_3 + \cdots + a_{2n} x_n (\leq, =, \geq) b_2$$
$$a_{31} x_1 + a_{32} x_2 + a_{33} x_3 + \cdots + a_{3n} x_n (\leq, =, \geq) b_3$$
$$\cdots$$
$$a_{m1} x_1 + a_{m2} x_2 + a_{m3} x_3 + \cdots + a_{mn} x_n (\leq, =, \geq) b_m$$
$$x_i \geq 0.$$

where

Z = objective function

x_i = decision variables

b_j = available resource for j^{th} constraint

c_i = objective function coefficients

a_{ij} = coefficient for i^{th} decision variable on j^{th} constraint.

Maximization Models

To illustrate these concepts in an example and build a linear programming model for it, consider the following maximization example.

EXAMPLE 10.1

An insurance company desires to enter the health care market and offer its potential customers both a staff model health maintenance organization (HMO) and commercial indemnity insurance. The company is deciding how to allocate its marketing efforts between those options to maximize its profits. The analysts have estimated that the company will realize a profit of $1,200 per enrollee from the HMO, and $600 per enrollee from commercial plans. Furthermore, for the coming year the company is forced to rely on its present resources in terms of sales force. The administrative support of the HMO will take two hundred hours, and the commercial administration will take, on average, four hundred hours; currently, the company can allocate 1.6 million hours to sales. To break even, the HMO requires that the contribution margins (contribution margin is sales revenue less variable costs; it is the amount available to pay for fixed costs and then provide any profit after variable costs have been paid) for enrollees must exceed $1.5 million. The estimated contribution margins are $500 and $300, for HMO and for commercial insurance enrollees, respectively. With a limited number of physicians participating in the staff model HMO at the present time, the HMO can handle at most 5,000 enrollees.

Solution

To formulate the model for this problem, first we must identify the decision variables. In this case the two options, HMO and indemnity insurance, are the decision variables. The number of enrollees required for profitable operations is determined by the level of activity in each of those variables. Let us assign a symbol of x_1 to indicate the potential number of HMO enrollees; similarly let x_2 represent the enrollees in the indemnity plan.

The next step is to express the objective function in a linear fashion to represent the maximum profits for each of those decision variables. Recall that the company was expecting, respectively, $1,200 and $600 profit from each HMO and each indemnity enrollee. The objective function is the summation of these expectations and can be formulated as:

$$\text{Maximize } Z \text{ (profit)} = 1{,}200x_1 + 600x_2.$$

Once the objective function is determined, the constraints it is subject to must be developed. It is indicated that the insurance company will use its existing resources to develop marketing campaigns for those new products, but the resources are limited by the parameters. For example, the available administrative support is limited to 1.6 million hours of staff time. We have to convert that information into a constraint; let us call it the administrative support constraint. To express the constraint as x_1, x_2, we must note the rate at which each product would consume the resource. In the problem those rates are given as two hundred hours for the HMO and four hundred hours for the indemnity plan, respectively. The formulation of the administrative support constraint is then:

$$200x_1 + 400x_2 \le 1{,}600{,}000 \text{ (administrative supported constraint)}.$$

This constraint indicates that the linear combination of enrollees from both plans can be administratively supported up to 1,600,000 hours from existing resources. The second constraint in the problem assures a minimum of $1,500,000 as the contribution margin, with $500 from each HMO enrollee and $300 from each indemnity enrollee, and is written as:

$$500x_1 + 300x_2 \ge 1{,}500{,}000 \text{ (contribution margin constraint)}.$$

It should be noted that this constraint has the sign greater than equal at the right end side of the equation indicating that expectation for the contribution margin is at minimum that amount ($1.5 million).

The final constraint of this problem is how many enrollees the company can handle at the start with the given resources. There is no restriction on indemnity enrollees, but for the HMO only 5,000 enrollees are permitted. Hence, this last equation can be expressed as:

$$1x_1 + 0x_2 \le 5{,}000 \text{ (enrollees constraint)}.$$

Since none of the decision variables can have a negative value, we must enforce a nonnegativity constraint on the variables as:

$$x_1, x_2 \ge 0.$$

Summarizing the development so far, we have a linear programming formulation of this problem:

$$\text{Maximize } Z \text{ (profit)} = 1{,}200x_1 + 600x_2$$

Subject to:

$$200x_1 + 400x_2 \leq 1{,}600{,}000 \text{ (administrative support constraint)}$$
$$500x_1 + 300x_2 \geq 1{,}500{,}000 \text{ (contribution margin constraint)}$$
$$1x_1 + 0x_2 \leq 5{,}000 \text{ (enrollees constraint)}$$
$$x_1, x_2 \geq 0.$$

The next step is to plot the constraints and identify an area that satisfies all the constraints, called the feasible solution space. Then one plots the objective function to determine the optimal solution in the feasible solution space. The following steps describe the graphical approach and the solution to this problem.

Step 1: Plot the identified constraints: determine where the line intersects each axis. Mark those intersections and connect them. Close attention must be placed to whether a constraint is a less-than or greater-than constraint. For instance, for the administrative support constraint, the intercepts are $x_1 = 8{,}000$ (determined by setting $x_2 = 0$ and solving for x_1: $1{,}600{,}000 \div 200 = 8{,}000$); and $x_2 - 4{,}000$ (determined by setting $x_1 = 0$ and solving for x_2: $1{,}600{,}000 \div 400 = 4{,}000$). Because it is a $\leq$ constraint, the area between the origin and this line is the feasible solution space.

Step 2: Continue plotting all constraints to identify the total feasible solution space.

Step 3: Plot the objective function and observe where it has the highest value (maximization) while still touching (tangent to) the feasible solution space. This is the location of the optimal solution.

The graphic presentation of this problem is shown in Figure 10.1. The first constraint, administrative support, is a $\leq$ type constraint, which means that the feasible solution must occur below the line and toward the origin point (0.0). On the other hand, the second constraint, contribution margin, is the $\geq$ type, which means that the feasible area must be above the line and away from the origin. Finally, the third constraint, enrollees, represents restriction in only one variable, and is a $\leq$ type constraint, so once again the feasible region must occur below the line and towards the origin.

The dashed parallel lines show the iso-profit (objective function) values. The goal is to maximize the profit by choosing the iso-profit line that has the highest value. In maximization problems, the iso-objective function line that is tangent to the feasible solution space at the farthest point yields the greatest value for the objective function, and provides the optimal solution.

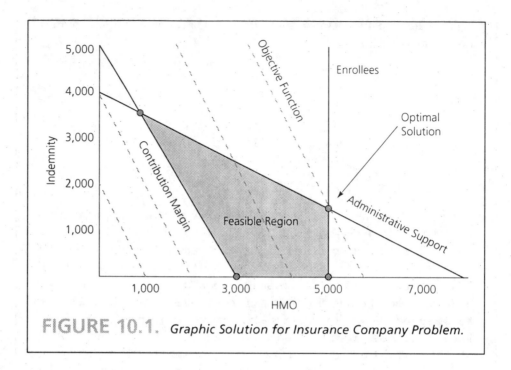

FIGURE 10.1. *Graphic Solution for Insurance Company Problem.*

The solution to this problem is also displayed in Figure 10.1, where resources are allocated to each program. That is, the insurance company should have 5,000 HMO and 1,500 indemnity enrollees to maximize its profit at $6,300,000 without violating any of the imposed constraints (limitations). It is noteworthy here that the solution to this problem occurs at the intersection of administrative support and enrollee constraints (first and third constraints). In linear programming terminology, a constraint that forms the optimal corner point of the feasible solution space is called the binding constraint. Here those two constraints are the binding constraints: any change in their right-hand side values, b_j, would immediately affect the objective function value and the solution. On the other hand, the nonbinding constraints, in this case the contribution margin constraint, do not affect the final solution unless a dramatic change occurs in the parameters.

Although the graphed solution to linear programming problems is illustrative and easy to understand, when there are more than two decision variables in the model, graphical solutions are no longer practical and linear algebraic methods are required. A method that is instrumental for obtaining optimal solutions to linear programming problems is the **simplex method.** This methodology is embedded in Excel, under "Tools" as an add-in tool called "Solver" (user can activate this by clicking on "Add-Ins").

Figure 10.2 depicts the Excel setup to this problem. Two decision variables, HMO and indemnity, are identified, and the first row of the data shows the objective function of the problem where maximization is sought. The coefficients (c_j) of each decision

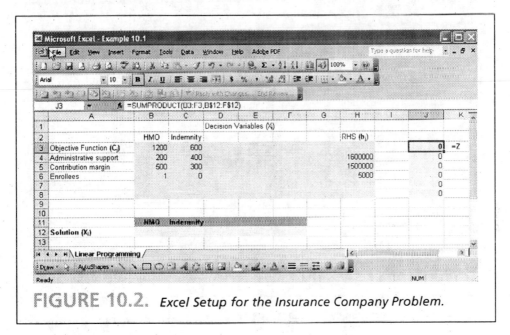

FIGURE 10.2.   *Excel Setup for the Insurance Company Problem.*

Source: Screen shots reprinted by permission from Microsoft Corporation.

variable (1,200 and 600) in the objective function are shown in the third row. The following three rows depict the constraints and right-hand side (RHS) values (b_j). The coefficients for each variable on a given constraint, a_{ij}, are also shown (for example, 200 and 400 for the administrative support constraint).

Figure 10.3 shows selection of "Solver" from the "Tools" menu, and Figure 10.4 displays the ensuing pop-up menus where the user can:

- Identify cell for objective function value (target cell (J3)),

- Select maximization (max) or minimization (min) from radio buttons,

- Identify solution cells (by changing cells box), and

- Add constraints (subject to the constraints box).

To add a constraint, the user can click on "Add," which activates another pop-up menu (Add Constraint, shown lower left section of the Figure 10.4) where cell references can be selected (for example, J4 for administrative support constraint). Additionally, type of equation ($\leq$, $=$, or $\geq$) and constant (RHS or b_j) value can be entered (H4). Once this setup is completed, clicking on "Solver" radio button provides results as shown in Figure 10.5. As the reader observes, another pop-up menu "Solver Results" appears to allow user to select various reports by clicking and highlighting each. These reports include "Answer, Sensitivity, and Limits." A final click on the "OK" button adds these reports as new spread sheets to the existing Excel file. These reports are shown in Figures 10.6 through 10.8, which require explanation to interpret them

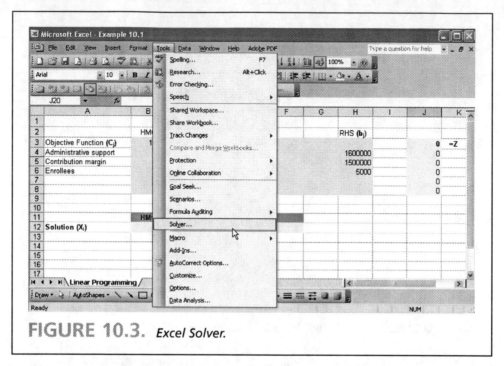

FIGURE 10.3. *Excel Solver.*

Source: Screen shots reprinted by permission from Microsoft Corporation.

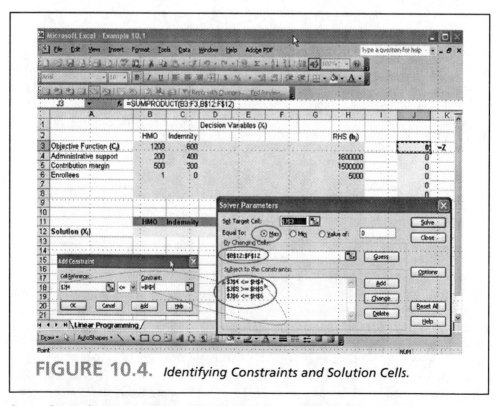

FIGURE 10.4. *Identifying Constraints and Solution Cells.*

Source: Screen shots reprinted by permission from Microsoft Corporation.

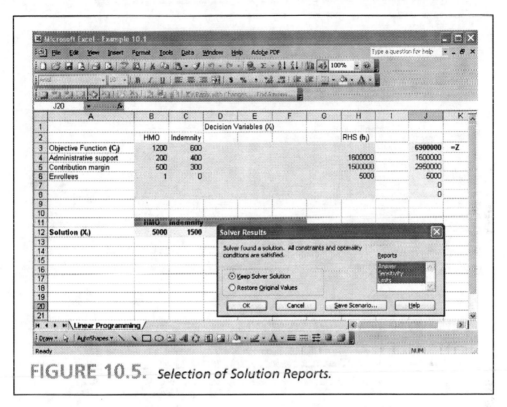

FIGURE 10.5. *Selection of Solution Reports.*

Source: Screen shots reprinted by permission from Microsoft Corporation.

and further analyze the problem. Observing from answer report, Figure 10.6, the solution value for each decision variable, the unit profit values, and the total contribution to the objective function are shown in the labeled columns. That is, with 5,000 enrollees at $1,200 per enrollee for the HMO, the total contribution to the objective function from this variable is $6,000,000. The remaining $900,000 is contributed by the indemnity product with 1,500 enrollees, each bringing $600 profit. Thus, the total profit amounts to $6,900,000 with this solution. Figure 10.7 displays sensitivity analysis for the model parameters. A "0" (zero) in the "Reduced Costs" column indicates that no further improvement is possible for the objective function from the associated constraint unless the right-hand side (resources) improves. "Final Value" column indicates that the particular decision variable is in the final solution and thus contributes to the objective function. There are instances in which not all decision variables contribute to the final solution. The "Allowable Increase" (c_j) and "Allowable Decrease (c_j) columns show the range of each decision variable for the objective function. In this example, profit per enrollee cannot be lower than $300 (1,200 − 900) for the HMO, but can be infinitely high (1E + 30 stands for a very large number). Similarly, for the indemnity product, profit can go as low as 0, but cannot be higher than $2,400 (600 + 1,800) per enrollee.

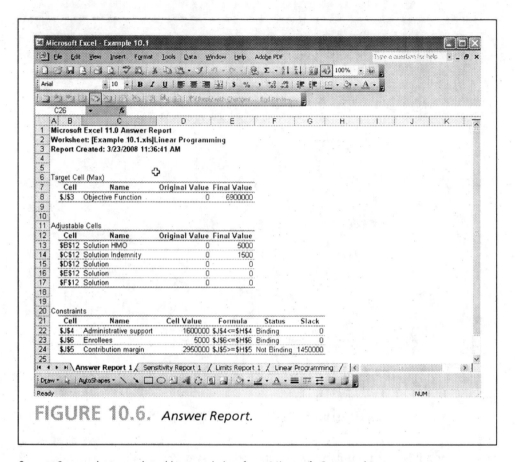

FIGURE 10.6. *Answer Report.*

Source: Screen shots reprinted by permission from Microsoft Corporation.

The last part of Figure 10.7 shows the constraints, their allowable values and their effects on the objective function. Recall that the intersection of the first and third constraints (administrative support, and enrollees) defined the optimal solution to this problem. These are binding constraints or tight constraints, which means that they cannot be moved to the left or right (in the graph) without affecting the solution. Notice that the values in the columns "Final Value" and "Right-Hand Side" for those two constraints are equal. However, the Final Value and RHS values are different for the non-binding constraint (contribution margin). These observations lead to a discussion of slack, surplus, shadow prices, and range of feasibility in linear programming. Let us define each of those concepts.

Slack—When the optimal values of decision variables are substituted into a ≤ constraint and the resulting value is less than the right-hand side value.

Surplus—When the optimal values of decision variables are substituted into a ≥ constraint and the resulting values exceed the right-hand side value.

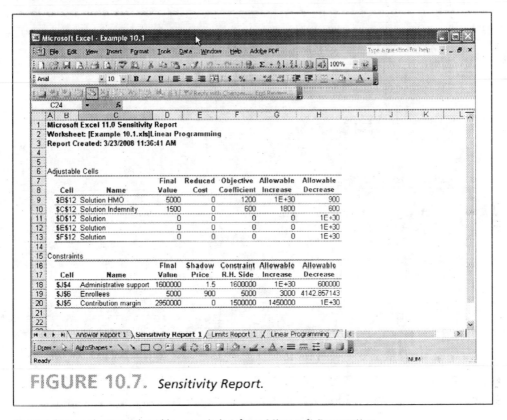

FIGURE 10.7. *Sensitivity Report.*

Source: Screen shots reprinted by permission from Microsoft Corporation.

Shadow Prices—How much a one-unit increase in the right-hand side of a constraint would increase the value of the objective function.

Range of Feasibility—The range of values for the right-hand side of a constraint over which the shadow price remains the same.

In Figure 10.6, the lower set of rows in the constraint section depicts the values of those concepts just defined. The second, and only nonbinding, constraint: "contribution margin," has 145,000 under the "Slack or Surplus" column. Since this constraint is a ≥ type constraint, that is the amount of surplus; one could increase the right-hand side of the equation by this amount (to 295,000) without violating the existing solution. In Figure 10.7, "Shadow Price" of enrollees appears as 900, indicating that every additional enrollee (beyond 5,000) can improve profits by $900. If the number of physicians to handle more than 5,000 HMO enrollees were not subject to restrictions, the insurance company could enroll up to 8,000 enrollees and generate additional 2,700,000 (3,000 * 900) profit.

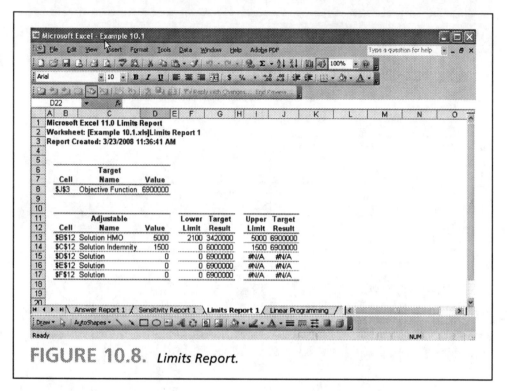

FIGURE 10.8. *Limits Report.*

Source: Screen shots reprinted by permission from Microsoft Corporation.

On the other hand, the company cannot afford to enroll fewer than 857 (5,000 − 4,142.8). The shadow price of administrative support is interpreted similarly, although the unit contribution to profit (objective function) is dramatically smaller at $1.50. Having said that, one should note that if the human resources are available (in hours), the contribution to profit is infinite. One then must make a cost-benefit analysis as to whether it is worthwhile to expand one extra hour of human resource to generate $1.50 in additional profit.

The Figure 10.9 displays the potential effect of relaxing the binding constraints and their impact on objective function (profits). For example, relaxing administrative support constraint (moving upward) can bring a new optimal solution at point B where objective function is marginally larger than original optimal solution (shadow price 1.5). However, relaxing the enrollees constraint (increasing RHS to 8,000) provides a new optimal solution at point A where objective function commands significantly higher profits (due to high shadow price). Of course, both constraints can be relaxed simultaneously producing yet another optimal solution at point C. Using the sensitivity analysis, a health care manager must assess cost and benefit of adding additional resources for increased profits. In this case, adding 3,000 more enrollees will require additional physicians, and the cost of adding physicians to this staff model HMO needs to be evaluated against the potential profits calculated in sensitivity analysis.

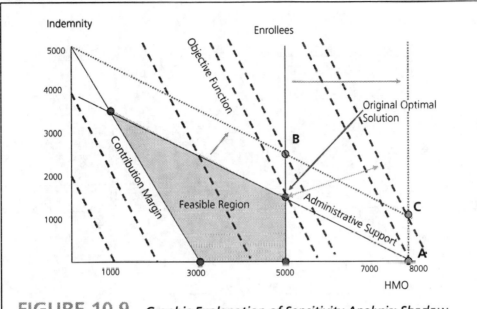

FIGURE 10.9. *Graphic Explanation of Sensitivity Analysis: Shadow Price and its Impact on Alternate Optimal Solutions.*

Minimization Models

When the measures in the objective function are costs, obviously health care managers seek to minimize those costs. Model setup follows the same steps, with one exception: in cost minimization problems, the constraints are generally the $\geq$ type. Thus, in the graphic solution, the feasible area is defined from infinity towards origin.

EXAMPLE 10.2

$$\text{Maximize } Z = 60x_1 + 30x_2$$

Subject to:

$$20x_1 + 40x_2 \geq 160 \text{ C1 (constraint 1)}$$
$$40x_1 + 30x_2 \geq 240 \text{ C2 (constraint 2)}$$
$$x_1, x_2 \geq 0$$

The graphical solution to this minimization problem is shown in Figure 10.10.

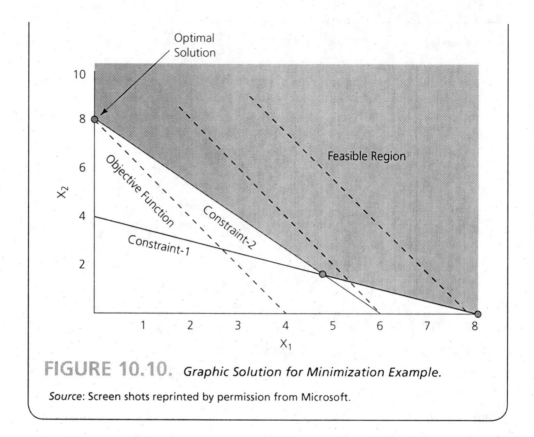

FIGURE 10.10. *Graphic Solution for Minimization Example.*

Source: Screen shots reprinted by permission from Microsoft.

Here, the optimal solution occurs at $x_2 = 8$ and $x_1 = 0$. The objective function, with its slope, just clears the feasible region (tangent) at this point. It should be noted that the objective function (the iso-cost lines) is coming down from higher values (cost) to this value, which is the minimum for this problem.

Finally, Figures 10.11 through 10.15 depict the Excel solution to the minimization example. The reader can observe from Figure 10.11 that "Min" option is selected at "Solver Parameters" menu to solve this problem.

Integer Linear Programming

In linear programming one of the assumptions is that decision variables are continuous. Therefore solutions can yield fractional values such as 4.3 patients, or 7.6 nurses. Such solutions are especially impractical, however, when linear programming is used for scheduling the clinical staff. Rounding off these values may generate infeasible or less optimal solutions. Integer programming is an extension of linear programming that eliminates the problem by enforcing integer decision variable outcomes.

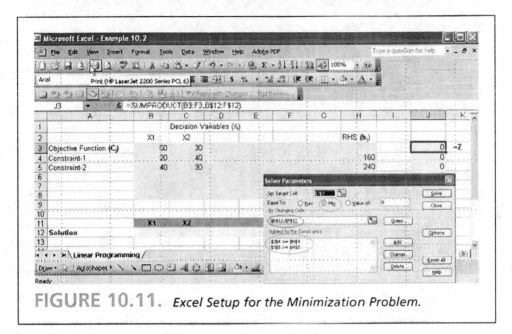

FIGURE 10.11. *Excel Setup for the Minimization Problem.*

Source: Screen shots reprinted by permission from Microsoft Corporation.

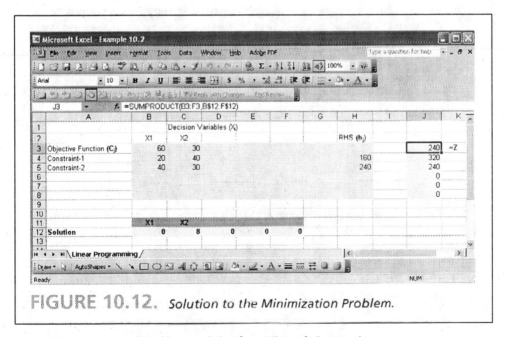

FIGURE 10.12. *Solution to the Minimization Problem.*

Source: Screen shots reprinted by permission from Microsoft Corporation.

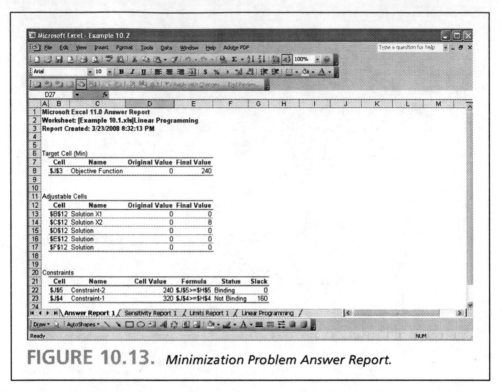

FIGURE 10.13. *Minimization Problem Answer Report.*

Source: Screen shots reprinted by permission from Microsoft Corporation.

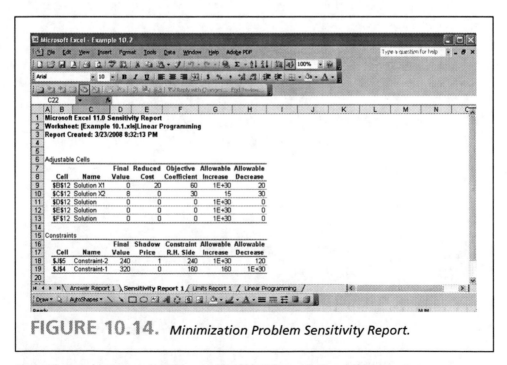

FIGURE 10.14. *Minimization Problem Sensitivity Report.*

Source: Screen shots reprinted by permission from Microsoft Corporation.

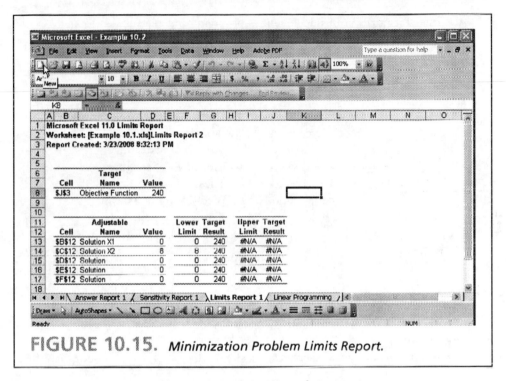

FIGURE 10.15. *Minimization Problem Limits Report.*

Source: Screen shots reprinted by permission from Microsoft Corporation.

Health care facilities usually provide service around the clock seven days a week, so scheduling staff is a significant operational task for clinic managers. Many factors must be included in the model so that an equitable schedule can be produced. A typical full-time employee works five days a week with two days off. Although the off days can be either consecutive or spread during the week according to resource availability, clinical staff generally prefer two consecutive days off, for rotating weekends. Each clinical unit has minimum staffing requirements (core staff) for each shift. The aim of management is to meet the core coverage of each day and shift while satisfying the schedule of five work days and two consecutive days off for each staff member.

Let us illustrate a simple version of staff scheduling. In linear integer programming, scheduling can be thought of as cycles (tours) of assignments. Since the most critical element of the scheduling is deciding on the off days, the decision variables can be conceptualized as the two off days that a staff member is assigned in a scheduling cycle. There are seven possible pairs of consecutive off days available: Saturday-Sunday, Sunday-Monday, Monday-Tuesday, Tuesday-Wednesday, Wednesday-Thursday, Thursday-Friday, and Friday-Saturday. If we can make the assignments to guarantee these off days to clinical staff while meeting the unit staffing level requirements for each day, we will have produced a satisfactory schedule.

A formal formulation of integer linear programming for staff assignments is as follows (adapted from Fitzsimmons & Fitzsimmons, 2004; p. 255):

$$\text{Minimize) } Z = x_1 + x_2 + x_3 + x_4 + x_5 + x_6 + x_7$$

Subject to:

$$x_1 + x_2 + x_3 + x_4 + x_5 \geq b_1 \text{ Saturday constraint}$$
$$x_2 + x_3 + x_4 + x_5 + x_6 \geq b_2 \text{ Sunday constraint}$$
$$x_3 + x_4 + x_5 + x_6 + x_7 \geq b_3 \text{ Monday constraint}$$
$$x_1 + x_4 + x_5 + x_6 + x_7 \geq b_4 \text{ Tuesday constraint}$$
$$x_1 + x_2 + x_5 + x_6 + x_7 \geq b_5 \text{ Wednesday constraint}$$
$$x_1 + x_2 + x_3 + x_6 + x_7 \geq b_6 \text{ Thursday constraint}$$
$$x_1 + x_2 + x_3 + x_4 + x_7 \geq b_7 \text{ Friday constraint}$$
$$X_i \geq 0 \text{ and integer}$$

where

Z = objective function

x_i = decision variables (x_1 = off on Saturday & Sunday, x_2 = off on Sunday & Monday, and so on)

b_j = minimum staff requirements for a day of the week (b_1 = required staff for Saturday).

To further illustrate staff scheduling, consider the following example:

EXAMPLE 10.3

A nurse manager must schedule staff nurses in a rehab unit. Nurses work five days a week with two consecutive off days. The staff requirements of the nursing unit are seven nurses for each day of the week. The nurse manager wants an equitable schedule for all the staff while meeting the unit staff requirements each day.

Solution

Since this problem has more than two decision variables, a graphic solution is not possible. A computer solution using Excel will be provided. Figure 10.16 displays the data entry and the setup for this problem. Figure 10.17 illustrates identification of constraints and integer values on "Solver Parameters" pop-up menus. Figure 10.18 displays solution and Figure 10.19 shows the answer report.

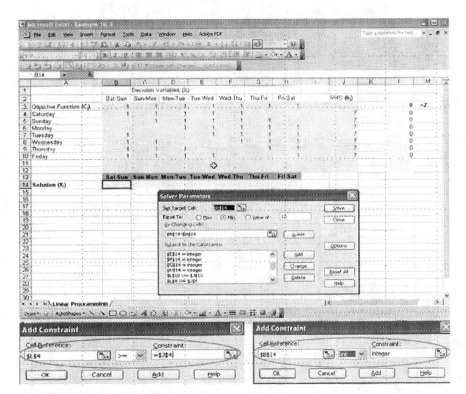

FIGURE 10.16. *Integer Programming: Excel Setup for the Staff Scheduling Problem.*

Source: Screen shots reprinted by permission from Microsoft Corporation.

FIGURE 10.17. *Identifying Constraints and Integer Values.*

Source: Screen shots reprinted by permission from Microsoft Corporation.

FIGURE 10.18. *Solution to the Staff Scheduling Problem.*

Source: Screen shots reprinted by permission from Microsoft Corporation.

FIGURE 10.19. *Answer Report for the Staff Scheduling Problem.*

Source: Screen shots reprinted by permission from Microsoft Corporation.

As the upper portion of the formulation depicts, the seven decision variables are the pairs of off days, and the right-hand side (RHS) of each day constraint shows the staff requirement for that day. It is more challenging to interpret the results, shown in the lower portion of the exhibit, to develop the schedule.

The solution for each decision variable indicates how many cycles (tours) are needed to satisfy the daily staffing requirement for the unit while assuring a pair of days off to each staff nurse. Explicitly, $x_1 = 2$ indicates that the nurse manager should assign two nurses with Saturday-Sunday off; $x_2 = 1$ indicates that one nurse should be assigned to have Sunday-Monday off; $x_3 = 2$ indicates that two nurses should be assigned to have Monday-Tuesday off. With that information, a nurse manager can draft a schedule.

Table 10.1 shows the resulting schedule, with A for assignments and O for days off. The last few rows of the table show the requirements and assignments, the total number of A's in a given day, and any excess assignment for a day. To implement this

TABLE 10.1. Nurse Scheduling with Integer Programming.

Nurse ID	Sat	Sun	Mon	Tue	Wed	Thu	Friday
1	O	O	A	A	A	A	A
2	O	O	A	A	A	A	A
3	A	O	O	A	A	A	A
4	A	A	O	O	A	A	A
5	A	A	O	O	O	A	A
6	A	A	A	O	O	A	A
7	A	A	A	A	O	O	A
8	A	A	A	A	A	O	O
9	A	A	A	A	A	O	O
10	O	A	A	A	A	A	O
Required	7	7	7	7	7	7	7
Assigned	7	7	7	8	7	7	7
Excess	0	0	0	1	0	0	0

schedule a total of 10 nurses are needed, which is the number given by the objective function value shown in the solution (Figures 10.18 and 10.19).

SUMMARY

Resource allocation can take the form of distribution of beds, products, staff, and other resources in various health services. Linear programming and its extensions provide optimal solutions to allocation problems. In practice, these methods often are imbedded into scheduling software that is used by divisional or departmental managers.

KEY TERMS

Linear Programming
Decision Variables
Objective Function
Constraints
Parameters
Feasible Solution Space
Maximization

Minimization
Optimal Solution
Slack
Surplus
Shadow Price
Range of Feasibility
Integer Programming

EXERCISES

10.1 Given the following linear programming formulation:

$$\text{Maximize} \, 1{,}600x_1 + 3{,}000x_2$$

Subject to:

$$40x_1 + 25x_2 \leq 80{,}000 \,(\text{constraint 1})$$
$$20x_1 + 30x_2 \leq 60{,}000 \,(\text{constraint 2})$$
$$x_i, x_2 \geq 0 \,(\text{non-negativity constrains}).$$

   a. Solve the problem graphically.

   b. Solve the problem using Excel solver.

   c. What is the total objective function value?

   d. Do both variables contribute to the solution? Why?

   e. Does any variable have a slack value? If so, what does it mean?

10.2 The cost of providing public services at a local hospital has been scrutinized by management. Although these services are used as marketing tools for the hospital, the cost and availability of scarce resources require their optimal allocation while minimizing costs.

Two popular programs being assessed for this purpose are "Family Planning" (FP) and "Health-Drive-Screenings" (HDS); their costs to the hospital for each offering are $200 and $400, respectively. The health care manager in charge of operations found three common patterns of resource consumption for each of these services and the available resources, shown in Table EX 10.2.

TABLE EX 10.2

Resource Type	FP	HDS	Available Resources per Month
Staff time	60	120	480 minutes
Materials	30	90	250 kits
Rent space		1	3 occasions

a. Formulate this as a linear programming problem.

b. Solve the problem graphically.

c. Solve the problem using Excel solver.

d. In a given month, how many FP and how many HDS should be offered?

e. With the proposed class offerings, how many kits will be left over (not distributed in the classes)?

f. What is the yearly cost of these two programs to the hospital?

10.3 A practice would like to allocate their resources optimally between the orthopedic and rheumatology departments. The revenues per case generated by orthopedics and by rheumatology are $2,000 and $1,000, respectively. The average number of visits, utilization of radiology resources per case, and available resources are in Table EX 10.3.

TABLE EX 10.3

	Orthopedics	Rheumatology	Available resources
Visits	2	3	600 hours MD time
Radiology	4	1	800 procedures

a. Formulate this as a linear programming problem.

b. Solve the problem graphically.

c. Solve the problem using Excel solver.

d. For the optimal solution, what should be the percentages of allocation between the two departments?

e. How much total combined revenue can be generated with this solution?

10.4 A hospital is evaluating the feasibility of offerings among three technologies, on the basis of what would make the most profit. These new technologies are:

1. Closed-chest cardiac bypass surgery with "daVinci Surgical Robot"

2. Gamma knife

3. Positron emission tomography (PET) scanner

Table EX 10.4 gives the information on profit, the amount of common resources used by each of the three technologies per case, and their available resources per month:

TABLE EX 10.4

	daVinci	Gamma Knife	PET	Available Resources
Profit $	2,000	3,500	2,000	
Total staff time	15	12	1.5	2,000 hours
Maintenance	25	25	22	1,500 minutes
Computer resources	20	25	10	3,000 minutes

a. Formulate this as a linear programming problem.

b. Solve the problem using Excel solver.

c. Based on optimal solution, which product(s) should be offered, and how many procedures can be offered in a month?

d. What is the expected contribution of new technology to the hospital's monthly profits?

10.5 A community hospital is planning to expand its services to three new service lines in the medical diagnostic categories (MDCs) and their corresponding diagnostic related groupings (DRGs) shown in Table 10.5.1

Five common resources must be allocated among these three new service lines according to which will bring the most revenue (using overall average DRG payments in a given MDC category). The resources are beds (measured as patient days), nursing staff, radiology, laboratory, and operating room (hint: constraints). The health care manager in charge of this expansion project obtained the average consumption patterns of these resources for each MDC from

TABLE EX 10.5.1.

MDC	DRGs	Description
2	36–47	Diseases and disorders of the eye
19	424–433	Mental diseases and disorders
21	439–455	Injury, poisoning, and toxic effects of drugs

other peer institutions, and estimated the resources that can be made available (per year) for the new service lines in Table EX 10.5.2:

TABLE EX 10.5.2

Resource Category	MDC-2	MDC-19	MDC-21	Available Resources
Length of stay (LOS)	3.3	6.1	4.4	19,710
Nursing hours	3	5	4.5	16,200
Radiology procedures	0.5	1.0		3,000
Laboratory procedures	1	1.5	3	6,000
Operating room	2		4	1,040

Average revenues from MDC-2, MDC-19, and MDC-21 are $8,885, $10,143, and $12,711, respectively.

    a. Formulate this as a linear programming problem.

    b. Solve the problem using Excel solver.

    c. To get the most revenue, which service(s) should be offered?

    d. What is the optimal volume(s)?

    e. What is the total expected revenue from the new services?

    f. Which resources should be expanded?

    g. How much additional revenue can be expected if resources are selected in part (f) for expansion without violating the current solution?

10.6 A regional laboratory that performs nontraditional tests is planning to offer new diagnostic tests for regional hospitals. Current analyzers and staff are capable of performing these tests. The laboratory manager assessed the required staff and analyzer times, as well as the chemical materials required for a bundle of 50 vials for each type of test listed in Table EX 10.6.

TABLE EX 10.6

Test Type →	I	II	III	IV	V	Available Resources
Profit ($)	8	10	8	7	10	
Staff (minutes)	15	15	15	20	25	3,400
Auto analyzer equipment (minutes)	20	40	40	60	45	6,000
Materials	12	15	16	14	14	2,700

    a. Formulate this as a linear programming problem.

    b. Solve the problem using Excel solver.

    c. For the optimal solution, in terms of profit, which test(s) should be offered?

    d. What is the optimal volume(s)?

    e. What is the total expected profit from the new tests?

    f. Which resources should be expanded?

How much additional revenue can be expected if the resources are selected in "f" for expansion without violating the current solution?

CHAPTER

SUPPLY CHAIN AND INVENTORY MANAGEMENT

LEARNING OBJECTIVES

- Describe the relationships of providers with the companies at the upstream source of medical supplies.
- Recognize the information sources for supply chain and inventory management in various health services operations.
- Review current use of just-in-time services and partnerships or alliances with suppliers for health care organizations.
- Describe the parameters involved in inventory management.
- Recognize the relationship between ordering costs and carrying costs.
- Develop A-B-C approach and EOQ models.
- Analyze an inventory management problem.

HEALTH CARE SUPPLY CHAIN

In health care organizations, supply chain is a new way of conceptualizing medical supply management. A supply chain is defined as "a virtual network that facilitates the movement of product from its production, distribution, and consumption"

(McFadden and Leahy, 2000). In considering supply chains, health care managers are not only concerned with how much of each type of supply, and when, they need to purchase and carry in their stockrooms (inventory) to effectively serve their patients; they also are concerned with their relationships with the companies at the upstream source of the products to minimize their overall costs in supply management. The health care manager, as a leader of the provider link in this chain, is in a strategic position and should facilitate collaborative partnerships with the adjacent links of the chain. Let us closely examine the various links in a supply chain from the prospective of a health care provider.

Figure 11.1 depicts the conceptualization of a health care supply chain identifying the upstream and downstream links with respect to providers. Upstream in the next place on the chain are distributors who purchase the drugs and medical and surgical devices from the manufacturers and who comprise wholesalers, group purchasing organizations (GPOs), and e-distributors. Downstream are the end users of, or payers for, the products. Providers are those who decide what to use and whom to use among all these products and secure their availability and end distribution.

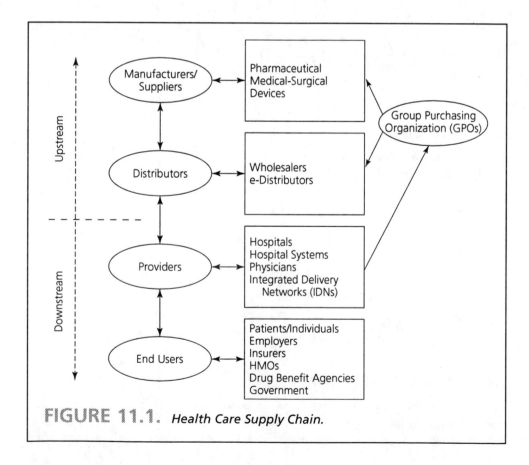

FIGURE 11.1. *Health Care Supply Chain.*

Manufacturers/Suppliers. Manufacturers of medical supplies can be classified in three categories: (1) drugs and pharmaceuticals; (2) medical-surgical supplies; and (3) devices. Some manufacturers produce supplies in more than one category or in all categories.

Pharmaceutical sales in the United States constitute about 8 percent of national health expenditures. Twenty-five percent of pharmaceutical products are distributed to providers (hospitals and other institutional settings) via distributors. Well-known pharmaceutical manufacturers include Abbott, Aventis Pharma, Bristol-Myers Squibb, Eli Lilly, GlaxoSmithKline, Hoffmann-La Roche, Janssen, Johnson & Johnson, Merck, Pfizer, Schering-Plough, and Wyeth.

Medical-surgical companies produce items such as injection syringes and needles, blood and specimen collection kits, hospital laboratory products, wound management products, and intravenous solutions. 3M, Abbott, Baxter, and Johnson & Johnson are a few of the well-known medical-surgical companies that sell the majority of their products through distributors.

Medical devices can be described as very high priced, technologically sophisticated and advanced apparatus that are used for diagnosis and therapies. The devices are produced and sold in low volumes, and their costs account for about 5 percent of national health expenditures in the United States (Burns, 2002; p. 243). Medical devices include surgical and medical instruments and apparatus, orthopedic, prosthetic and surgical appliances (for example, shoulder, knee, and hip replacements), X-ray apparatus, tubes, irradiation apparatus, electromedical and electrotherapeutic devices. Dupuy, Ortho Biotech, Medtronic, and Zimmer are examples of the companies that manufacture such devices (Burns, 2002; p. 244).

Distributors, Wholesalers, and Electronic Data Interchange (EDI). Distributors for medical-surgical supplies are independent intermediaries who operate their own warehouses; they purchase the products from manufacturers and suppliers to sell to providers. Similarly, pharmaceutical intermediaries purchase the drugs and pharmaceuticals from manufacturers and wholesale them to pharmacies or to providers. The intermediaries are called distributors or wholesalers depending on whether the products' final resale has another layer before reaching the customer (Burns, 2002; p. 127). Distributors in the United States sell products from a wide range of manufacturers and manage over 100,000 different items (p. 244). Burns states: "One of the most significant contributions of distributors to the health care supply chain was the deployment of electronic order-entry systems to their customer base" (p. 129). Linking providers through electronic communication to their distributors is formally defined as electronic data interchange (EDI). EDI provides direct, real time computer to computer electronic transmission of purchase orders, shipping notices, invoices, and the like between providers and distributors. Over 75 percent of distributors use EDI, and 70 to 80 percent of their business volume is handled through EDI (pp. 130–131). EDI is also proliferating to manufacturer transactions with other parts of the health care supply chain; more than one-third of their business transactions use EDI. The cost for standardized EDI transactions for a purchase order, as compared to costs with manual systems, saves operational costs for both providers and distributors. For example, a purchase order with standardized EDI costs the provider $11.20, whereas with a manual system it costs $40–$150. For the distributors or suppliers these costs are $3.20 versus $30–$150 per purchase, for EDI and manual systems, respectively. Put together, the total costs for both parties are $14.40 versus $70–$300, a savings of 500 percent to 2,000 percent (Burns, 2002; p. 134).

Well-known distributors of pharmaceuticals include AmeriSource/Bergen Brunswig, Cardinal Health/Bindley Western, and McKesson, whose market shares are 32, 29, and 27 percent, respectively (Burns, 2002; p. 146).

Medical-surgical supply distributors, with approximately $20 billion in sales, distribute their products to three major provider organizations: hospital/hospital systems, physician offices, and long-term care organizations. Hospital/hospital systems consume 60 percent of medical-surgical supplies, while physician offices consume 25 percent, and long-term care and other facilities consume the remaining 15 percent.

Cardinal Health, Owens & Minor, and McKesson are major distribution companies in the hospital medical-surgical market with their combined market share amounts to 92 percent. Henry Schein and McKesson serve the physician office market, as do PSS, PHCC, and AEH/BBMC. Collectively these distributors cover about 65 percent of the physician market. Over 50 percent of the long-term care market is served by the following distributors: McKesson, Gulf South/Gateway, Medline, and AEH/BBMC (Burns, 2002, p. 154).

Group Purchasing Organizations (GPOs). Group purchasing organizations provide a critical financial advantage to providers, especially hospitals and hospital systems, by negotiating purchasing contracts for products and nonlabor services. A typical GPO has many hospital organizations as its members and uses this as collective buying power in negotiating contracts with many suppliers: of pharmaceuticals, medical-surgical supplies, laboratory, imaging, durable medical equipment, facility maintenance, information technology, insurance, and food and dietary products and services. The contracts usually last three to five years, giving providers price protection (Burns, 2002; pp. 60–64).

The overwhelming majority of hospitals participate in group purchasing. Often a hospital belongs to one or more GPOs. The GPOs can be either for-profit and investor owned, or nonprofit. They differ in geographic coverage, size, and scope. Over six hundred GPOs operate in the United States; perhaps half of them focus their business on hospitals. It is estimated that GPOs mediate contracts for two-thirds of the $50 billion spent by hospitals on medical-surgical supplies. The contract negotiations for pharmaceuticals cover almost 90 percent of what hospitals spend on them, or nearly $13 billion (Burns, 2002; p. 70).

Five major nonprofit and two investor-owned for-profit GPOs capture 72 percent of the hospital market among them. The two largest GPOs are Novation and Premier, which are nonprofit. The scope of the contracts maintained by GPOs can be exhaustive, especially for large GPOs like Novation. According to Burns (2002), Novation, with 2,100 members, maintains 1,600 contracts covering nearly 900,000 items for $14 billion in value. Premier has over 1,800 members and commands contracts for $13 billion in value (p. 60). The three other nonprofit GPOs of similar size (in terms of annual revenue of $3–5 billion) are AmeriNet, HSCA, and Consorta (which serves mostly Catholic hospital systems). The major investor-owned for-profit GPOs are HCA/Health Trust, MedAssets, and Broadlane.

Although GPOs function more on the upstream with suppliers, their downstream relationship with their provider membership makes possible clinical standardization, rationalization in stock keeping units (SKU), product bundling, and reduction of utilization and cost (Burns, 2002; p. 59).

E-Distributors. E-commerce in health care can be viewed from different perspectives. Here we will concentrate on two aspects: business-to-business (B2B) commerce and business-to-customer (B2C) commerce. B2B e-distribution provides efficiencies in many areas for providers, GPOs, and suppliers in the chain through reduced transaction costs and prices, reduced cycle times with automatic replenishments, deliveries on a just-in-time (JIT) basis, and dynamic planning—all the way to upstream forecasting for pull-demand, rather than push-demand sales by suppliers.

Examples of B2B firms are: GHX, Neoforma, OmniCell, and Promedix. These firms provide e-Catalog, e-Request for Proposal (eRFP), e-Auction, and e-Specials (limited discounts on some items), which emulate traditional systems on-line and are available to both hospitals and physician offices. Since the mid-1990s, the e-companies have gone through various acquisitions and mergers and have started carving out parts of the traditional systems' market share with their on-line systems. However, their future effects on the medical supply trade remain uncertain (Burns, 2002; pp. 297–301).

Flow of Materials

It is important to note that depending upon the type of medical supply, the flow of materials in the supply chain may take more direct routes to providers or end users. Suppliers may bypass GPOs by not contracting or negotiating price arrangements. High-end implants and medical devices, specialty items of low volume but high price, are good examples of such medical supplies for which suppliers use direct delivery, usually via express services (like FedEx, UPS, or DHL) or have their own local/regional sales representatives make the JIT delivery and serve as consultants to physicians. In some cases, the company's representatives provide technical participation with surgeons in implanting devices surgically. Other cases in which suppliers may bypass GPOs in contracting are for small-volume, esoteric items, and for the brand-name, specialty drugs used to treat cancer and cardiovascular problems. Those, however, would not be delivered directly, but by a wholesaler or distributor.

Supply Chain Management Issues for Providers

As was mentioned above, the providers decide, for all products, what to use and whom to use and secure their availability and end distribution of these products. This function of providers in the supply chain link can be characterized as inventory management. Good inventory management is essential to the successful operation of any health care organization, for a number of reasons. One of the most important is the proportion of the organizations' budget that represents money spent for inventory. Although the amounts and dollar values of the inventories carried by different types of health care providers vary widely, in a typical hospital's budget 25 to 30 percent goes for medical supplies and their handling. On the national scene, health care supplies constitute 8 to 9 percent of health care expenditures. According to Burns (2002, p. 34), of supply costs, 15 to 23 percent is for pharmacy, 30 to 50 percent is for medical-surgical supplies, and 11 to 24 percent is for equipment. Clearly, medical supplies require significant attention in health care budgeting. Furthermore, a widely used measure of managerial performance is the return on investment (ROI), which is profit after taxes, divided by total assets. Because the inventory of medical supplies may comprise a significant portion of a health care organization's total assets, reducing its inventories significantly raises its ROI, and hence its position in the financial markets. Health care managers must be able to manage the inventory of medical supplies effectively. This chapter presents concepts that support good inventory management.

Contemporary Issues in Medical Inventory Management

In the current era of health care delivery, when cost-effectiveness is the key measure of performance, health care managers have a number of inventory management options available: traditional inventory management, just-in-time or stockless inventory systems, single or multiple vendor relationships, and partnerships with suppliers and GPOs.

A system that is highly effective in one health care organization could be disastrous in another. Familiarity with the systems in use makes it easier to determine which one(s) will be effective for a particular organization.

Regardless of what inventory system and practices an organization uses, certain fundamental changes can optimize the cost-effectiveness of the inventory function. Such changes include the computerization of material functions, integration of clinical and financial systems, bottom line measurement, and decentralization of the inventory management function. The advent of microcomputers has created opportunities for restructuring routine tasks to improve productivity and performance. For example, orders from institutional users are now transferred via computer, and then go to vendors that can provide on-line confirmations. And these ongoing routine operations create databases of utilization, price, and other information that will facilitate future decision making (for pull-demand on upstream in the supply chain).

The linkage of inventory databases with other clinical and financial data systems in an institution can identify utilization patterns by patient groups, DRGs, physicians, and others. Data analysis, by indicating where large amounts of material resources are being used, can focus review efforts. Quantitative measures of utilization patterns are used to assess whether or not cost objectives are being met. Benchmarking the institutions' costs against other providers' costs can identify problem areas where efforts should be made to improve performance. Using comparative data from other institutions, health care managers may identify practice patterns or utilization trends that could cut costs.

A computerized inventory management system frees health care managers from traditional routine tasks to focus on material utilization review. Having administrative and clinical personnel review how they use goods when providing health care facilitates a common goal of reducing, altering, or even eliminating items of the mix used, although a specified level of quality should be maintained. A new operating philosophy can emerge: the best way to save money on inventory is to decide whether some products or services are even needed. Savings that have been realized by such decisions have ranged from a few thousand dollars on syringes to hundreds of thousands of dollars on specialty beds (Sanders, 1990).

Just-in-Time (JIT) and Stockless Inventories. Inventory management in health care organizations is becoming increasingly decentralized. JIT means that goods arrive just before they are needed. An organization practicing JIT places orders and receives deliveries frequently and stores virtually no inventory in a warehouse or stockroom. Hospitals have extended JIT principles to include programs known as stockless inventories. Stockless inventory means obtaining most supplies from a single source (a prime vendor) in small packaging units ready to be taken to the user departments. A stockless system uses little or no space, inventory, or storeroom staff, because the vendor's warehouse doubles as the partnering hospital's warehouse. Some vendors even deliver specific quantities of a good directly to the department that ordered it. JIT and stockless inventory require sophisticated management, however, of the data moving between institution and vendor. Computers help to minimize on hand quantities and automatically generate reorders. The best applications of JIT systems in health care are for highly expensive implants and medical devices. Use of prime vendor purchasing facilitates the process by committing the vendor to the service levels dictated by management in terms of inventory holdings, stock-outs, and deliveries (Krumrey and Byerly, 1995).

Stockless inventory in hospitals parallels JIT programs in industry. Many hospitals use the concept at a lesser level in specific areas; for example, surgical carts that have all the supplies necessary for a procedure arrive just before it is scheduled to begin. Unit dose medication carts are used to refill individual patient bins just before the next dose is needed. Substantial long-term savings can result from applying stockless inventory to these supply groups: computer equipment and supplies, food supplies, housekeeping supplies, linen, maintenance supplies, office supplies, and X-ray supplies.

Advantages and Disadvantages of JIT and Stockless Inventory. It should be noted that a stockless inventory program substantially affects many facets of a hospital's purchasing operations. An advantage is that a supplier may agree to lower unit product prices because of increased volume from a hospital. Besides that, inventory service should improve because of the mutual commitment with suppliers and the intensity of the services provided. Stockless inventory also reduces the number of supplies and the total orders processed. However, the number of staff hours and salary expenses in a purchasing department may not be significantly reduced because only a portion of FTE time is saved by automation (Kowalski, 1991).

Stockless inventory systems typically do not involve all products. They may not reduce total supply expenses because consumption rates by user departments may remain the same, regardless of who supplies them. Another limitation is that since hospitals typically have from three to ten times the investment in user department inventory that they have in a storeroom, stockless inventory does not necessarily affect most of a hospital's inventory. Moreover, a stockless inventory is not free. While the hospital may reduce staff, inventory, and space costs, suppliers must be paid for their value-added services, which can range from 3 to 13 percent of the price of a product.

Single Versus Multiple Vendors. The essence of the purchasing function is to obtain the right equipment, supplies, and services, and of the right quality, in the right quantity from the right source at the right price at the right time. Keeping that in mind, the health care manager has to decide whether to use a single source for supplies (if possible) or many different vendors. Each relationship has advantages and disadvantages.

A single source will almost guarantee better pricing, because, as the exclusive supplier the source will have higher volume. If the hospital runs into an unexpected shortage, the vendor will adjust shipping priorities to ensure that the hospital, as a major account, does not get into a stock-out situation. Purchasing from a single source increases the health care organization's influence on that vendor; the health care manager's ideas and suggestions are valued far more. Single sourcing may also allow a health care manager to negotiate small purchases that could not normally be made without paying exorbitant premiums. As a buyer, the manager will be able not only to negotiate with the supplier, but to protect sensitive information, as well. Should the organization become aware of new items or processes, the supplier can obtain and provide such information without revealing to the manufacturer or the distributor who the ultimate customer might be. Finally, because the single source supplier has a much better idea of what an organization's total requirements are, it can recommend more cost-effective ways to handle shipments (Sheehan, 1995).

There are also advantages to multiple sourcing. For one thing, vendors are always looking for steps they can take to encourage customer hospitals to purchase products from them. Most importantly, however, multiple sources protect the hospital's supply lines, since the need for a product can literally mean life or death. A disadvantage of single sourcing is that, in a crisis, a health care organization may feel at the mercy of its supplier. Another important reason for using multiple sources is to encourage competition among them. Notwithstanding rapidly changing technology, few products come on the market without a competing product existing somewhere. Competition at the top of a supply chain creates pressure to improve the product's quality and availability. And of course, competition helps a health care organization to get the best price from the vendor they eventually choose.

Traditional Inventory Management

Any discussion on inventory management must begin with a working definition of what inventory is. **Inventory** can be defined simply as a stock or store of goods, or stock keeping items (SKUs). Hospitals stock drugs, surgical supplies, life—monitoring equipment, sheets and pillowcases, food supplies, and more. Inadequate controls of inventories can result in both under- and overstocking of items. Understocking can result in lost sales because of the dissatisfaction of the physicians or surgeons. For example, physicians could take their patients elsewhere for procedures because the needed supplies—whether brand names or specific items—have been unavailable. More important than lost sales is the risk that understocking might cause a patient death. From a simply practical viewpoint, on the other hand, overstocking unnecessarily ties up funds that might be more productive elsewhere. Overstocking appears to be the lesser of the two evils. However, for excessive overstocking, the price tag can be staggering for interest, insurance, taxes (in some states), depreciation, obsolescence, deterioration, spoilage, pilferage, and breakage. Those costs, known as **holding** or **carrying costs,** can be overwhelming if you are dealing with high-priced inventory such as pharmaceuticals. As an example of excessive overstocking, it is not unusual for health care managers to discover that their facility has a ten-year supply of an item.

Inventory management has two main concerns: (1) the level of service, that is, having the right goods, in sufficient quantities, in the right place, and at the right time; (2) the costs of ordering and carrying inventories. Any prudent health care manager aims to both maintain a high level of service and minimize the costs of ordering and carrying inventory. In other words, the two fundamental decisions are when to order and how much to order. Welcome to the exciting world of inventory management!

Inventories have several functions. Among the most important are to: (A) meet anticipated patient demand for medical supplies; (B) communicate demand information upstream on the supply chain (to distributors, then to suppliers) in order to smooth manufacturers' production requirements; (C) to protect against stock-outs; (D) to take advantage of order cycles; (E) to hedge against price increases or to take advantage of quantity discounts; and—most fundamental—(F) to permit a health care organization's operations to continue.

Let's put these basic inventory functions into perspective with an example of what any health care manager would not want to have happen on her or his watch. Imagine the following scenario, in which the health care supply chain manager has to explain to a member of senior management why the emergency room found itself without the syringes.

"Sorry sir, but when she (the patient) came into the ER, we were out of syringes. Our anticipation stocks were depleted because we hadn't corrected the ordering patterns for seasonal variations. Then, the snow delayed shipments from supplier, and our safety stocks just weren't good enough! You know we usually order in bulk to take advantage of large economic lot size and lower our ordering cycle. Our last order was especially large because we wanted to hedge against predicted price increases! In the final analysis, our inventory just wasn't sufficient to permit smooth operations."

Requirements for Effective Inventory Management

Besides the basic responsibilities of deciding when and how much to order, the other basic responsibility is to establish a system for keeping track of items in inventory. These, then, are the requirements for effective inventory:

- A system to keep track of the inventory in storage and on order

- A reliable forecast of demand

- Knowledge of lead times and lead time variability

- Reasonable estimates of inventory holding costs, ordering costs, and shortage costs

- A classification system for inventory items in terms of their importance

Inventory Accounting Systems

Inventory accounting systems can be periodic or perpetual. Under a **periodic system,** items in inventory are physically counted either daily, weekly, or monthly, for the purpose of deciding how much to order of each. An advantage of the periodic system is that orders for many items occur at the same time, which reduces the processing and shipping of orders. However, this system can also produce dilemmas. In addition to a lack of control between reviews, the need to protect against shortages between review periods means carrying extra stock. Health care managers also must decide on order quantities at each review.

A **perpetual system** continuously keeps track of removals from inventories, so it can always give the current level of inventory for each item (Stevenson, 2002; pp. 545–546). When the amount on hand reaches a predetermined minimum, a fixed quantity, Q, is ordered. An obvious advantage of this system is the control provided by the continuous monitoring of inventory withdrawals. Another major advantage is the fixed order quantity; managers can identify an **economic order size** (discussed later in this chapter). However, even in a perpetual system, a periodic physical count of inventory must still be performed to verify that the reported inventory levels equal the effective inventory levels. The difference between what is reported and what is actually on hand is caused by errors, theft, spoilage, and other factors. For perpetual systems, a disadvantage is the added cost of record keeping and information systems.

Perpetual systems can be either batch or on-line. In batch systems, inventory records are collected periodically and entered into the system. In on-line systems, the transactions are recorded instantaneously.

An example of a perpetual on-line system is the computerized checkout system in grocery stores, where a laser scanning device reads the Universal Product Code (UPC), or bar code, on an item. Such a system also is now used in many health care organizations to track inventories as items are used or dispensed for patients. A brief discussion of such systems will help understanding of their importance to a health care organization.

Universal Product Codes (UPCs). The UPCs have been around since late 1970s and are used in industry. A UPC can have up to twenty character numbers that uniquely identify a product, for example, of pharmaceutical or medical-surgical supply, using bars with different variety and thickness that can be read by scanners. The order of the information in UPCs identifies the type of product, its manufacturer, and the product itself. In health care, the source of UPCs can be either the Health Industry Business Communications Council (HIBCC) or the Uniform Code Council (UCC). UPCs can be assigned at unit dose, package, or case level. The pharmaceutical numbering system for UPC codes is based on universally recognized National Drug Codes (NDCs). UPCs are an essential part of an electronic data interchange (EDI) system to create efficiencies in materials ordering, handling, and charging, as well as relatively error-free processing. With UPCs, it is reported that distributors can increase their deliveries sixfold and with half the manpower needed with non-bar-coded systems. Although an overwhelming number of consumer products contain UPC codes, their implementation in health care lags behind the retail and industrial sectors (Burns, 2002; pp. 140–144). Only 26 percent of medical-surgical products can be scanned on nursing units, and only 50 percent of drugs have bar codes for unit doses.

According to the final regulation issued by the Food and Drug Administration (FDA) in 2004, drug manufacturers must adopt bar-coding to single-dose units within two years, and hospitals must eventually implement bedside scanning systems. The FDA estimates, however, that it may take up to two decades for all hospitals to implement such systems because of their high costs: from $500,000 to $1 million. Only a few more than 100 hospitals currently use them. Yet bar code systems would significantly improve the quality of patient care through reduction of medication errors. It is estimated that over a twenty-year period, fully implemented bar code systems would prevent about 0.5 million medical errors. Moreover, by improving the cost-efficiency of medical supply management, hospitals would also reap $90 billion in savings, which would help to pay for the technology (Becker, 2004).

While health care facilities are catching up with this efficient system of supply management, the remaining materials must be handled the old-fashioned way, entered to ordering systems manually; and their management must be carried in house (by providers) using traditional inventory management methods.

Lead Time

Inventories are used to satisfy demand requirements, so reliable estimates of the amounts and timing of demand are essential. It is also essential to know how long it will take for orders to be delivered (Stevenson, 2002; p. 547). Now that health care organizations increasingly rely on their vendors to maintain adequate inventory levels in their facilities, their data relevant to demand must be transferred to their vendors. Health care managers also need to know the extent to which demand and lead time (the time between submitting an order and receiving it) may vary; the greater the potential variability, the greater the need for additional stock to avoid a shortage between deliveries.

Cost Information

Three basic costs are associated with inventories: holding, ordering, and shortage costs. Holding or carrying costs, as mentioned earlier, relate to physically having the medical supplies in storage. Such costs include interest on the money borrowed to buy the items, insurance, warehousing, security, compliance with industry and government requirements (for example, HIPPA), obsolescence, outdated medications, deterioration, spoilage, pilferage (for example, of IV bags), theft (for example, of narcotics), and depreciation. Holding costs can be calculated either as a percentage of unit price or as a dollar amount per unit. In any case, typical annual holding costs range from 20 to 40 percent of the value of an item. In other words, to hold a $10 item for one year could cost from $2 to $4 (Stevenson, 2002; p. 547–548).

Ordering costs include the time and effort spent to calculate how much is needed, prepare invoices, inspect goods upon arrival for quality and quantity, and move goods to temporary storage or the appropriate diagnostic and therapy units. Because those costs are incurred for each order, they are generally expressed as a fixed dollar amount per order, regardless of order size (Stevenson, 2002; p. 548).

Shortage costs result when an appropriate medical supply is not on hand. They range from the opportunity cost of losing a patient's or physician's goodwill, to the risk of lawsuits and even the death of a patient. Such costs could be extremely high, even threatening the financial viability of a health care organization. Shortage costs are usually difficult to measure and are often subjectively estimated.

Classification System

An important element of inventory management deals with classifying the items in stock according to their relative importance in terms of dollars invested, volume, utilization, and profit potential—to say nothing of the disastrous financial consequences that could result from allowing a stock-out to occur. For instance, a typical hospital carries items such as drugs, biomedical equipment, and linens for beds; it would be unrealistic to devote equal attention to each. Obviously, control efforts should be based on the relative importance of the various items in inventory.

A classic method of classifying inventory is the **A-B-C approach.** Inventory items are placed in one of three classes: A (very important), B (important), and C (somewhat important), according to a measure of importance such as annual dollar value. That measure is simply the dollar value per unit multiplied by the annual usage (demand) rate. Health care managers can of course create many categories, depending on the extent to which they want to differentiate control efforts.

With three classes of items, A items generally account for 15 to 20 percent of the items in total inventory, but for two-thirds of dollar usage. B items are moderate in terms of inventory percentage and dollar usage. Finally, the C items may represent two-thirds of the items, but only 10 percent of dollar usage. Although those percentages may vary, for most facilities relatively few items will account for a large share of the value or cost associated with an inventory, and it is those items that should receive a high share of control efforts. Because of their high dollar value per unit, A items should receive the most attention, through frequent reviews of the amounts in stock, as well as close monitoring of their withdrawals from inventory. The C items should receive looser control, and B items be controlled with efforts between those two extremes. The health care manager's A-B-C analysis should not overemphasize minor aspects of customer service at the expense of major aspects. For example, one would be unlikely to change the importance of a health care item from C to B or A, despite its low cost, if it serves a crucial need of patient care. Table 11.1 illustrates an example of the A-B-C concept.

TABLE 11.1. A-B-C Classification Analysis.

Item	Annual Demand	Unit Cost	Annual Costs	Percent of Total	A-B-C Classification
1	20,800	2.50	52,000	1.2%	C
2	83,200	0.50	41,600	1.0%	C
3	9,100	37.50	341,250	8.0%	B
4	13,000	3.50	45,500	1.1%	C
5	13,000	1.75	22,750	0.5%	C
6	790	1,290.00	1,019,100	24.0%	A
7	78,000	2.25	175,500	4.1%	B
8	114,400	0.65	74,360	1.8%	C
9	66,040	0.95	62,738	1.5%	C
10	6,240	12.50	78,000	1.8%	C
11	11,440	2.00	22,880	0.5%	C
12	18,200	1.50	27,300	0.6%	C
13	910	1,300.00	1,183,000	27.9%	A
14	315	2,700.00	850,500	20.1%	A
15	65,000	3.75	243,750	5.7%	B
Total Annual Costs			4,240,228		

In this example, items 6, 13, and 14 have relatively high dollar values, so it seems reasonable to classify them as A items. That classification is supported by the calculation of percentage shares in annual dollar volume from all the items. Those three items collectively constitute about 72 percent of the annual expenditure on all items. Items 3, 7, and 15 are moderate in their percentage values and could be classified as B items. The remaining items could be classified as C items for their relatively low shares in annual dollar value.

Economic Order Quantity Model

The economic order quantity (EOQ) model is frequently used to answer the question of how much to order. EOQ calculates optimal order quantity in terms of minimizing the sum of certain annual costs that vary with the order costs—namely, inventory's holding and ordering costs. A few assumptions are important for this model: that for an individual item the demand for a period (week, month, or year) is known, and that the demand rate is constant throughout the period; that purchase price of the item does not affect order quantity (no high quantity discounts) and that delivery of the item (in quantity) is received at once with a constant lead time.

Before we proceed through the EOQ process, it is important to understand the **inventory cycle.** As Figure 11.2 illustrates, the cycle begins when an order for Q units is received. These units are withdrawn from inventory at a constant rate over time

FIGURE 11.2. *The Inventory Order Cycle for Basic EOQ Model.*

(depletion or demand rate). When the quantity on hand is just sufficient to meet the anticipated demand during the lead time, a new order for Q units is submitted to the vendor; that occurs at quantity R, called the reorder point (ROP). Under the assumption that lead time and usage rate are constant, the order will be received at the precise instant that the inventory on hand falls to zero units. Thus orders are timed to avoid both excess stock and stock-outs. However, if those conditions were not the case or if deliveries were expected to be late, as illustrated in cycle 2, the health care manager should keep safety stocks on hand so operations could safely continue until the order is received.

The optimal order quantity reflects a trade-off between carrying costs and ordering costs: as the order size increases, its associated holding cost also increases; on the other hand, ordering costs decrease when keeping higher quantities on hand reduces frequent ordering. Looking at this issue in another way, if the order size is relatively small, its average inventory will be low, and hence have low carrying costs; but the small order size will necessitate frequent orders, which will drive up annual ordering costs. Figure 11.3 shows the relationship between ordering and holding costs with respect to the order quantity, Q.

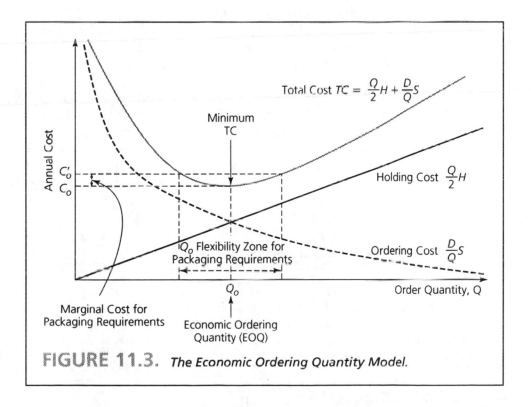

FIGURE 11.3. *The Economic Ordering Quantity Model.*

After observing these two extremes, it should be clear that the ideal solution is an order size that avoids either a few large orders or many small orders. The basic EOQ model serves that purpose, but the exact amount to order nevertheless will depend on the relative amounts of holding and ordering costs for a particular item, as well as the packaging requirements of its manufacturers and distributors.

The first step of the model is to identify the holding and ordering costs associated with an item, while keeping the model assumptions in mind. Annual holding cost is computed by multiplying the average amount of inventory in stock by the cost to carry one unit for one year. The average inventory is one half of the order quantity. As can be observed from Figure 11.2, the amount on hand depletes at a constant rate from Q to 0 units; here we make one observation at full quantity (Q) and one at zero quantity, when all items are depleted. However, at any given time the average inventory for a cycle can be calculated by taking the average of these two observations as $[(Q + 0)/2]$, or $Q/2$. The symbol H is commonly used to represent the average holding cost per unit; thus the total annual holding cost can be expressed as:

$$\text{Annual holding cost} = \frac{Q}{2}H \qquad (11.1)$$

Holding costs are a linear function of Q: holding costs increase or decrease in direct proportion to changes in the order quantity Q, as shown in Figure 11.3.

Ordering costs, commonly labeled as S, are inversely and nonlinearly related to order size Q. As Figure 11.3 shows, annual ordering costs will decrease as order size increases. For a given annual demand level, the larger the order size, the fewer the orders needed. For instance, if annual demand for knee joints is 200 units and the order size is ten units per order, there must be twenty orders over the year. But if we order Q = 40 units, only five orders will be needed, and for Q = 50 units, only four orders will be needed. In general, the number of orders per year, or order frequency, is computed by dividing annual demand (D) by order quantity (Q), D/Q. Ordering costs are relatively insensitive to order size and pretty much fixed, because regardless of the amount of an order, certain activities (for example, preparing invoices, checking samples for quality) must be done for each order. Total annual ordering cost is a function of the number of orders per year and the ordering cost per order and can be expressed as:

$$\text{Annual ordering cost} = \frac{D}{Q}S \qquad (11.2)$$

If we add holding and ordering costs for every point in their respective graphs, we can determine the total annual cost (TC) associated with inventory management. Figure 11.3 shows this as the TC curve where holding and ordering inventory for a given order quantity (Q) ordered each time. The total cost can be expressed as the sum of annual holding cost and annual ordering cost:

$$TC = \frac{Q}{2}H + \frac{D}{Q}S \qquad (11.3)$$

where
  D = demand, usually in units per year
  Q = order quantity, in units
  S = ordering cost, in dollars
  H = holding cost, usually in dollars per unit per year.

(Note: D and H must be in the same units, such as months or years.)

We see in Figure 11.3 that the total cost curve is U-shaped and that **it reaches its minimum at the quantity where carrying and ordering costs are equal.** The mathematical solution to find this minimum point requires differentiating TC with respect to Q.

$$\frac{dTC}{dQ} = \frac{dQ}{2}H + d\left(\frac{D}{Q}\right)S = \frac{H}{2} - \frac{DS}{Q^2} \qquad (11.4)$$

The next step is to set the right hand side of this equation to zero. We can solve for the value of Q as:

$$\frac{H}{2} - \frac{DS}{Q^2} = 0,$$

and rearranging the equation, we get

$$Q^2 = \frac{2DS}{H} \quad \text{and}$$

$$Q_o = \sqrt{\frac{2DS}{H}}. \qquad (11.5)$$

That is the optimum solution for Q, given by the minimum total cost of the TC curve. We will call the point where both costs equal each other, as derived by the above equations, Q_o. And that is the EOQ formula (11.5). It can be used when given annual demand, the ordering cost per order, and the annual holding cost per unit. One can also compute the minimum total cost by substituting Q_o for Q in the TC formula. Once Q_o is known, the length of an order cycle (the length of a time between orders), or order frequency, can be calculated as:

$$Length\,of\,order\,cycle = \frac{Q_0}{D} \qquad (11.6)$$

Holding cost is sometimes stated as a percentage of the purchase price of an item, rather than as a dollar amount per unit. However, as long as the percentage is converted into a dollar amount, the EOQ formula is still appropriate. One final important point regarding the EOQ model: since the holding and ordering costs are estimates, EOQ is an approximate quantity rather than the exact quantity needed. An obvious question one may ask is, Given the use of estimates, how stringent is the EOQ measure as an optimal number in minimizing total cost? Figure 11.3 shows us that the total cost curve is relatively flat near the EOQ, especially to the right of the EOQ, which provides flexibility for the Q value to be higher or lower than Q_o with marginal change in total cost, expressed as $\Delta C = C_o' - C_o$. Thus, health care managers can adjust their order sizes around Q_o according to manufacturers' or distributors' packaging requirements without incurring significant increases in total inventory management costs.

Although beyond the scope of this text, there are other, more complicated EOQ models, such as the EOQ model with non-instantaneous delivery and the quantity discount model. For such models, readers are referred to texts that specialize in operations management. What follows is a typical, basic EOQ model.

EXAMPLE 11.1

An orthopedic physician group practice uses 12cc syringes from Sherwood for its cortisone injections. During each of the last two years, forty thousand of the syringes were used in the office. Each syringe costs $1.50. The physician's office annually discards, on average, five hundred of the syringes that have became inoperable (broken, wrong injection material, lost). The syringes are stored in a room that occupies 2 percent of the storage area. The storage area constitutes 10% of the leased space. The annual office lease costs $60,000. The group practice can secure loans from a local bank at 6% interest to purchase the syringes. For each placed order, it takes about three hours for an office assistant (whose hourly wage is $9.00 and who receives $3.25 in fringe benefits) to prepare and communicate the order and place its shipment in storage. In addition, each order's overhead share of equipment and supplies (phone, fax, computer, stationery paper) is approximately $4.50. In the past, the office assistant always placed 5,000 syringes in each order. The deliveries are made in boxes of one thousand syringes and are always received three working days after the order is placed.

What should be the EOQ for the 12cc syringe?

What are the inventory management costs for these syringes?

What are the investment costs?

How many times in a year should an order be placed?

Solution

To calculate EOQ, we need to estimate the holding and ordering costs.

Annual holding cost

1.   Cost of inoperable syringes: $1.50 \times 500 = \$750$.

2.   Storage cost: (60,000 Lease) $\times$ 0.10 (storage area) $\times$ 0.02 (syringe) = $120.

3. Interest on a loan used to purchase 5,000 syringes: 5,000 × 1.5 × 0.06 = $450.

   Total annual holding costs = 750 + 120 + 450 = 1,320.

   Annual holding cost per syringe: $1,320 ÷ 40,000 = $.033.

Ordering cost

   Office assistant's time: 3 hours × (9.00 + 3.25) = $36.75.

   Overhead: $4.50.

   Total ordering cost: $36.75 + $4.50 = $41.25.

Using formula (11.5) the EOQ:

$$Q_o = \sqrt{\frac{2DS}{H}} = \sqrt{\frac{2 \times 40,000 \times 41.25.}{.033}} = 10,000.$$

Total inventory management cost calculated using formula (11.3):

$$TC = \frac{10,000}{2}.033 + \frac{40,000}{10,000}41.25$$

   TC = $165.00 + $165.00 = $330.00.

Investment cost:

Investment costs = Order quantity × Price of the item, or

   $Q_o p = 10,000 \times 1.50 = \$15,000.00.$

Investment cost is the amount committed to purchase the syringes. It is cycled as the cost of the syringes is recovered from patients and third party payers.

Order frequency is calculated using formula (11.6):

$$Length\,of\,order\,cycle - \frac{Q_o}{D} = \frac{10000}{40000} = .25\,years\,or\,every\,three\,months.$$

In other words, order frequency is four times a year.

Excel Solution

We will seek and demonstrate the solutions for the syringe problem using Excel. The Excel setup and results for analyzing and solving this problem are provided in Figure 11.4. Reader can observe the EOQ formula at cell D3. Multi-item EOQ models can be solved in Excel (assuming independence among the items), and ABC status of

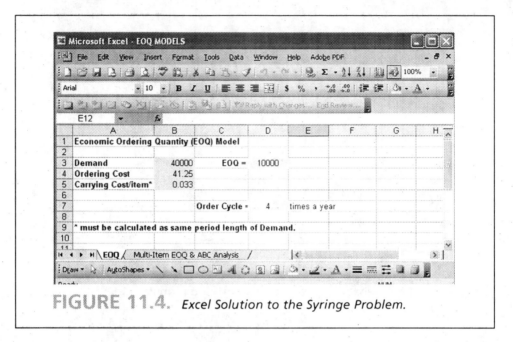

FIGURE 11.4. *Excel Solution to the Syringe Problem.*

Source: Screen shots reprinted by permission from Microsoft Corporation.

each item can be determined. Figure 11.5 illustrates an example for 15-item inventory problem. Reader can observe the formula for ABC classification at cell "O8."

When to Reorder

We used the EOQ model to answer the question of how much to order, but not the question of when to order. We will now look at a new model that identifies the **reorder point** (ROP) in terms of the quantity of an item currently in stock. The reorder point occurs when the quantity on hand drops to a predetermined amount (see Figure 11.2 and ROP level). This trigger amount usually includes the expected demand during the lead time. There are four conditions that affect the reorder point quantity: (1) the rate of forecast demand; (2) the length of lead time; (3) the extent of variability in lead time and demand; and (4) the degree of stock-out risk acceptable to management.

When demand rate and lead time are constant, there is no risk of a stock-out created by increased demand or lead times longer than expected. Therefore, no cushion stock is necessary, and ROP is simply the product of usage rate and lead time as:

$$ROP = D \times L \tag{11.7}$$

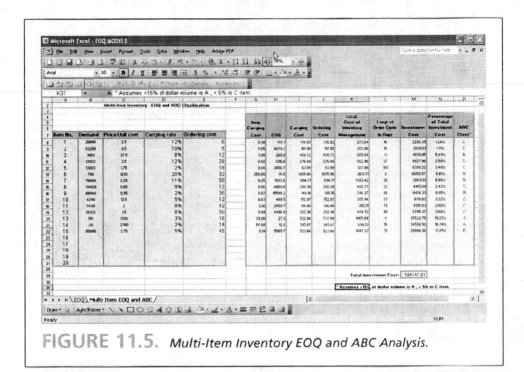

FIGURE 11.5. *Multi-Item Inventory EOQ and ABC Analysis.*

Source: Screen shots reprinted by permission from Microsoft Corporation.

Where

D = demand per period, and
L = lead time; demand and lead time must be in the same units.

Example 11.2 illustrates an ROP with constant demand rate and lead time.

EXAMPLE 11.2

An orthopedic surgeon replaces two hips per day. The implants are delivered two days after an order is placed, via express delivery. When should the supply chain manager order the implants?

Solution

Usage = 2 implants daily.
Lead time = 2 days.
ROP = Usage × Lead time = 2 × 2 = 4.

Thus, order should be placed when four implants are left!

When demand or lead time is not constant, the probability that actual demand will exceed the expected demand increases. In that situation, health care providers may find it necessary to carry additional inventory, called safety stock, to reduce the risk of running out of inventory (a stock-out) during lead time. In variable situations, the ROP increases by the amount of the safety stock:

$$\text{ROP} = \text{expected demand during lead time} + \text{safety stock} \quad \textbf{(11.8)}$$

Here, the expected demand is indicated as an average, so variability of demand is present. Similarly, the expected lead time is variable. Hence the health care facility may run out of stock because of either more than expected demand or more than expected lead time for the shipment's arrival. The only way to ensure the continuity of operations is to keep an appropriate level of safety stock.

For example, if the expected demand for implants during lead time is ten units, and the management keeps a safety stock level of twenty units, the ROP would be thirty units. The following example illustrates this concept.

EXAMPLE 11.3

A dentist office uses an average of two boxes of gloves (100-glove boxes) per day, and lead times average five days. Because both the usage rate and lead times are variable, the office carries a safety stock of four boxes of gloves. Determine the ROP.

Solution

Using formula (11.8),

ROP = 2 boxes/daily × 5 day lead time + 4 boxes = 14 boxes.

Because of the cost of holding safety stock, a provider must balance that cost with the reduction in stock-out risk that the safety stock provides, bearing in mind that the service level increases as the risk of stock-out decreases. Service level is defined as the probability that the amount of stock on hand is enough to meet demand. A service level of 95 percent means that there is a 95 percent probability that patient demand will not exceed the provider's supply of service during lead time, or that patient demand will be satisfied in 95 percent of such instances. In other words, service level is the complement of stock-out risk: A 95 percent service level implies a 5 percent stock-out risk. The greater the variability in either demand rate or lead time, the more safety stock is needed to achieve a given service level.

$$\text{Service Level} = 100 \text{ percent} - \text{Stock-out Risk} \qquad (11.9)$$

SUMMARY

The providers decide, for all medical-surgical products, what to use and whom to use and secure their availability and end distribution. This function of providers in the supply chain link can be characterized as inventory management. Good inventory management is essential to the successful operation of any health care organization.

Because the inventory of medical supplies may comprise a significant portion of a health care organization's total assets, health care managers must be able to manage the inventory of medical supplies effectively to enhance their position in the financial markets. This chapter presented concepts that support good inventory management.

KEY TERMS

Supply Chain
Electronic Data Interchange (IDE)
Group Purchasing Organizations (GPOs)
Just-in-Time (JIT)
Stockless Inventory
Multiple Sourcing
Inventory

Holding Cost
Economic Order Quantity (EOQ)
Lead Time
Inventory Cycle
Reorder Point
Safety Stock.

Satja . EOQ excel
green areas . input
yellow areas outcomes

EXERCISES

(11.1) A product used in a laboratory of the hospital costs $60 to order, and its carrying cost per item per week is one cent. Demand for the item is six hundred units weekly. The lead time is three weeks and the purchase price is $0.60.

D = 600 × 52
S = 60
H - 0.52

a. What is the economic order quantity for this item?

b. What is the length of an order cycle? *EOQ/D   watch frequency*

c. Calculate the total weekly costs. *TC = Annual holding costs + Annual order costs/52*

d. What is the investment cost for this item? *Oq × 0.60*

e. If ordering costs increase by 50 percent, how would that affect EOQ? *S= $90*

f. What would be the reorder point for this item if no safety stocks were kept? *D × L*

g. What would be the reorder point if one thousand units were kept as safety stock? *D × L + stock*

(11.2) The CHEMSA chemical supply center provides popular sterilization materials for hospitals. The weekly demand for sterilization materials is two hundred packages. This center is functional for fifty-two weeks a year. The unit purchase cost of the sterilization materials is $15 per package. There are no discounts available for ordering large quantities. A cost

D = 200 × 52

study finds that the average cost of placing an order is $50 per order, and the weekly carrying cost is $0.60 per package.

$D = 200$
$S = 50$
$H = 0.6$
$P = 15$

a. Determine the economic order quantity. $EOQ = 183$

EOQ/2 b. Determine the average number of packages on hand. 91

c. Determine the number of orders per year.

d. Calculate the total cost of ordering and carrying for sterilization packages.

11.3 A medical supply distributor needs to determine the order quantities and reorder points for the various supplies. A particular item of interest costs $30 to order. The yearly carrying cost of the item is 20 percent of the product cost, and the item's cost is $250. Annual demand for the item is eight hundred units. Lead time for delivery is eight days and constant.

a. What is the EOQ for this item?

b. What is the total inventory management cost for this item?

c. What is the investment cost for the item?

d. What is the reorder point?

11.4 WE CARE ASSOCIATES (WCA), a local physician practice group, orders supplies from various distributors. Order quantities of fifteen items have been determined based on the past five years of usage. Other relevant information from the practice's inventory records is depicted in Table EX 11.4. The practice is functional for fifty-two weeks a year.

TABLE EX 11.4

Item No.	Weekly Demand (Unit/Week)	Unit Cost in $	Yearly Carrying Rate of Each Item	Ordering Cost in $
1	400	2.50	15%	12.00
2	1,600	0.50	16%	6.00
3	175	37.50	20%	32.00
4	250	3.50	12%	50.00
5	250	1.75	18%	12.00
6	32	2,300.00	2%	35.00
7	1,500	1.25	14%	10.00
8	2,200	0.65	17%	6.00
9	1,270	0.95	21%	5.00
10	120	12.50	12%	12.00
11	220	2.00	15%	28.00
12	350	1.50	14%	18.00
13	18	5,000.00	2%	25.00
14	6	6,700.00	2%	50.00
15	1,250	2.60	22%	19.00

a.   Determine the basic EOQ on each item.

b.   Provide the ABC classification of these items.

c.   Calculate the yearly cost of inventory management.

d.   Calculate the investment cost (per cycle) for each item.

e.   Explain the difference between inventory management cost and investment cost.

11.5 A portion of a hospital pharmacy formulary contains the twenty medications listed in Table EX 11.5.

Ordering cost of items is $30 and yearly carrying cost is 5 percent of the unit price.

a.   Determine basic the EOQ on each item.

b.   Provide the ABC classification of these items.

c.   Calculate the yearly inventory management cost.

d.   Determine the investment cost (per cycle) for each item.

TABLE EX 11.5 - will upload Template - EOQ template

Item No.	Description	Unit Price	Weekly Demand ×52
1	Albuterol 0.083% 3ml	7.83	25
2	Alprazolam 1mg	3.15	35
3	Bumetanide 0.5 mg	7.42	40
4	Captopril 50mg	29.66	10
5	Cerumenex	9.98	15
6	Clotrimazale crm 1%	4.38	100
7	Deltason 20mg	11.89	30
8	Diflunisal 250mg	15.43	15
9	Fluocinonide 0.05%	9.85	140
10	Intron A 5ml	32.23	45
11	Lanoxin 0.25mg 2ml	36.90	9
12	Morphine 25mg 10ml	32.21	12
13	Mucosil 10% 10ml	8.64	20
14	Mycelex 1%	6.78	215
15	Propulsid 10mg	22.90	50
16	Retin-A 0.1%	19.90	15
17	Succinylcholn 10ml	10.65	25
18	Sucralfate 1Gm	114.00	65
19	Theophylline	9.80	350
20	Triamterene	30.81	245

11.6 SURGERY ASSOCIATES, a local surgery practice group, orders implants from device manufacturers. Order quantities for ten items have been determined based on the past two years of usage. Other relevant information from the practice's inventory records is depicted in Table EX 11.6. The practice is functional for fifty-two weeks a year.

   a.   Perform basic EOQ analysis for each item.

   b.   Classify the implant inventory items according to the ABC analysis.

   c.   Calculate the yearly inventory management cost.

   d.   Determine the investment cost (per cycle) for each item.

TABLE EX 11.6

Implant Item No.	Yearly Demand (Unit/Year)	Unit Cost	Yearly Carrying Rate of Each Item	Ordering Cost
1	104	2,225	12%	6.00
2	260	5,000	10%	5.00
3	728	3,550	8%	12.00
4	1,248	1,205	12%	28.00
5	104	11,100	2%	18.00
6	1,040	1,500	20%	32.00
7	780	1,900	11%	50.00
8	884	3,700	9%	12.00
9	780	6,400	2%	35.00
10	520	2,700	5%	12.00

CHAPTER

QUALITY CONTROL

LEARNING OBJECTIVES

- Describe the meaning of quality and quality control in health care.
- Review measures of quality in various health care operations.
- Recognize process variability and randomness concepts.
- Develop quality monitoring and control charts.
- Analyze quality control chart for a health care situation.
- Describe and analyze control chart patterns.
- Describe quality improvement techniques.

QUALITY IN HEALTH CARE

Quality in general terms means meeting and exceeding customer expectations. In health care, the definition of customer and the criteria for quality are complicated matters in comparison to the meaning of those terms in industry. Obviously, it is patients who receive health care services. However, what they receive is often not understood by them, when diagnosis and therapy are purchased on their behalf by providers. Hence, quality in health care is evaluated from differing perspectives of recipients and third-party payers.

Most clinicians accept the Institute of Medicine (1990) definition: "Quality is the extent to which health services for individuals and populations increase the likelihood of desired health outcomes and are consistent with current professional knowledge." In accordance with this definition, health care organizations have developed many valid technical measures to evaluate diagnostic and therapeutic clinical processes. A different set of measures is based on health care outcomes that become available or are obtained at the same time or after health services were rendered. If the outcomes can be related to a process or series of processes known to improve outcomes, they also are considered to be valid measures of quality. However, an outcome measure that is related to patients' or clinicians' experience, particularly their feelings about processes (collected using satisfaction surveys), is defined as a subjective perception about the quality of care (Chassin, 1998).

Figure 12.1 illustrates Donebedian's structure-process-outcome conceptualization extended to health services. The input-throughput-output sequence facilitates conceptualizing measurements that can be taken at various stages of providing health care services production. Applying Donebedian's concepts, inputs are part of structure, comprising patients' requests for services from providers who have facilities, staff, equipment, and materials to serve them. At the next stage, the conversion process (for example, from ill health to good health) encompasses diagnostic and therapeutic procedures. At the third stage, outputs, patients exit the system, at which point we assess their conditions as either treated successfully, treated with morbidity, or mortality. Patient satisfaction surveys with follow-up give health care managers feedback on how a patient assessed the treatment process, the overall experience, and the final outcome.

A health care system that has less than acceptable patient satisfaction reports, repeated morbidity, and unacceptable mortality must examine its conversion process.

FIGURE 12.1.   *Quality Measurement.*

That is, the health care managers must investigate what mistakes and errors were committed systematically to produce the undesirable outcomes.

Another way to look at the maintenance of quality is how mistakes are to be avoided—design mistake-proof processes across the whole spectrum of care, to reduce undesired outcomes. Variance in diagnostic and therapeutic interventions and the associated errors hamper the delivery of safe, effective patient care and add to poor outcomes. To minimize the variation and the errors—sometimes euphemistically called "quality gaps"—and work toward completely eliminating them are major goals for health care systems. Chassin (1998) classifies the underlying causes of "quality gaps" into three categories: (1) overutilization, (2) underutilization, and (3) misutilization.

(1) **O**verutilization—when the potential benefit of a therapy is less than its risk, overuse of health services affects the quality of care. Pressures for overuse of services may come from either providers or patients. Pressures from the provider side are: physician ownership in facilities or equipment and consequent self-referrals, the zeal and enthusiasm of a physician to perform a procedure, specialists performing procedures because they are expected to by their referring primary care colleagues, and providers' fear of malpractice suits. Pressures from the patient side are cultural factors: expectations for physicians to perform and the desire to have the latest, most publicized, and technologically advanced treatment.

(2) **A** patient's lack of insurance or insurance that has high copayments and deductibles can cause underutilization of necessary health care. A lack of standardization for various procedures, due to their complexity and also the overwhelming amount of information on therapies, creates selection bias in physicians' choices of treatment.

(3) **A**voidable complications, negligent care, mistakes, and mishaps create misutilization of services. Health care providers who generate such conditions harm the quality of patient care and produce poor outcomes; they also waste the organization's resources and increase lengths of stay (Chassin, 1998).

It is not uncommon to learn from the media about mistakes that occur in health care facilities: patients undergoing second surgeries because something was left in their bodies during the previous one; chemotherapy overdoses; the wrong organs being removed; or organ transplants done with mismatched blood or tissue donors. What shows up in the media are the high profile cases, yet mistakes occur continuously in health care organizations, and, especially in medications, with the wrong medications given to patients or medications given before checking allergies or interactions. Some of those errors occur because appropriate existing technologies are not in place; for example, in a hospital pharmacy, use of drug interaction software; bar coding technology to match unit dose medications to patients; and proper measurements of weight, height, age, and other conditions of a patient to avoid mistakenly calculated doses. Of course, despite the presence of sophisticated systems, everyone must still be on guard against human error or negligence causing such mishaps as delivering medication to a patient without scanning, mislabeling blood tubes, ignoring the alarm sound from an IV dropper, or not checking a patient's oxygen supply.

Health care providers do have an arsenal of methods to deal effectively with the problems affecting quality of care. They include the programs called quality control (QC), total quality management (TQM), continuous quality improvement (CQI), reengineering, and Six Sigma. All of these programs include data gathering, analysis and statistical monitoring to identify the problem and its cause. Nevertheless, the crux of the solution to quality problems lies in changing human behavior; changing minds to perform care in new ways. That is a colossal task in health care, especially as it involves clinicians. The hopeful aspect is that when evidence is provided, clinicians are more willing to adopt and follow changes. Thus health care managers and leaders should provide such evidence.

Quality Experts

The ideas behind the methodological programs listed above emanated from various experts who have contributed to and shaped contemporary methods for improving quality. W. Edwards Deming is known for his list of fourteen items to achieve quality in organizations. The main message of the list is that poor quality occurs as a result of the system and so should be corrected by the management. Deming also stressed that variation in output should be reduced by identifying particular causes that differ from random variation. Later in this chapter we will examine statistical methods for identifying such causes in output variation. Joseph M. Juran's thought was geared towards what the customer wanted, and he asserted that 80 percent of quality gaps can be corrected by management through quality planning, control, and improvement. Philip B. Crosby introduced the concept of zero defects and stressed prevention. He pointed out that the cost of achieving higher quality also reduces costs, hence the quality is free (Stevenson, 2002; pp. 402–406).

Quality Certifications and Awards

Like many other organizations, health care facilities seek certifications and hope to win prestigious quality awards so that they can gain a larger share of the market and confidence of their patients and also of other customers. Such awards are given annually to raise awareness of the desirability of quality and to recognize those institutions that successfully pursue good quality management in their operations. The Baldrige Award is given annually, up to two awards, for large service organizations as well as for large manufacturers and small businesses in the United States. The Deming Prize is given by Japan for organizations' successful efforts to demonstrate quality.

Apart from awards, organizations can seek quality certification through the International Organization for Standardization (ISO). The ISO is an amalgamation of national standardization institutes from 91 countries. The American National Standards Institute (ANSI) is the U.S.-based participant in ISO. ISO 9000 are a set of international standards on quality management and quality assurance; it takes one to one-and-a-half years to go through the process of documentation and on-site assessment to obtain such certification (Stevenson, 2002; pp. 407–410).

Organizations can earn awards or achieve certifications and accreditations by international organizations or by their own trade organizations; for instance, hospitals are evaluated periodically by the Joint Commission on Accreditation of Health care Organizations (JCAHO). For the medical group practices, the Medical Group Management Association (MGMA) is the principal voice. "MGMA's 19,000 members manage and lead 11,500 organizations in which approximately 237,000 physicians practice. MGMA leads the profession and assists members through information, education, networking and advocacy" (Medical Group Management Association, 2004). Quality is always a major concern in those advocacy and accreditation bodies.

To comply with known standards or to establish new benchmarks, health care providers can implement well known quality methods to improve or overhaul their clinical care and management processes. As noted, such methods include QC, TQM and CQI as well as the more contemporary Six Sigma programs. We will discuss the nature of those programs and examine the tools used to implement them in health care organizations.

Total Quality Management (TQM) and Continuous Quality Improvement (CQI)

TQM combines certain concepts introduced by the quality experts mentioned previously, to create a systematic approach for achieving better outcomes of care and also more patient satisfaction through an organization's continual efforts. Many successful applications of TQM in health care have been conducted as the projects of various provider institutions. Often the projects sought to improve the "conversion process" through care pathways and disease management, identification of the causes and prevention of medical errors, risk management in nursing units or in ambulatory health care, and so on.

As a systematic approach, TQM requires the dedication and combined effort of every person in the health care organization. The success of a TQM program depends upon how well the following steps are taken: (1) measuring patient wants as well as needs from the providers, through surveys and focus groups; (2) designing a process for health care service process that will meet and even exceed patient expectations; (3) designing process for health care services that is fail proof ("pókayoke") or fail-safe—that is, systems are designed so that they can work only one way, the safe way (the medication system), so human error is eliminated; (4) monitoring the results and using that information to improve the system; and (5) benchmarking the system by comparisons to peer providers (Stevenson, 2002; pp. 470–472).

TQM is achieved through a team approach that creates synergies among clinicians, administrators, and all the support staff involved in health care delivery. TQM projects have often failed for a variety of reasons: lack of motivation, communication, dedication, plan, leadership, or hodgepodge implementation of the project. To implement successful TQM projects, health care managers see to it that standardized problem-solving techniques are adopted across the organization and for all processes. A framework for problem solving and improvement activities is identified by the Deming wheel/ Shewhart cycle which contains these activities: Plan-Do-Study-Act (PDSA).

Figure 12.2 displays the PDSA cycle, in which each step can be broken down to more detailed steps. In general, the planning activity would comprise recognition and definition of the problem in a current process by health care management, followed by forming teams that include clinical and administrative personnel to document and detail the problem. The team would develop performance measures to evaluate the problem, and identify goals (benchmark), collect data and analyze. In the "Do" cycle, the possible causes of the problem are identified and the solution to fix the problem is implemented. Then, in the "Study" cycle, the solution is monitored, evaluated, and compared against available benchmarks to ensure that performance is acceptable. If implementation has proved successful, the health care manager's action, in the "Act" cycle, includes standardization of the procedures, making them formal through training and communication across the organization. Otherwise, to further improve the process, revision of the plans and a repeat of the process are required. Even when targets have been achieved, the health care quality team can continue the process to set a new benchmark; that is known as continuous quality improvement (CQI). Some health care managers, though, may choose to stop the process at this point and pursue other methods (Stevenson, 2002; pp. 475–477).

Continuous quality improvement (CQI) of various clinical and administrative processes is a systematic approach that also involves documentation, measurement, and analysis. The objective for CQI is to increase patients' and clinicians' satisfaction, while achieving higher quality, reducing waste and cost, and increasing productivity. The CQI is a detailed version of a PDSA cycle that is composed of: (1) selecting a process that needs an improvement; (2) studying and documenting the current process; (3) seeking ways to improve it; (4) designing an improved process; (5) implementing the new process; (6) monitoring and evaluating (7) documenting the process if it

FIGURE 12.2.   *The Deming Wheel/Shewhart Cycle.*

worked successfully and publicizing it through the health care organization; and (8) if it did not achieve its goals, restarting from step 1.

Six Sigma

Six Sigma is one of the latest quality improvement concepts to have emerged during the 1990s. Its name comes from the measure of variation from the normal distribution (six standard deviations). General Electric and Motorola are major companies that have successfully adopted a Six Sigma quality strategy and been examples for other organizations that followed. Adopting a Six Sigma strategy as a quality goal sets tolerance levels for errors (defectives) to levels that occur only 3.4 times per million observations. The defect rates in health care can be defined in such distinct areas as public health, inpatient care, ambulatory care, and so on. For example, infant mortality rates can be considered as defects per million population. Similarly, rate of deaths caused by anesthesia during surgery or of injuries to patients due to negligence are measures of defects for inpatient facilities (Chassin, 1998). According to Chassin, health care organizations have reduced the deaths caused by anesthesia from twenty-five to fifty per million cases to five per million cases since the 1980s through improved monitoring techniques, adaptation of practice guidelines, and other systematic approaches to reduce errors. Hence, this is one area that comes very close to Six Sigma standards. That example portrays the essence of the Six Sigma method: the defects are measured in terms of deviation from the norm, and strategies are adopted to eliminate them through a process and get as close to zero defects as possible.

Adopting Six Sigma strategies in service systems, especially in health care, has lagged by about a dozen years. According to various sources, about 1 percent of health care providers in the United States have deployed Six Sigma methods. It is expected that the adoption rate will increase (Redinius, 2004).

Deployment of Six Sigma to improve the quality of health care and delivery performance can be considered in the following areas: clinical excellence, service delivery, service costs, and customer satisfaction. The deployment can use either of these methodological sequences: DMAIC—define, measure, analyze, improve, and control; or DMADV—define, measure, analyze, design, and verify. DMAIC is generally used to improve existing systems that have fallen below Six Sigma levels, DMADV is used to design and develop new processes or products at Six Sigma levels (Stahl, Schultz, and Pexton, 2003).

The essence of Six Sigma methodologies is both improvement of the knowledge and capability of employees, and also behavior changes through training. Thus, Six Sigma employs a classification system that identifies education and training for employees, project managers and executives. Emulating karate honors, certification is granted at Green Belt (GB), Black Belt (BB), and Master Black Belt (MBB) levels. Green Belts are the employees who have taken the training courses on implementing the projects. Black Belts are the project leaders, whose training may be more intensive; they may complete several projects a year depending upon their size and scope.

Master Black Belts are generally assigned to an area that needs improvement (for example, human resources), to ensure that objectives are set, targets are identified, plans are made, and resources are secured to implement the projects in their assigned area. MBBs may oversee many Six Sigma projects at a time, working with various BBs.

Six Sigma projects require BBs and MBBs to have expertise in basic statistical tools such as Pareto Diagrams, descriptive and higher level statistics including regression, and statistical modeling techniques as well as control processes. In addition to statistical concepts, they are expected to understand project management, finance, leadership, measurement through sociometric (survey) analysis, reliability, and validity.

Examples of successful Six Sigma deployments in health care include reduction of emergency room diversions, fewer errors in operating rooms' cart materials, reduced bloodstream infections in an ICU, and improved radiology turnaround time (Stahl, Schultz, and Pexton, 2003). As health care organizations increase scrutiny in monitoring clinical outcomes, health care managers must develop and adopt fail proof systems to achieve the desired quality levels (Morrisey, 2004).

In order to define, measure, analyze, and monitor systems in health delivery, managers need various quality deployment tools. These tools are useful whether the program used is quality management through TQM or DMAIC, or quality improvement through CQI or DMADV.

QUALITY MEASUREMENT AND CONTROL TECHNIQUES

Process Variability

In the delivery of health care, there are many occasions when an error can happen in the tasks performed by physicians, nurses, or allied health professionals such as radiation or physical therapists. Often the same task may not even be performed the same way for all patients, though minor alterations within defined limits can be acceptable. When, however, provider performance falls beyond acceptable limits, the errors that occur require investigation and correction. In order to detect noteworthy variations in process, or tendencies that may cause unacceptable levels of errors, health care managers must monitor the processes for quality, using various charts. The intent of the monitoring is to distinguish between **random** and **nonrandom variation.** The common variations in process variability that are caused by natural incidences are in general not repetitive, but various minor factors due to chance and are called random variation. If the cause of variation is systematic, not natural, and the source of the variation is identifiable, the process variation is called nonrandom variation. In health care, nonrandom variation may occur by not following procedures, using defective materials, fatigue, carelessness, or not having appropriate training or orientation to the work situation, among many reasons.

Process variation is the range of natural variability in a process for which health care managers use control charts to monitor the measurements. If the natural variability or the presence of random variation exceeds tolerances set by control charts, then the process is not meeting the design specifications.

Figure 12.3 shows a chart with design specifications to achieve a certain level of quality as determined by the lower confidence level (LCL) and the upper confidence level (UCL). (We will show later how the LCL and UCL can be determined.) From this chart, three possible outcomes can be seen to occur. First, the actual outcomes can be so good that process variability would be contained in a narrower band than the design specifications. That may be due to an excellent quality program, or on the other hand, to design specification being too lax. In the second scenario outcomes could occur within LCL and UCL so that the expected quality would be achieved. However, in the third scenario, outcomes could occur beyond the design specifications, not meeting the expected quality outcomes. Then, health care managers should focus on the causes that create such variation by conducting investigations. Such outcomes are generally not random but systematic, and the sources in systematic factors must be found and corrected. In such situations, the health care manager usually must consider redesigning the system that causes such nonrandom outcomes. For example, high turnover and improperly trained new staff could be one of the sources for the process variation in nursing care units. Therefore, the health care manager may have to redesign and enforce the in-service training as well as having to attack problems causing high staff turnovers.

Monitoring Variation Through Control Charts

A control chart is a tool to display in graphic form the control limits on process outcomes. In the hospitals, the outcomes can be staff response to patient requests, accuracy

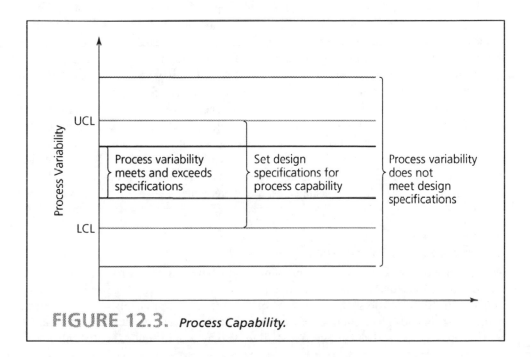

FIGURE 12.3. *Process Capability.*

of medications, infections, accuracy of laboratory tests, and expedience of admissions and discharge processes, to name just some among the many that can be monitored with control charts. The health care manager has to use the appropriate type of control chart for the process being monitored, and that depends on how the process is measured. For example, how many times a staff member did not respond within the appropriate time to a patient request is a counting process, and the variables used to measure this outcome are attributes. Thus a **c-chart** for attributes is the appropriate control chart for such count-type measurements. Similarly, if the process is measured by the percentage of the responses received by patients that were inappropriate, or the percentage of design specifications that were not met (for example, percentage of discharges that are not processed within two hours of discharge orders), then the appropriate attribute-based control chart is a **p-chart.** The other two commonly used charts are **mean** and **range charts,** which monitor process mean and range. Note that mean and range charts must be used together to monitor process variation.

Although the construction of control charts depends on the measurement variable (monitoring attribute versus process mean/range), all control charts have common characteristics. Each chart has a process mean and lower and upper control limits that are calculated according to the type of measurement variable. The control limits theoretically separate random variation from nonrandom variation. Samples taken from the process in a time order are shown in Figure 12.4, where the variation within ±2 sigma level—95.5 percent probability—can be described as random variation.

However, we must approach this determination with caution. If all points appear within the LCL-UCL, we are sure about this with only 95.5 percent confidence; that means there is a 4.5 percent chance that we may be erroneously concluding the process is random, when it is not. This is called **Type II error.** Similarly, consider the two points (samples 5 and 8) beyond the UCL in the graph, where we conclude the variation is nonrandom. Again, we are able say this with only 95.5 percent confidence, and 4.5 percent of the time we may commit the error of concluding nonrandomness when randomness is present; that is called **Type I error,** or α risk. Since Type I error can occur above or below the confidence levels, the risk is divided evenly for each part, $\alpha/2$. One can reduce Type I error by using wider limits such as ±3 sigma. However, then detection of nonrandom variations would become more difficult, leading to greater Type II error of concluding that nonrandom variations are random. In practice, ±2 sigma level is usually used to determine LCL and UCL for control charts.

Control Charts for Attributes

When process characteristics can be counted, attribute-based control charts are the appropriate way to display the monitoring process. However, counting can be conceptualized in different ways. If the number of occurrences per unit of measure can be counted, or there can be a count of the number of bad occurrences but not of nonoccurrences, then a c-chart is the appropriate tool to display monitoring. Counting also can

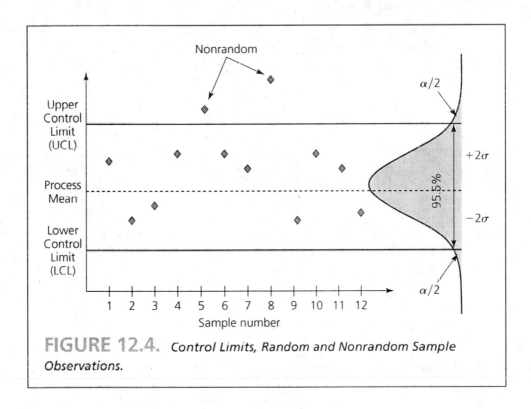

FIGURE 12.4. *Control Limits, Random and Nonrandom Sample Observations.*

occur for a process with only two outcomes, good or bad (defective); in such cases, p-chart is the appropriate control chart. The p-chart arises from binomial distribution where only two outcomes are possible.

c-Chart. Certain processes require counting bad occurrences as quality defects. For example, the number of wrong medications delivered in one thousand patient days or the number of infections occurring during a month are such occurrences. Remember that counting occurs over a sample or over time and that occurrences can be counted per unit of measure. The theoretical conceptualization of this process is described by Poisson distribution, with a mean of c and standard deviation of $\sqrt{c}$. When there are enough samples in the quality control process, by invoking central limit theorem we can use normal approximation to Poisson and define the control limits of the c-chart as follows:

$$UCL = c + z\sqrt{c} \qquad (12.1)$$

$$LCL = c - z\sqrt{c} \qquad (12.2)$$

where c represents the population mean for the number of defects over a unit (or time period). In the absence of population parameters, estimates of the sample mean and standard deviation can be used by replacing c with $\bar{c}$, and confidence limits can be established as:

$$UCL = \bar{c} + z\sqrt{\bar{c}} \qquad (12.3)$$

$$LCL = \bar{c} - z\sqrt{\bar{c}}. \qquad (12.4)$$

If LCL values are negative, for practical reasons they should be set to zero.

EXAMPLE 12.1

The number of infections from the Intensive Care Unit (ICU) at the ABC Medical Center over a period of twenty-four months is obtained. These numbers are the counts of stool assay positive for toxin, segregated by month. The patient population and other external factors such as change in provider have been stable.

Months	Infections in ICU	
	Year 1	Year 2
January	3	4
February	4	3
March	3	6
April	4	3
May	3	4
June	4	3
July	5	5
August	3	6
September	4	3
October	3	3
November	7	6
December	4	3
Total	47	49

The nurse manager who serves on the quality team wants to discover whether the infections are in control within 95.5 percent confidence limits.

Solution

If we consider each month as a sample of bad quality outcomes, for twenty-four samples we have a total of ninety-six quality defects (infections), and the average would be:

$$\bar{c} = 96 \,/\, 24 = 4.0.$$

Since the z-value for 95.5 percent confidence level is equal to 2, using formulas (12.3) and (12.4), we obtain

$$UCL = \bar{c} + z\sqrt{\bar{c}} = 4 + 2\sqrt{4} = 4 + 2 \times 2 = 8.$$
$$LCL = \bar{c} - z\sqrt{\bar{c}} = 4 - 2\sqrt{4} = 4 - 2 \times 2 = 0.$$

The corresponding control chart for ICU at ABC Medical Center is shown in Figure 12.5.

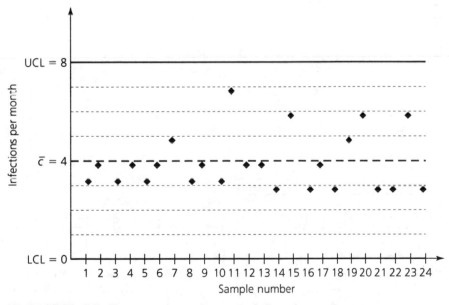

FIGURE 12.5. *ABC Medical Center Infection Control Monitoring.*

p-*Chart*. The proportion of defects in a process can be monitored using a p-chart that has binomial distribution as its theoretical base. The center of the p-chart represents the average for defects and LCL and UCL are calculated as:

$$UCL = p + z\sigma_p \tag{12.5}$$

$$UCL = p - z\sigma_p \tag{12.6}$$

where

$$\sigma_p = \sqrt{\frac{p(1-p)}{n}}.$$

If the average proportion of defects is not known, then the sample average for the proportion of defects ($\bar{p}$) can be used and the above formulas can be rewritten for sample proportions as:

$$UCL = \bar{p} + z\sqrt{\frac{\bar{p}(1-\bar{p})}{n}} \tag{12.7}$$

$$LCL = \bar{p} - z\sqrt{\frac{\bar{p}(1-\bar{p})}{n}}. \tag{12.8}$$

Here also, the negative LCL values for practical reasons should be set to zero.

EXAMPLE 12.2

The indicator Family Satisfaction, which is part of the National Hospice and Palliative Care Organization's survey, reflects the percentage of respondents who would not recommend the hospice services to others. The following data are from Holistic Care Corporation's completed surveys from two hundred families each month during a year, showing the number of respondents each month who expressed dissatisfaction with the organization's services.

Months	Dissatisfied Patient Families	Percent Dissatisfied
January	12/200 =	0.060
February	14	0.070
March	16	0.080
April	14	0.070
May	25	0.125
June	14	0.070
July	15	0.075
August	16	0.080
September	14	0.070
October	14	0.070
November	24	0.120
December	14	0.070
Total	192 /240 =	0.080 ~ P̄

The manager in charge of quality wishes to construct a control chart for these data within 95.5 percent confidence intervals.

Solution

First, we need to estimate the proportion mean,

$$\bar{p} = \frac{Total\ number\ of\ quality\ in\ fractions}{Total\ number\ of\ observed} = \frac{192}{12(200)} = \frac{192}{2400} = .08$$

Since the z value for the 95.5 percent confidence level is equal to 2.0, using formulas (12.7) and (12.8), we obtain:

$$UCL = .08 + 2\sqrt{\frac{.08(1-.08)}{200}} = 0.118.$$

$$LCL = .08 - 2\sqrt{\frac{.08(1-.08)}{200}} = 0.042.$$

The corresponding control chart for the Holistic Care Corporation data is shown in Figure 12.6.

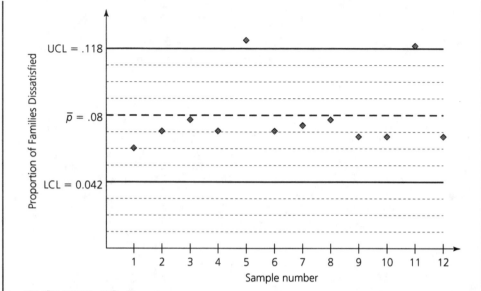

FIGURE 12.6. *Holistic Care Corporation's Quality Monitoring.*

As can be observed from the chart, the percentages of families dissatisfied with the care in samples #5 and #11 are over the control limit.

Control Charts for Variables

Mean and range charts are for variables measured continuously, such as "time" it takes to admit or discharge a patient. Mean charts monitor a central tendency or process average, and range charts monitor the dispersion of a process. These two charts are used together to determine whether a process is in control.

Figure 12.7 displays two situations where neither chart alone can detect anomalies in the process quality. The upper chart in the figure shows that the process mean is stable but that dispersion (variability) in the process is increasing. In this situation the mean chart would not detect the shift in process variability, but the range chart would, as the range indicator increases steadily. The lower chart shows a process with stable range; however, the process mean increases. In this situation, the range chart would not detect the increasing trend in the process average; however, the mean chart would.

Mean Charts. Depending upon the available information, a mean chart can be constructed using either standard deviation or range information.

Standard Deviation Approach. In general the population standard is unknown, and so the average of sample means $\bar{\bar{x}}$ and the standard deviation of sample distribution $\sigma_{\bar{x}}$ are used to construct the confidence limits as:

$$UCL = \bar{\bar{x}} + z\sigma_{\bar{x}} \qquad (12.9)$$

$$LCL = \bar{\bar{x}} - z\sigma_{\bar{x}} \qquad (12.10)$$

where

$$\sigma_{\bar{x}} = \frac{s}{\sqrt{n}}.$$

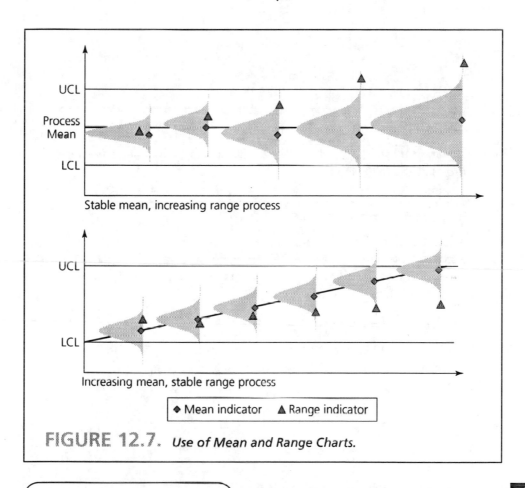

FIGURE 12.7. *Use of Mean and Range Charts.*

EXAMPLE 12.3

With a time-motion study, the IV startup process has been examined in a medical center nursing unit for five weekdays to determine whether in the future, additional training of nurses is required. Each day nine new patients' IV startups were observed and the measurements recorded in minutes, as shown below. Construct 99.7 percent (z = 3) confidence limits for IV startup times.

Observation	Day 1	Day 2	Day 3	Day 4	Day 5
1	5.1	4.9	5.5	6.1	6.0
2	5.4	5.7	5.6	5.8	5.2
3	5.5	6.3	5.3	5.9	6.3
4	5.8	7.5	4.9	6.0	5.0
5	5.6	5.8	5.2	6.2	5.5
6	5.8	5.9	5.4	5.7	5.1
7	5.3	5.5	6.4	4.8	5.9
8	4.9	5.8	7.5	6.3	5.3
9	6.2	5.5	5.8	5.9	4.8

Solution

Observation means, $\bar{x}$, for each day (sample) are calculated and shown in the last rows of the following table.

Sample	Day 1	Day 2	Day 3	Day 4	Day 5
$\bar{x}$	5.51	5.88	5.73	5.86	5.46
s-overall	0.6				

The sample standard deviation (s), for the nine observations over five days is calculated to be 0.6 as shown above. The grand mean, $\bar{\bar{x}}$, calculated over five days of observations

$$\bar{\bar{x}} = \left(5.51 + 5.88 + 5.73 + 5.86 + 5.46\right) \div 5 = 5.69.$$

Using formulas (12.9) and (12.10), $UCL = \bar{\bar{x}} + z\,\sigma_{\bar{x}}$, $LCL = \bar{\bar{x}} - z\,\sigma_{\bar{x}}$ with $z = 3$, $n = 9$ observations per sample (day), and $s = 0.6$, we obtain:

$$UCL = 5.69 + 3\left(0.6 / \sqrt{9}\right) = 5.69 + 3\left(0.2\right) = 6.29.$$
$$LCL = 5.69 - 3\left(0.6 / \sqrt{9}\right) = 5.69 + 3\left(0.2\right) = 5.09.$$

Note that on the following days the specific observations are beyond the control limits.

Day 1: observation 8.
Day 2: observation 1, 3, and 4.
Day 3: observations 4, 7, and 8.
Day 4: observations 7 and 8.
Day 5: observations 3 and 9.

Managers responsible for quality would investigate the variations to determine whether they are caused by one or more individuals who need additional in-service training.

Range Approach. Another way to construct a mean chart is to use the average of sample distribution ranges, $\bar{R}$. This approach requires a factor to calculate the dispersion of the control limits.

$$UCL = \bar{\bar{x}} + A_2\bar{R} \qquad (12.11)$$

$$LCL = \bar{\bar{x}} - A_2\bar{R} \qquad (12.12)$$

Where A_2 is a factor from Table 12.1.

TABLE 12.1. Factors For Determining Control Limits for Mean and Range Charts (for Three-Sigma or 99.7 Percent–Confidence Level).

Sample Size n	Factor for Mean Chart, A_2	Factors for Range Chart	
		LCL, D_3	UCL, D_4
5	0.58	0	2.11
6	0.48	0	2.00
7	0.42	0.08	1.92
8	0.37	0.14	1.86
9	0.34	0.18	1.82
10	0.31	0.22	1.78
11	0.29	0.26	1.74
12	0.27	0.28	1.72
13	0.25	0.31	1.69
14	0.24	0.33	1.67
15	0.22	0.35	1.65
16	0.21	0.36	1.64
17	0.20	0.38	1.62
18	0.19	0.39	1.61
19	0.19	0.40	1.60
20	0.18	0.41	1.59

Source: Adopted from R. S. Russell & B. W. Taylor, *Operations Management, 2nd Ed.* (Upper Saddle River, NJ: Prentice-Hall), 1995.

EXAMPLE 12.4

During five weekdays, each day the number of minutes spent for each of ten patient registration operations were observed in a time study as follows:

Observation	Day 1	Day 2	Day 3	Day 4	Day 5
1	10.2	10.3	8.9	9.5	10.5
2	9.7	10.9	10.5	9.7	10.2
3	10.3	11.1	8.9	10.5	10.3
4	8.9	8.9	10.5	9.8	10.9
5	10.5	10.5	9.8	8.9	11.1
6	9.8	9.7	10.2	10.5	9.8
7	10.0	8.9	8.9	10.4	9.5
8	11.3	10.5	10.5	8.9	9.7
9	10.7	9.8	9.7	10.5	10.5
10	9.8	11.3	10.5	9.8	8.8

Solution

The overall mean for each sample and range is required to apply the formulas (12.11) and (12.12), using the range approach. Here each day is considered as a sample. The range is calculated by taking the difference between the maximum and minimum of each sample (day). The, mean for each day also is calculated and shown as follows:

Sample	Day 1	Day 2	Day 3	Day 4	Day 5
Maximum	11.3	11.3	10.5	10.5	11.1
Minimum	8.9	8.9	8.9	8.9	8.8
Range	2.4	2.4	1.6	1.6	2.3
$\bar{x}$	10.12	10.19	9.84	9.85	10.13

Before the step of using the formulas, calculation of the averages of sample means, $\bar{x}$, and ranges, $\bar{R}$, is required.

$$\bar{\bar{x}} = (10.12 + 10.19 + 9.84 + 9.85 + 10.13) \div 5 = 10.03.$$

$$\bar{R} = (2.4 + 2.4 + 1.6 + 1.6 + 2.3) \div 5 = 2.06.$$

Finally, using the formulas (12.11) and (12.12), we get

$$UCL = \bar{x} + A_2\bar{R} = 10.03 + 0.31(2.06) = 10.67.$$

$$LCL = \bar{x} - A_2\bar{R} = 10.03 - 0.31(2.06) = 9.39.$$

where A_2 is a factor selected as n = 10 from Table 12.1.

There are observations, in Day 1 and Day 2, and Day 5 with values above the mean chart in this example.

Range Charts. Process dispersion is best monitored by range charts. The control limits for range charts are constructed using factors. To calculate LCL, factor score D_3 is obtained from a factor chart based on the number of observations in the sample distributions. Similarly, to calculate UCL, factor score D_4 is required. Control limits for range charts using these factor scores are then constructed as follows:

$$UCL = D_4\bar{R} \tag{12.13}$$

$$LCL = D_3\bar{R}. \tag{12.14}$$

EXAMPLE 12.5

Use the information provided in example 12.4 to construct a range chart.

Solution

For $n = 10$, D_3 and D_4 from Table 12.1 are 0.22 and 1.78, respectively. Using formulas (12.13) and (12.14), we obtain:

$$UCL = D_4\bar{R} = 1.78(2.06) = 3.67$$
$$LCL = D_3\bar{R} = 0.22(2.06) = 0.45.$$

stop notes

Investigation of Control Chart Patterns

It is necessary to evaluate control chart patterns for anomalies, even though the observations stay within the confines of control limits. Although quality managers expect the sample variations to occur around the average line, sometimes consistent patterns can occur within control limits that are due to nonrandom causes and may require investigation. Such behavior can be characterized as consistent observations above or below the average (or centerline); persistent zigzagging above and below the centerline may signal disturbances in the system. Furthermore, high magnitude jumps from LCL to UCL or even beyond those limits may suggest nonrandomness and invokes investigation.

Run-Based Pattern Tests. A pattern in a control chart described by a sequence of observations that have similar characteristics is called a "run." A simple classification of sample observations with respect to the centerline that identify consecutive patterns is called an Above/Below run, or A/B run. For example, twelve observations shown in Figure 12.8 are classified as being above or below (A/B) the centerline (CL). If their

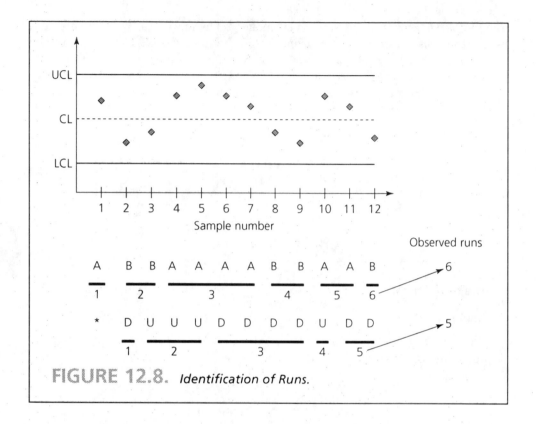

FIGURE 12.8. *Identification of Runs.*

classification is consecutive, it constitutes a run. In this example, an above (A) observation is followed by two consecutive below (B) observations, which are followed by four consecutive above observations, and so on. Whenever there is a switch in a classified observation, a new run starts. Hence there are six such A/B runs in this chart.

Up (U) and down (D) runs is another way to classify and observe patterns. To classify sample observations as U or D, the first observation is used as a reference point, shown with "*" in Figure 12.8. Starting with the second observation one can classify each observation with respect to its predecessor. Here the second observation as compared to the first observation has a lower value, so its position is classified as down (D). The third observation as compared to the second observation has a higher value, so its position is classified as up (U). Ensuing observations are classified similarly. Once all observations are classified, the runs are identified by checking the consecutive patterns. In this example, the second observation is a stand-alone run. The next three observations are classified as up and constitute another run. The third run is a down run containing four observations. In total, there are five observed U/D runs in this example.

Control chart patterns identified by runs require statistical testing of whether the runs are within expectations and hence the patterns are random, or beyond expectations and hence nonrandomness is present. It has been shown that runs are distributed approximately normally (Stevenson, 2002; p. 436) and using the z-test the significance of too few or too many observed runs can be determined as follows:

$$z = \frac{Observed\ runs - Expected\ runs}{Standard\ deviation\ of\ runs}.$$

(12.15)

A z-value within ± 2, which provides 95.5 percent confidence level, would show that the runs are random; however, beyond these values $\leq \pm 2 \geq$, a nonrandom presence would be shown. We already know how to determine observed runs, from an earlier discussion (Figure 12.8). It is necessary to calculate the expected runs and their standard deviations. The formulas for expected A/B or U/D runs and their standard deviations are as follows:

$$E(run)_{A/B} = \frac{N}{2} + 1$$

(12.16)

$$\sigma(run)_{A/B} = \sqrt{\frac{N-1}{4}}$$

(12.17)

$$E(run)_{U/D} = \frac{2N-1}{3}$$

(12.18)

$$\sigma(run)_{U/D} = \sqrt{\frac{16N-29}{90}}.$$

(12.19)

EXAMPLE 12.6

Determine the presence or absence of nonrandomness for the example presented in Figure 12.8, with 95.5 percent confidence limits.

Solution

The example has twelve observations, so N = 12. Using the formulas (12.15) through (12.19) above, we get:

$$E(run)_{A/B} = \frac{12}{2} + 1 = 7.0; \quad \sigma(run)_{A/B} = \sqrt{\frac{12-1}{4}} = \sqrt{\frac{11}{4}} = \sqrt{2.75} = 1.66;$$

$$E(run)_{A/B} = \frac{(2 \times 12) - 1}{3} = 7.67; \quad \sigma(run)_{U/D} - \sqrt{\frac{(16 \times 12) - 29}{90}} - \sqrt{\frac{163}{90}} - \sqrt{1.81} - 1.35$$

$$z_{A/B} = \frac{6-7}{1.66} = -0.60;\ \text{conclude that the A/B runs exhibit randomness.}$$

$$z_{U/D} = \frac{5-7.67}{1.35} = -1.98;\ \text{conclude that U/D runs exhibit randomness.}$$

However, this particular case is a close one, the quality manager should be on the lookout in the future, and compute the z-test again after collecting more observations.

Zone Tests. An alternative method that is often used by quality control software packages is called the "zone test." The essence of the zone test rests on deviation from the centerline by one-sigma, two-sigma, or three-sigma limits. Zone C, Zone B, and Zone A are identified by these limits, respectively. To create the zones, the formulas for constructing mean chart with range approach, (12.11) and (12.12) are used. Those formulas, presented earlier, use A_2 from Table 12.1, and the values for this table were calculated for three-sigma levels (or 99.7 percent confidence level). Thus, in constructing the zones, one must reduce the A_2 factor proportionately, according to the sigma level. Since A_2 is designated for three-sigma, for two-sigma 1/2 of A_2, and for one-sigma 1/3 of A_2 would be appropriate. The zone formulas can be written as:

$$Zone\,A = \bar{\bar{x}} \pm A_2\bar{R} \tag{12.20}$$

$$Zone\,B = \bar{\bar{x}} \pm \frac{1}{2}A_2\bar{R} \tag{12.21}$$

$$Zone\,C = \bar{\bar{x}} \pm \frac{1}{3}A_2\bar{R}. \tag{12.22}$$

Figure 12.9 displays the zones constructed this way. After determining the zones, quality managers may use various guidelines associated with the zones to determine whether there are any nonrandom patterns in the control chart.

Sensitizing Rules for Control Charts. These rules determine whether the process is statistically out of control. The most commonly suggested rules for detecting nonrandom patterns are:

- Single point outside of three-sigma limits
- Two out of three consecutive observations above two-sigma limits
- Four out of five consecutive observations above one-sigma limits
- Eight consecutive observations are one side of the centerline
- Eight consecutive observations are in up or down pattern

- Fourteen points alternating up and down
- Single observation jumps four-sigma (Russell and Taylor 1995, p. 150; Chang, 2004)

FIGURE 12.9. *Zone Test.*

EXAMPLE 12.7

Apply the pattern rules to the observations displayed in Figure 12.9.

Solution

Rule 1: no violation
Rule 2: violation: samples #10 and #12 are over 2-sigma limits in Zone A
Rule 3: samples #5,#6,#7,#8 and #9; four out of five above one-sigma limits
Rule 4: no violation
Rule 5: no violation
Rule 6: no violation
Rule 7: violation: sample #2 is down by 4-sigma, from Zone B above CL to Zone C below CL
According to the pattern rules there are two violations, and nonrandomness may be present. Hence an investigation is required.

Process Improvement

Health care quality managers often face circumstances that require improvement or reengineering of care processes. Methods and tools used in reengineering processes are available to accomplish difficult and costly improvement tasks. One group of methods is for generating new ideas. Another group of tools are used to measure and display the findings for decisions on actions.

Methods for Generating New Ideas

The 5W2H Approach. This approach takes its name from five questions starting with "W" and two questions starting with "H." Health care managers can generate questions related to quality problems by asking "What?" (subject); "Why?" (purpose); "Where?" (location); "When?" (timing sequence); "Who?" (people); "How?" (method); and "How much?" (cost) (Stevenson 2002; pp. 487–489). The answers to the questions can be sought using such methods as brainstorming or quality circles and such tools as cause-and-effect diagrams or Pareto charts, all of which are discussed below.

Brainstorming. This is a group process: discussion to generate free-flowing ideas that might identify causes and generate solutions to a problem. The guidelines are that each member of the group expresses her or his ideas without receiving criticisms from the others and that no member should be allowed to dominate the discussion. This approach works by focusing on a problem and coming up with very many radical solutions. Ideas should be developed as fast as possible, to facilitate generating a wide spectrum and should be very odd. The generated ideas can be evaluated after the brainstorming session, perhaps by using nominal group technique.

Nominal Group Technique. This technique is similar to brainstorming, but the session is led by an assigned moderator who presents the topic (problem) to session participants. Participants may ask questions and briefly discuss the topic; then they think of ideas and write them down. The moderator asks each participant to read and elaborate on one of their responses. The responses usually are summarized on a flip chart. After everyone has given a response, participants are asked for second and then third responses, until all their ideas have been recorded on flip chart sheets posted around the room.

In the next step the moderator, working with the participants, eliminates redundant or similar responses. Session participants are then asked to choose five to ten responses that they feel are the most important and rank them according to their relative importance. If necessary, the moderator can give the results back to the participants to stimulate further discussion for a possible readjustment of the overall rankings of the responses. That is done, however, only when consensus about the ideas' ranking is important to the topic or the problem. The nominal group technique is an alternative to both the focus group and the Delphi techniques. It has more structure than the focus group does but still takes advantage of the synergy created by group participants.

Interviewing. Keeping patient satisfaction as a goal, rich information about quality defects can be obtained from interviews of patients, in addition to satisfaction surveys.

Benchmarked provider staff also can be interviewed for their insights about the quality of care.

Focus Groups. Focus groups are in-depth, qualitative interviews of small groups of carefully selected people who have been brought together to discuss a problem. Unlike a one-to-one interview, focus groups generate data through the give-and-take of group discussion, as people share and compare their different points of view. The focus group participants not only express what they think about the problem, but explain why they think that way. The composition of a focus group is usually based on the homogeneity or similarity of the group members. Bringing people with common interests or experiences together makes it easier for them to carry on a productive discussion. When there are different issues, different groups should be used for each issue.

Quality Circles "Kaizen Teams." As for a focus group, a group of employees in a health care organization come together to address issues about quality in their facility. Their focus in the health care organizations is to improve processes so that the best quality of care can be achieved. The strategy involved is to bring the employees' own ideas into play to improve quality. The group works as a team (the term Kaizen Teams was adopted from Japanese management practice), and its results are based on consensus. The employees joining the team do so voluntarily and participate under the leadership of their supervisor during normal work hours. The team meets regularly and makes recommendations to management. There are no formal rules for organizing a quality circle. However, meetings should take place away from work areas to minimize distractions, and should be held for at least one hour per week with clear agendas and objectives. The quality circles must be of manageable size. When needed, outside experts can be brought in (for example, a quality circle member from a different provider).

Benchmarking. The purpose of benchmarking is to identify the best in health care processes and try to match that level. Examining the processes of the best providers reveals invaluable information for health care managers trying to improve their own organizations. As mentioned above, Six Sigma quality, which many industries have adopted as a benchmark goal, has now been applied in health care as well.

Tools for Investigating the Presence of Quality Problems and Their Causes

Health care managers who are responsible for the quality of care and their team can use the approaches explained above to begin to understand a problem, but they also need tools to develop a detailed analysis of it. That effort requires quantification and visualizations to develop alternative plans for a solution. The following are tools that are essential for the effort.

Check Sheet. This is a tallying tool used for fact finding or problem identification. It provides a format for health care managers to count the defects in the process for a list of the causes such as have been identified earlier while generating the ideas. For example, in an emergency room, long waiting times are recognized by the patients as defects in quality. However, the cause of the delays may arise from (1) the wait time for registering; (2) the registration process itself; or (3) the wait time to see a doctor. Figure 12.10 illustrates a check sheet developed to investigate the causes of long emergency room wait times.

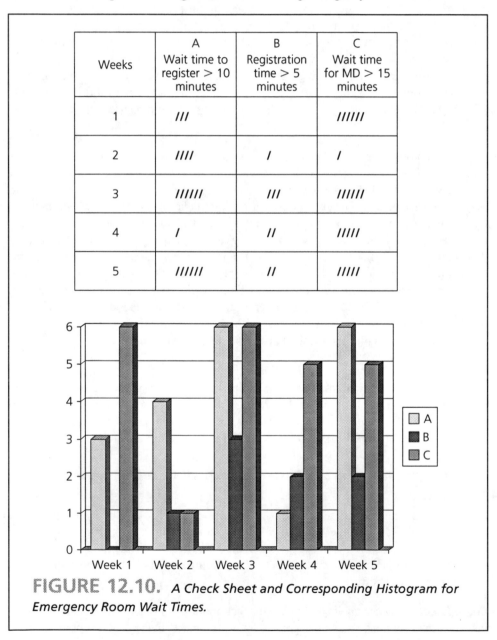

Weeks	A Wait time to register > 10 minutes	B Registration time > 5 minutes	C Wait time for MD > 15 minutes
1	///		//////
2	////	/	/
3	//////	///	//////
4	/	//	/////
5	//////	//	/////

FIGURE 12.10. *A Check Sheet and Corresponding Histogram for Emergency Room Wait Times.*

Histogram. This is a chart that displays empirical (collected) data, the frequency distribution of a process. Examining the chart, health care managers can identify extremes (outliers at tail ends), as well as peak occurrences (mode) in the data. Histograms can be used to display the count data from check sheets.

Scatter Diagram. This diagram displays the possible relationships between two variables, to identify a pattern that constitutes a problem for the quality of care. For example, medication errors or infection rates may correspond to hospital mortality or morbidity rates. Figure 12.11 displays a scatter diagram illustrating the correspondence between the number of infections per month and the hospital's morbidity rate.

Flow Chart. As also discussed in Chapter Six, flow charts could provide a chronological execution of processes in which a decision point—shown by a diamond symbol—may indicate a bottleneck in the process. Rectangular shape shows procedures, and arrows show the flow of the process. A good process would minimize the decision points without sacrificing necessary auditing requirements. Figure 12.12 is an example of a flow chart for the X-ray order process in an emergency department.

Cause-and-Effect Diagram. Also known as a fishbone diagram or an Ishikawa chart, a cause-and-effect diagram displays the structured results of the ideas generated from brainstorming, the nominal method, interviewing, focus groups, and quality circles. The main causes of the problem are displayed on ticker lines or bones (such as methods or processes); then specific causes are displayed within on thinner lines (such as, too many steps).

FIGURE 12.11. *Scatter Diagram.*

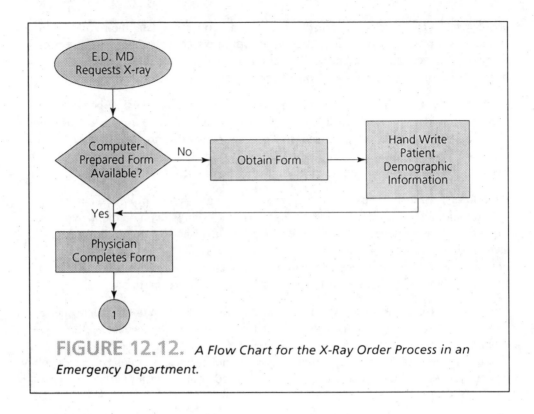

FIGURE 12.12. *A Flow Chart for the X-Ray Order Process in an Emergency Department.*

Pareto Diagram. The next step in analyzing the problem is a Pareto diagram. Quality managers using nominal technique can prioritize the importance and contribution of each cause to the problem. The aim is to identify 80 percent of the causes and start working on the solutions. Figures 12.13 and 12.14 show a cause-and-effect diagram and the corresponding Pareto diagram, respectively.

SUMMARY

Quality in health care is evaluated from differing perspectives of recipients and third-party payers. A health care system that has less than acceptable patient satisfaction reports, repeated morbidity, and unacceptable mortality mwust examine its conversion process. That is, the health care managers must investigate what mistakes and errors were committed systematically to produce the undesirable outcomes.

To comply with known standards or to establish new benchmarks, health care providers can implement well known quality methods to improve or overhaul their clinical care and management processes. As noted, such methods include quality control, total quality management, and continuous quality improvement as well as the more contemporary Six Sigma programs.

FIGURE 12.13. *Cause-and-Effect Diagram.*

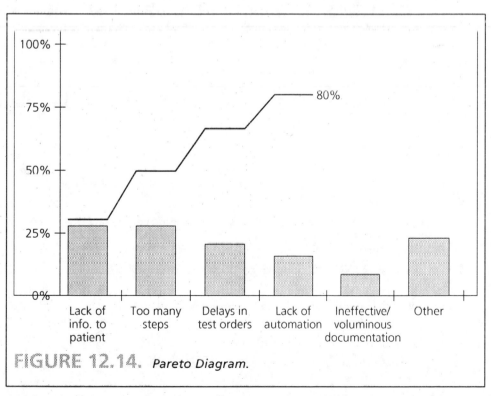

FIGURE 12.14. *Pareto Diagram.*

In health care delivery, to detect note-worthy variations in process, or tendencies that may cause unacceptable levels of errors, health care managers must monitor the processes for quality by using various charts. If they encounter repeated anomalies in the process, health care quality managers should take steps to improve or reengineer the care processes. As discussed in this chapter, there are many methods and tools available to health care managers for generating new ideas, measuring and displaying the findings, and for making decisions to improve quality of care.

KEY TERMS

Total Quality Management (TQM)
Continuous Quality Improvement (CQI)
Six Sigma
Process Variability

Random Variation
Control Chart
Process Improvement.

EXERCISES

12.1 The Chief Nursing Officer (CNO) is concerned about medication errors in two hospital units. Collection of data over a year resulted in Table EX 12.1.

$$UCL = \bar{c} + z\sqrt{\bar{c}} \qquad z = 2$$

TABLE EX 12.1
$$LCL = \bar{c} - z\sqrt{\bar{c}}$$

(handwritten margin note: simple C-chart for each unit)

Medication Errors	Jan	Feb	Mar	Apr	May	Jun	Jul	Aug	Sep	Oct	Nov	Dec
Unit A	4	6	2	5	3	6	3	4	5	3	7	4
Unit B	3	4	6	5	4	7	3	4	6	4	5	4

a. Using a 95.5 percent confidence level, calculate the UCL and LCL for an appropriate control chart for each unit.

b. Construct the charts and identify any observations that are beyond the control limits.

12.2 The data in Table EX 12.2 records the patient falls in three care units over a seventeen-week period. $z = 2$

(handwritten margin note: multiple C-chart)

a. For each unit, calculate LCL and UCL for an appropriate control chart, using 95.5 percent confidence limits.

b. Construct a control chart for each unit.

(handwritten margin note: non-random variation)
c. Are any observations in violation of the control limits for the unit?

TABLE EX 12.2

Patient Falls	Unit-I	Unit-II	Unit-III
Week 1	2	1	3
Week 2	1	2	1
Week 3	2	3	0
Week 4	2	2	2
Week 5	3	1	2
Week 6	1	0	1
Week 7	2	2	2
Week 8	1	0	1
Week 9	0	1	4
Week 10	1	1	3
Week 11	2	2	1
Week 12	1	0	2
Week 13	0	1	1
Week 14	2	2	2
Week 15	2	1	0
Week 16	1	0	2
Week 17	2	1	3

12.3 Using samples of 200 observations each, a quality inspector found the results shown in Table FX 12.3.

complaints = # of defectives
sample = 200

TABLE EX 12.3

P-chart

Sample = 200	1	2	3	4	5	6
Number of Defectives	4	2	5	8	6	5
fraction defective	*0.02*	*0.01*	*0.025*	*0.04*	*0.03*	*0.025*

$\bar{x} = 0.025$

a. Determine the fraction defective in each sample. */200*

b. Estimate the mean and standard deviation of the sampling distribution of fractions defective.

c. Determine the control limits that would give an alpha risk of .025 for this process.

$-\frac{P}{\&} \mp$
TO
1- 0.025

d. Construct an appropriate control chart and identify any observations that are not within control limits.

Random vs. nonrandom distribution

12.4 A medical center routinely conducts patient satisfaction surveys upon discharge and follows up with another survey within three months. The discharge and follow-up surveys, conducted on samples of five hundred discharges per month and identifying the number of patients dissatisfied with their care, are shown in Table EX 12.4.

TABLE EX 12.4

Dissatisfied Patients	Jan	Feb	Mar	Apr	May	Jun	Jul	Aug	Sep	Oct	Nov	Dec
At discharge	24	44	36	18	16	19	17	18	27	26	29	26
3-month follow-up	17	24	15	8	11	7	11	9	10	15	12	11

a. Determine the fraction of dissatisfied patients at discharge and on follow-up, for each month.

b. Estimate the mean and standard deviation of the sampling distribution of dissatisfied patients at discharge and at follow-up.

c. For both surveys, determine the control limits for 95 percent confidence limits.

d. For both surveys, construct appropriate control charts and identify any observations that are not within the control limits.

12.5 Complaints of late responses to patient calls in a nursing unit trigger a study by the decision support department, requested by the nursing manager. A time study team made observations and compiled the data in Table EX 12.5.

TABLE EX 12.5

Observation	Day 1	Day 2	Day 3	Day 4	Day 5	Day 6	Day 7
1	3	6	2	4	5	3	4
2	6	5	3	7	3	4	1
3	4	2	5	3	5	3	6
4	7	6	5	9	2	5	4
5	8	3	3	3	4	3	2
6	12	8	4	2	3	7	6
7	5	6	5	6	5	7	4
8	6	4	8	5	8	4	7
9	8	7	6	4	3	6	2

10	9	6	7	3	4	11	2
11	6	3	3	8	4	4	5
12	4	7	4	3	3	2	9
13	7	2	5	5	5	3	3
14	11	4	7	3	2	1	3
15	7	6	3	2	3	4	2

The measurements are recorded in minutes (rounded to the nearest minute) of response time once the patient has pressed the call button.

    a. Using the standard deviation approach, construct 99.7 percent confidence limits for patient call response times.

    b. Develop an appropriate control chart for the days.

    c. Are there any days in violation of the confidence limits?

12.6 Using the information in Exercise 12.5:

    a. Calculate the range for each day and calculate LCL and UCL for a mean chart, using the range approach.

    b. Construct a corresponding control chart and identify any violations of the limits.

12.7 Using the information in Exercise 12.5:

    a. Calculate LCL and UCL for a range chart.

    b. Construct a corresponding control chart and identify any violations of the limits.

12.8 Consider the control chart in Exercise 12.1, part (b):

    a. Perform a median run test and an up/down run test, using 95.5 percent confidence intervals.

    b. Are the medication error patterns random?

12.9 Consider the control chart in Exercise 12.2, part (b), for Unit-III:

    a. Perform a median run test and an up/down run test, using 95.5 percent confidence intervals.

    b. Are the patient fall patterns random in this unit?

12.10 Analyze the control chart in Exercise 12.3, part (c), using a median run test and an up/down run test. What can you conclude?

12.11 Consider the control chart in Exercise 12.4, part (d):

   a. Perform a median run test and an up/down run test, using 95.5 percent confidence intervals.

   b. Are the dissatisfaction patterns random?

12.12 Consider the control chart in Exercise 12.5, part (b):

   a. Perform a median run test and an up/down run test, using 95.5 percent confidence intervals.

   b. Are the response patterns to patient calls random?

12.13 The graph in Figure EX 12.13 represents sample means of delays on laboratory reports at periodic intervals, plotted on a control chart.

   a. Is the output random? Why?

   b. Perform run tests for randomness using a 95.5 percent confidence interval, and interpret the results.

12.14 A hospital has identified nonrandom variations in medication errors. These errors can emanate along a process from prescription orders to delivery to a patient. Hence, consider the departments involved in the process such as nursing, pharmacy, and others as appropriate, to:

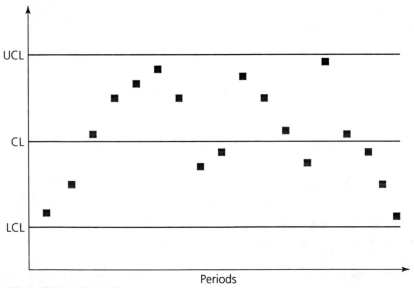

FIGURE EX 12.13.

a. Draw a flow chart for the medication process.

b. Construct a cause-and-effect diagram showing the potential causes of errors.

c. Develop a Pareto diagram to prioritize the causes (problems), for planning to solve them.

12.15 A hospital has identified nonrandom variations in patient falls.

a. Draw a flow chart showing under what circumstances a patient might fall.

b. Construct a cause-and-effect diagram showing the potential causes of falls.

c. Develop a Pareto diagram to prioritize the causes of falls for planning to solve the problem.

CHAPTER

13

PROJECT MANAGEMENT

LEARNING OBJECTIVES

- Describe the need for project management and its use for administrative and clinical operations.
- Review the information sources for project management in various health services operations.
- Evaluate projects with PERT/CPM techniques.
- Recognize risk in project completion, and develop probabilistic methods.
- Describe the concept of project compression.
- Evaluate the cost/benefit of project compression.

Health care managers typically oversee a variety of operations intended to deliver health services. Besides those, health care managers may work on projects that are unique and nonroutine, designed to accomplish a specified set of objectives in a limited time. Projects can be viewed as temporary endeavors undertaken to create new products and services (Klastorin, 2004; p. 3). Typical examples of such nonroutine projects are moving a hospital to a new location by a certain date or renovating an outpatient facility to meet changing demand patterns. Projects like these have considerable costs. They involve a large number of activities that must be carefully planned and coordinated to achieve the desired results, and may take a long time to complete (Stevenson, 2002; pp. 766–767 and Kerzner, 2004; pp. 179–180).

Project management is an approach for handling these unique, one-time endeavors that may have long or short time horizons, significant costs, and significant effects on the organization's operation. Since these projects include many separate activities, planning and coordination are essential to complete them on time, within cost constraints, and with a high quality result.

Most projects are expected to be completed within time, cost, and performance guidelines, meaning that goals must be established and priorities set. Tasks must be identified and time estimates made. Resource requirements for the entire project have to be projected. Budgets have to be prepared. Once under way, progress must be monitored to make sure that project goals and objectives are met. Through the project approach, the organization focuses attention and concentrates efforts on accomplishing a narrow set of objectives within a limited time and budget.

Project management can be handled by assigning existing staff to the project for its duration. However, problems arise if the project manager lacks expertise or continues to have responsibility for other assignments, and also later when the individual or team must be reintegrated into routine operations. For these and other reasons, often independent consultants are hired to take over project management for the health care providers. Whether projects are managed internally or externally, however, it is still important for the managers in health care organizations to understand project management concepts, in order to successfully manage internal projects and to understand the information presented to them by outside consultants.

THE CHARACTERISTICS OF PROJECTS

Projects have phases: planning, execution of planned activities, and phase-out. Those phases are known as a project's life cycle, and typically consist of four stages:

1. **Formulation and Analysis:** The organization recognizes the need for a project (for example, the need to replace a health care facility with a more modern one) or responds to a request for a proposal from a potential customer or client (for example, expanding health care services to secure a new third-party contract). The expected costs, benefits, and risks of undertaking the project must be analyzed at this stage.

2. **Planning:** At this stage, details of how the work will flow are hammered out and estimates are made of necessary human resources, time, and cost.

3. **Implementation:** The project is undertaken; most of the time and resources for a project are consumed at this stage.

4. **Termination:** The project is completed; tasks include reassigning personnel and dealing with leftover and excess materials and equipment.

During the project's life cycle, a project brings together people with expertise and diverse skills, who each become associated with only a portion of the project, rather than its full scope. Their involvement relates to their specialized skills. To manage these diverse, skilled personnel is a challenge that is the responsibility of the project manager.

The Project Manager

The central figure in a project is the project manager, who bears the ultimate responsibility for its organization and completion. A project manager must be able to communicate effectively among project team members and coordinate their activities to accomplish the objectives.

Once the project is underway, the project manager oversees a range of support activities. Both time constraints and costs must be managed so that the project is completed within the projected time frame and budget. Open channels of communication must be maintained so that everybody has the information they need to do their work. The quality of the work done must be assessed constantly to ensure that performance objectives are realized. Workflow must be managed so that activities are accomplished in the necessary sequence. Meanwhile, the project manager must also communicate with external constituencies such as regulatory boards, potential patients, subcontractors, and so on. Finally, it is important to direct and motivate the diverse people working on the project, as well as coordinate their activities (Stevenson, 2002; p. 769).

Managing Teams and Relationships on Projects

A project manager's job has its share of headaches as well as rewards. Personnel who are loyal to their bosses in their own functional areas have to be motivated by the project manager towards the project's unique goals. Since the team members report both to the project manager and to their functional bosses, the task of managing personnel with two or more bosses can be challenging indeed, especially with the dynamic and intelligent workforce in health care. Supervisors often are reluctant to allow their employees to interrupt their normal responsibilities to work on a project because their absence necessitates training replacements. Training costs may be incurred for a replacement who will work only over the project's life span, until the incumbent employee returns. In any case, supervisors are reluctant to lose the output of valuable employees. The employees themselves are not always eager to participate in projects because of the potential strains of working under two bosses in a matrix type of organization. From the employee's perspective, working on a project may disrupt daily routines and personal relationships. It also raises a risk of being replaced in the original position.

Another potential strain arises from the fact that the personnel who work on a project frequently possess specialized clinical knowledge and skills that the project manager lacks. Yet, the project manager is expected to guide their efforts and evaluate their performance. Apart from all these particular challenges, the environment in which project managers in health care facilities work is constantly changing and filled with uncertainties, in spite of which they must meet budgets and time constraints.

A project manager can, however, anticipate important rewards from adapting to and overcoming the unique challenges of the job: the career benefits of being associated with a successful project and the personal satisfaction of seeing it through to its conclusion. Many people embrace the dynamic environment of a project as a welcome diversion from routine tasks. They welcome the challenge of working under pressure and solving new problems. Projects may also present opportunities to meet new people and increase future job opportunities through networking. Project participants can point to a successful project as a source of status among their fellow workers. Finally, projects frequently generate a team spirit that increases the satisfaction of achieving project goals (Stevenson, 2002 pp. 770–772).

Although project managers aim to have smooth operations, conflicts can occur in various areas: (A) priorities in scheduling and sequencing the tasks; (B) among the team members; (C) budget and costs; and (D) other administrative and technical issues.

Planning and Scheduling Projects

Planning a project starts once its objectives have been established and the project manager and major players of the team have been identified. For planning and scheduling the project there are useful methodologies available. The Gantt chart, the Program Evaluation and Review Technique (PERT), and the Critical Path Method (CPM) give project managers graphic displays of project activities and allow calculation of a time estimate for the project. Activities are project steps that consume resources and time. The crucial activities that require special attention to ensure on-time completion of the project can be identified, as well as the limits for how long others' start can be delayed.

The Gantt Chart

The Gantt chart is useful for scheduling project activities in the planning stage and then monitoring them by comparing their actual progress to planned progress. We will illustrate a Gantt chart, launching a new radiation oncology service, with the list of necessary activities and their duration, in Exhibit 13.1.

The Gantt chart depicts the duration of this project as sixty-four weeks; however, not all the activities occur at the beginning. For example, contractor selection—activity C—does not start until land has been acquired and a radiation oncologist hired—activity B. For certain decisions, the input of key personnel for the new service must be considered; dependency relationships exist among the activities. Some activities cannot start until after others are finished. Yet certain activities can be carried out parallel with others. For example, activities D and E can be carried out during the same time frame. What other activities in this example can be carried out simultaneously? Since a Gantt chart displays the information on a time scale, project managers can report the activities to their internal and external constituencies during their implementation. They also can monitor the work of the subcontractors for conformity to the schedule.

The Gantt chart's display of the schedule of activities is based on their sequential relationships, and those are identified during the formulation phase of the project. They are called dependency or precedence relationships. The activity precedence relationships for the example of the radiation oncology facility are identified in Table 13.1.

EXHIBIT 13.1. Gantt Chart for Launching a New Radiation Oncology Service.

Activity	Time
A. Land acquisition	4 weeks
B. Hire a radiation oncologist	16 weeks
C. Select contractor and develop a construction plan	8 weeks
D. Build the facility	24 weeks
E. Acquire equipment	28 weeks
F. Hire technical staff	4 weeks
G. Purchase and set up information systems and software	8 weeks
H. Testing of equipment	4 weeks

This table displays the crucial information that structures the project, so that an activity cannot be started until after a previously necessary activity has been done. Similarly, those activities that can be performed simultaneously are identified.

Table 13.1 shows that activities A and B start around the same time and are followed by activity C. Activities D and E follow activity C and also should start at around the same time. Those two activities are followed by activities F and G, which should start simultaneously. Finally, activities F and G lead to activity H, the last activity, which will complete the project.

TABLE 13.1. **Activity Precedence Relationships.**

Activity	Predecessor
A	
B	
C	A, B
D	C
E	C
F	D, E
G	D, E
H	F, G

An obvious advantage of a Gantt chart is its simplicity, which makes it a very popular management tool. However, Gantt charts cannot depict other chronological relationships among the activities that also affect whether the project is done on time and successfully. For example, a Gantt chart cannot show a health care manager how a delay in one of the early activities will affect later activities. Conversely, some activities may be safely delayed without affecting the overall project schedule, but the health care manager cannot see that from a Gantt chart. This tool is most useful, then, for simple projects or for the early planning on more complex projects.

PERT and CPM

Program Evaluation and Review Technique (PERT) and the Critical Path Method (CPM) are tools for planning and coordinating large projects. Project managers can graph the project activities, estimate the project's duration, identify the activities most critical to its on-time completion, and calculate how long any activity can be delayed without delaying the project (Stevenson, 2002; p. 775).

PERT and CPM were developed independently in the late 1950s. Initially, PERT was developed by the U.S. government and private contractors in order to speed up weapons development, because it was believed then that the Soviet Union was ahead of the United States in their missile programs. CPM was developed by Du Pont and Remington Rand Corporation to plan and coordinate maintenance projects in chemical plants (Stevenson, 2002; pp. 770–772). PERT considers the probabilistic nature of completion times. CPM is used mostly for deterministic problems. Both methods, however, have common features for scheduling project tasks. For instance, the project manager must use the precedence information to visualize a network of activities, which can be accomplished in a couple of ways.

The Network

A network is a diagram of project activities and their precedence relationships, as shown with arrows and nodes. An activity represented by an arrow is called activity on arc (arrow), or AOA. An activity also can be represented by a node (a circle) and is then called an activity on node, or AON. Although in practice both representations are used, most project management computer programs are designed using an AON network because of its simplicity. To represent certain precedence relationships in AOA networks, a dummy arc with no time (or resource) must be used, which certainly may confuse nontechnical users.

Figure 13.1 illustrates the conventions used for activity on arc and activity on node networks. Three activities, A, B, and C are to be completed for the project. Activities A and B start and finish at the same time; activity C cannot start until A and B have been finished. In Figure 13.1, diagram (a) shows the conceptualization of these activities; diagram (b) represents the activity on arc (AOA); and diagram (c) represents the activity on node (AON). The activities in the AOA diagram show the consumption of resources and time. Nodes that appear in the AOA approach represent the beginnings and completions of activities, which are called events; since events are points in time,

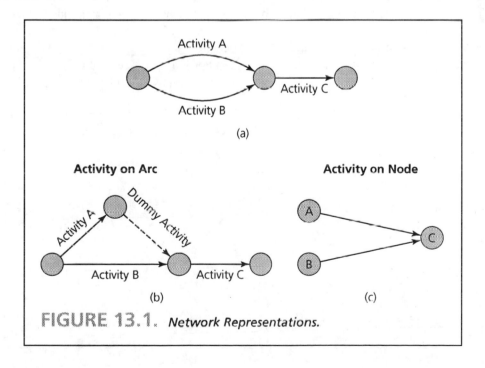

FIGURE 13.1. *Network Representations.*

they do not consume resources or time. However, when the events are represented by nodes in the AON diagram, they do represent resource and time consumption.

Most computer programs identify activities by their endpoints; so without dummy variables, activities sharing the same endpoints could not be separated, even if they had quite different expected durations. The AON approach usually uses more nodes, but it eliminates the need for dummy activities. In practice, both approaches are used; neither is more effective than the other. Most PERT/CPM computer programs can process either method. Often the choice depends on personal preference or established procedures. However, the AON convention is probably simpler for nontechnical users and is used in this text.

Projects are analyzed on the basis of the information that is available. If activity times and resource consumption are fairly certain, a deterministic analysis called the critical path method would be appropriate. On the other hand, if the activity times and resources are subject to variation, that leads also to variation in the project's completion, so in that case a probabilistic approach must be used.

Critical Path Method (CPM)

Let us consider the radiation oncology example presented earlier to illustrate the CPM method. Figure 13.2 displays the network diagram of this project using the activity on node convention and the precedence relationship displayed in Table 13.1.

One of the main features of a network diagram is that it shows the sequence in which activities must be performed. On AON networks, it is customary to add a start node preceding the activities to mark the start of the project, and an end node to mark its conclusion. Figure 13.2 shows that activities A and B must be completed before activity C can begin, and activities D and E cannot be started until activity C is finished. In ensuing sections, activities F and G cannot start before activities E and D are finished. Finally, activity H can start once activities F and G are finished.

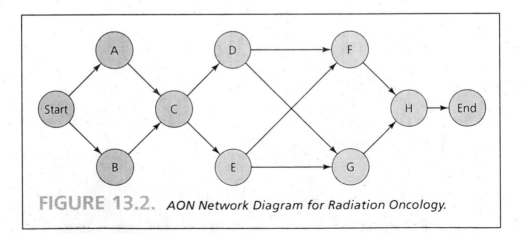

FIGURE 13.2. *AON Network Diagram for Radiation Oncology.*

A **path** is a sequence of activities that leads from the start node to the end node. The radiation oncology project has eight paths, as follows:

1) A-C-D-F-H

2) A-C-D-G-H

3) A-C-E-F-H

4) A-C-E-G-H

5) B-C-D-F-H

6) B-C-D-G-H

7) B-C-E-F-H

8) B-C-E-G-H

The length of time for any path is found by summing the times of the activities on that path. The time lengths for these eight paths, using times from Exhibit 13.1, are calculated and shown in Table 13.2.

The **critical path,** or the path with the longest time, is the most important: it defines the expected project duration. Paths that are shorter than the critical path could

TABLE 13.2. **Path Lengths for the Radiation Oncology Project.**

Paths and Activities	Path Time Length
1) A-C-D-F-H	4 + 8 + 24 + 4 + 4 = 44 weeks
2) A-C-D-G-H	4 + 8 + 24 + 8 + 4 = 48 weeks
3) A-C-E-F-H	4 + 8 + 28 + 4 + 4 = 48 weeks
4) A-C-E-G-H	4 + 8 + 28 + 8 + 4 = 52 weeks
5) B-C-D-F-H	16 + 8 + 24 + 4 + 4 = 56 weeks
6) B-C-D-G-H	16 + 8 + 24 + 8 + 4 = 60 weeks
7) B-C-E-F-H	16 + 8 + 28 + 4 + 4 = 60 weeks
8) B-C-E-G-H	16 + 8 + 28 + 8 + 4 = 64 weeks

encounter some delays without affecting the overall project completion time, as long as the highest possible path time is defined by the length of the critical path.

In this example, path 8 (B-C-E-G-H) is the critical path, with a total project completion time of sixty-four weeks. All activities on the critical path are known as **critical activities.**

The path sequences given in the above example would not be apparent in a computer program. In order for a program to identify paths, an algorithm is used to develop four critical pieces of information about the network activities:

ES: the earliest time an activity can start, if all preceding activities started as early as possible

LS: the latest time the activity can start and not delay the project

EF: the earliest time the activity can finish

LF: the latest time the activity can finish and not delay the project

Figure 13.3 shows that nomenclature, which this text uses to display those four times in a network diagram.

By computing the ES, LS, EF, and LF, one can determine the expected project duration, critical path activities, and slack time.

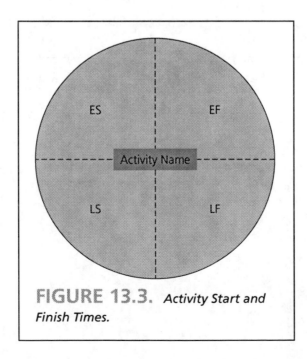

FIGURE 13.3. *Activity Start and Finish Times.*

Computing ES and EF Times. Two simple rules compute the earliest start and finish times:

1. The earliest finish time (EF) for any activity is equal to its earliest start time plus its expected duration, *t:*

$$EF = ES + \text{Activity time } (t). \qquad (13.1)$$

2. The earliest start time (ES) for activities at nodes with one entering arrow is equal to the earliest finish time (EF) of the entering arrow (the preceding activity). ES for activities leaving nodes with multiple entering arrows is equal to the largest EF of the entering arrow.

Computing LS and LF Times. The two rules for computing the latest starting and finishing times are as follows:

1. The latest starting time (LS) for each activity is equal to its latest finishing time minus its expected duration:

$$LS = LF - \text{Activity time } (t). \qquad (13.2)$$

2. For nodes with one leaving arrow, the latest finish time (LF) for arrows entering that node equals the LS of the leaving arrow. For nodes with multiple leaving arrows, LF for arrows entering that node equals the smallest LS of the leaving arrows.

To find ES and EF times, move forward from left to right through the network; to find LS and LF times, move backward from right to left through the network. Begin with the EF of the last activity and use that time as the LF for the last activity. The LS for the last activity is found by subtracting its expected duration from its LF. Figure 13.4 shows the calculated ES, LS, EF, and LS times for each activity. All project management software reports these values; nevertheless, the reader is encouraged to calculate a few to gain practical experience.

The allowable slippage of time for an activity, as well as for a path, is called **slack.** The slack for an activity is the difference between the latest start time and the earliest start time. It can also be computed by taking the difference between the latest finish time and the earliest finish time. Slack for a path is the difference between its length and the length of the critical path. The critical path has zero slack: all activities must start and finish at their allotted times. Formally, two ways to compute slack time are:

$$\text{Slack} = LS - ES \qquad (13.3)$$

or

$$\text{Slack} = LF - EF. \qquad (13.4)$$

Microsoft Excel - Project Management

File Edit View Insert Format Tools Data Window Help Adobe PDF

E29

	A	B	C	D	E	F	G	H
1		CPM - Deterministic				Length of Project =		64
2						Number of Critical Path(s) =		1

Activity Name	Description	Time	Predecessor
A	Land acqusition	4	
B	Hire radiation oncologist	16	
C	Select contractor & plan	8	A,B
D	Build facility	24	C
E	Acquire equipment	28	C
F	Hire technical staff	4	D,E
G	Setup software	8	D,E
H	Test equipment	4	F,G
I			
J			
K			
L			
M			
N			
O			
P			
Q			
R			
S			
T			
U			
V			
W			
X			
Y			
Z			

Activity Name	On Critical Path	Earliest Start	Latest Start	Earliest Finish	Latest Finish	Slack (LS-ES)
A	No	0	12	4	16	12
B	Yes	0	0	16	16	0
C	Yes	16	16	24	24	0
D	No	24	28	48	52	4
E	Yes	24	24	52	52	0
F	No	52	56	56	60	4
G	Yes	52	52	60	60	0
H	Yes	60	60	64	64	0

CPM-Deterministic / PERT-Probabilistic / GANTT-CHART-CPM / GANTT-CHART-PER

Draw AutoShapes

Ready NUM

FIGURE 13.4. *Excel Setup and Solution to the Radiation Oncology Project, CPM Version.*

Source: Screen shots reprinted by permission from Microsoft.

The four algorithms discussed previously can be used to find the critical path of a network diagram. Any activities with zero slack time are on the critical path. Knowledge of slack times lets project managers plan with more flexibility as well as detail for how to allocate scarce resources. They can focus efforts on those critical path activities that have the greatest potential for delaying the project. It is important to recognize that activity slack times are calculated on the assumption that all the activities on the same path will start as early as possible and not exceed their expected durations. Figure 13.4 depicts the Excel solutions to the example of the radiation oncology project.

Probabilistic Approach

Many real-life project networks are much larger than the simple network illustrated in the preceding example; they often contain hundreds or even thousands of activities. Because the necessary computations can become exceedingly complex and time-consuming, large networks are usually analyzed by computer programs rather than manually.

Often situations arise when health care managers cannot estimate activity times with certainty. Such situations require a probabilistic approach, which uses three time estimates for each activity instead of one:

1. **Optimistic time (o):** the length of time required under the best conditions.

2. **Pessimistic time (p):** the length of time required under the worst conditions.

3. **Most likely time (m):** the most probable length of time required.

These time estimates can be made by health care managers or by others knowledgeable about the project: contractors, subcontractors, and other professionals who have completed similar tasks or project components. They also could provide time and cost estimates for each task they are familiar with. Care should be taken to make the estimates as realistic as possible. The values can then be used to find the average or expected time for each activity t_e, and the variance of each activity time, σ^2. That calculation uses a **beta distribution,** where the expected time (mean) is computed as a weighted average of the three time estimates:

$$t_e = \frac{o + 4m + p}{6}. \tag{13.5}$$

The standard deviation of each activity's time is estimated as one-sixth of the difference between the pessimistic and the optimistic time estimates. The variance is then found by squaring the standard deviation:

$$\sigma^2 = \left[\frac{(p-o)}{6}\right]^2 \text{ or } \sigma^2 = \frac{(p-o)^2}{36}. \tag{13.6}$$

The size of the variance reflects the degree of uncertainty about an activity's time; the larger the variance, the greater the uncertainty. After completing the average time estimates and the variances for each activity, the analysis returns to the paths in the project network, since completing a project on time depends on the path completion times. The completion time for any path is a simple sum of all activity time estimates:

$$t_{path} = \sum t_e. \tag{13.7}$$

The standard deviation of the expected time for each path can also be computed, by summing the variances of the activities on a path and then taking the square root of that number:

$$\sigma_{path} = \sqrt{\sum \sigma^2_{path\ activities}}. \tag{13.8}$$

Once the probabilistic expected path times and their standard deviations are determined, a health care manager can calculate the probability that the project will be completed by a specified time, as well as the probability that it will take longer. Probabilistic estimates in network diagrams are based on the assumption that the duration time of a path is a random variable that is normally distributed around the expected path time. That follows from the fact that activity times (random variables) are being summed and that sums of random variables tend to be normally distributed when the number of items (here, project activities) is large, as is frequently the case with PERT projects. Even when the number of items is relatively small, the normal distribution provides a reasonable approximation of the actual distribution.

$$z = \frac{Specified\ Time - Expected\ Time}{Path\ Standard\ Deviation}$$

$$z = \frac{t_s - t_e}{\sigma_{path}} \qquad (13.9)$$

For probabilistic time estimates, it is assumed that path duration times are **independent** of each other, meaning activity times are independent of each other and that each activity is on only one path. The reason for using the independence assumption is simple: finding the probability of when an individual path will be completed makes sense only if that path's activities are independent of other paths. In a large project with many paths, the independence assumption is considered to be met if only a few activities are shared among paths. Project managers use common sense to decide whether the independence assumption is justified.

One final, important point before looking at a probabilistic network example: sometimes a path other than the critical path takes longer to complete, making the project run longer than expected. Therefore, it can be risky to focus exclusively on the critical path. Health care managers must always consider the possibility that at least one other path will delay the overall completion of the project beyond the expected time. They therefore should compute the probability that all paths will finish by a specified time. To do that, find the probability for each path finishing by its specified time and multiply the resulting probabilities to find the **joint probability** of timely completion.

The probabilistic PERT concepts are illustrated in Example 13.1 using the earlier radiation oncology case adapted to probabilistic time outcomes.

EXAMPLE 13.1

In planning for a new radiation oncology clinic, project managers determined that due to the nature of some of the activities, time estimates vary. After consulting with experts in each of the activity areas, they have calculated the optimistic, pessimistic, and most likely time estimates, in weeks, as shown in Table 13.3.

TABLE 13.3. Probabilistic Time Estimates for Radiation Oncology Clinic.

Activity	Optimistic (o)	Most Likely (m)	Pessimistic (p)
A	2	4	8
B	8	16	24
C	4	8	16
D	12	24	36
E	16	28	36
F	2	4	12
G	4	8	12
H	2	4	6

The network diagram for this project was shown in Figure 13.2, and the paths and activities for each path were shown in Table 13.2. In order to calculate project completion time probabilities, first we must calculate the expected time and variance for each activity and path. Table 13.4 displays the calculations for each activity and path: the means (t_e) and standard deviations (s) for all eight possible paths for the project. Given this information, the health care project manager can develop probabilistic estimates for the completion of the project, for various specified opening times or target dates (t_s). The expected completion times of paths (t_{path}) vary from forty-six (ACDFH) to sixty-four (BCEGH) weeks. Therefore, in calculating the project completion probabilities for a target date, all paths must be considered, especially those closest to the critical path.

Although we computed each activity's mean and variance using a beta distribution, path means and variances, on the other hand, are normally distributed (having many activities approximates to normality by invoking the central limit theorem). The critical path in this example is path 8 (BCEGH), which has the longest expected completion time. Besides that, the expected time can go beyond sixty-four weeks because of variation (standard deviation of approximately five weeks). That is, if sixty-four weeks is the average completion time (t_e), that indicates 50 percent completion probability under the normal curve. For an additional five weeks (one standard deviation, or

TABLE 13.4. Calculation of Expected Time and Standard Deviations on Each Path for the Radiation Oncology Clinic.

Paths	Activities	o	m	p	$t_e = \dfrac{o+4m+p}{6}$	$t_{path} = \Sigma t_e$	$\sigma^2 = \dfrac{(p-o)^2}{36}$	$\Sigma\sigma^2$	σ_{path}
1	A	2	4	8	4.33		1.00		
	C	4	8	16	8.67		4.00		
	D	12	24	36	24.00	46.00	16.00	24.22	4.92
	F	2	4	12	5.00		2.78		
	H	2	4	6	4.00		0.44		
2	A	2	4	8	4.33		1.00		
	C	4	8	16	8.67		4.00		
	D	12	24	36	24.00	49.00	16.00	23.22	4.82
	G	4	8	12	8.00		1.78		
	H	2	4	6	4.00		0.44		
3	A	2	4	8	4.33		1.00		
	C	4	8	16	8.67		4.00		
	E	16	28	36	27.33	49.33	11.11	19.33	4.40
	F	2	4	12	5.00		2.78		
	H	2	4	6	4.00		0.44		
4	A	2	4	8	4.33		1.00		
	C	4	8	16	8.67		4.00		
	E	16	28	36	27.33	52.33	11.11	18.33	4.28
	G	4	8	12	8.00		1.78		
	H	2	4	6	4.00		0.44		
5	B	8	16	24	16.00		7.11		
	C	4	8	16	8.67		4.00		
	D	12	24	36	24.00	57.67	16.00	30.33	5.51
	F	2	4	12	5.00		2.78		
	H	2	4	6	4.00		0.44		
6	B	8	16	24	16.00		7.11		
	C	4	8	16	8.67		4.00		
	D	12	24	36	24.00	60.67	16.00	29.33	5.42
	G	4	8	12	8.00		1.78		
	H	2	4	6	4.00		0.44		
7	B	8	16	24	16.00		7.11		
	C	4	8	16	8.67		4.00		
	E	16	28	36	27.33	61.00	11.11	25.44	5.04
	F	2	4	12	5.00		2.78		
	H	2	4	6	4.00		0.44		
8	B	8	16	24	16.00		7.11		
	C	4	8	16	8.67		4.00		
	E	16	28	36	27.33	64.00	11.11	24.44	4.94
	G	4	8	12	8.00		1.78		
	H	2	4	6	4.00		0.44		

$z = 1$), or specifically by week sixty-nine (t_y), the project completion probability can be improved to 84 percent. Figure 13.5 illustrates this concept. Completion probability nears 100 percent when the standard deviate z is 3.5 or more.

Again, note that each path's expected duration time is assumed to be independent, that is, each activity is on one path, and activity times are independent of each other. However, if a few activities are on multiple paths, we can assume a weak independence.

Table 13.5 depicts the calculation of z-values for each path in the example, for sixty-five weeks as the targeted completion time. As can be observed, paths 1 through 4 have z-values greater than 2.5, so those paths should have no significance for completion of other paths. To observe the impact of the remaining four paths (5 through 8), we can calculate the probabilities, as shown in Figure 13.6.

The last step in the analysis is the computation of joint probability, that is, we are interested in the joint effect of all the paths on the completion of the project. This is a simple multiplication of the completion probabilities of the significant paths (paths 5 through 8). The probability of completion of this project within sixty-five weeks is:

P (completion by sixty-fifth week) = .9082 $\times$ .7881 $\times$ .7852 $\times$ .5793 = .3255 or 32.5 percent.

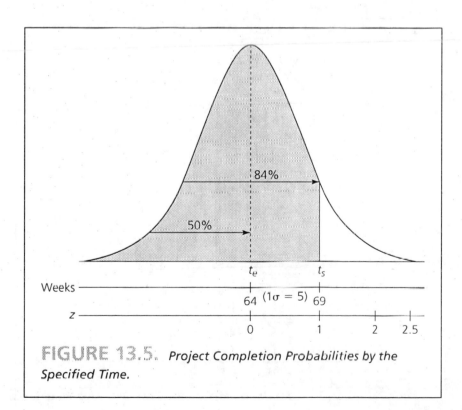

FIGURE 13.5. *Project Completion Probabilities by the Specified Time.*

TABLE 13.5. Path Completion Probabilities.

Path	t_{path}	σ_{path}	$z = \dfrac{t_s - t_e}{\sigma_{path}}$
1) ACDFH	46.00	4.92	3.86
2) ACDGH	49.00	4.82	3.32
3) ACEFH	49.33	4.40	3.56
4) ACEGH	52.33	4.28	2.96
5) BCDFH	57.67	5.51	1.33
6) BCDGH	60.67	5.42	0.80
7) BCEFH	61.00	5.04	0.79
8) BCEGH	64.00	4.94	0.20

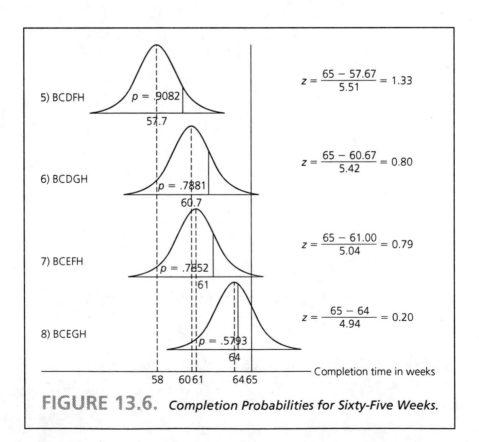

FIGURE 13.6. *Completion Probabilities for Sixty-Five Weeks.*

Similarly, one can compute the probability of completion for other target days such as sixty-six, sixty-seven, and seventy weeks.

P (completion by sixty-sixth week) = .9345 × .8365×.8389 × .6700 = .4394 or 43.9 percent.

P (completion by sixty-seventh week) = .9545 × .8770×.8830 × .7486 = .5533 or 55.3 percent.

P (completion by seventieth week) = .9871 × .9573×.9625 × .8869 = .8066 or 80.7 percent.

The Case of a Dominant Critical Path

If a critical path is dominant (no other paths are significant for completion probabilities), then joint probabilities need not be calculated. In such a case, software programs can calculate the completion probabilities for any number of targeted completion times. The Excel solution to the probabilistic radiation oncology project is shown in Figure 13.7. Figure 13.7 also depicts the solution for P (completion by the sixty-fifth week) as 58% and the completion time for target probability of 95% as about seventy-two weeks.

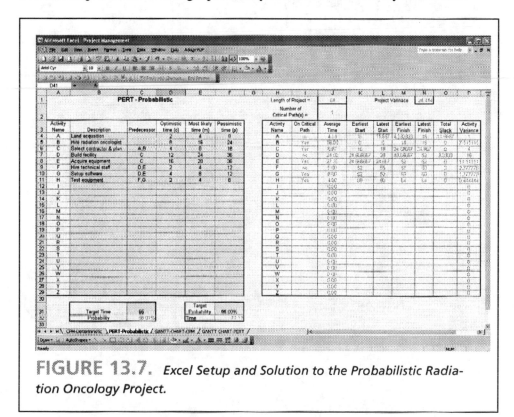

FIGURE 13.7. *Excel Setup and Solution to the Probabilistic Radiation Oncology Project.*

Source: Screen shots reprinted by permission from Microsoft Corporation.

Using this platform, a range of values for desired completion time in weeks can be evaluated, and a summary for decision makers can be tabulated as shown in Table 13.6.

Using this information, health care managers can assess how much risk they can tolerate in making firm commitments for the opening date. In particular, a manager who can assume a 5 percent noncompletion risk can set the opening date about seventy-two weeks after start of the project.

Project Compression: Trade-Offs Between Reduced Project Time and Cost

Today's health care environment offers many opportunities due to rapidly changing technologies. In a competitive market environment, these opportunities provide

TABLE 13.6. **Project Completion Probabilities.**

Desired Completion Time in Weeks	Critical Path	Probability
64	B-C-E-G-H	0.5000
65	B-C-E-G-H	0.5801
66	B-C-E-G-H	0.6571
67	B-C-E-G-H	0.7280
68	B-C-E-G-H	0.7908
69	B-C-E-G-H	0.8441
70	B-C-E-G-H	0.8876
71	B-C-E-G-H	0.9216
72	B-C-E-G-H	0.9472
73	B-C-E-G-H	0.9656
74	B-C-E-G-H	0.9784
75	B-C-E-G-H	0.9869
76	B-C-E-G-H	0.9924

incentives for early completion of projects. The strategic importance of market share gain with early product entry to the market often justifies consideration of earlier project completion. However, such opportunities do not come without added costs. Reducing project completion time requires shortening activity times, especially for activities on the critical path. A reduced activity time means more resources must be spent on that activity, raising its cost. Keeping this in mind, health care project managers must inform themselves of the costs of reduced activity times and perform a cost-benefit analysis for early project completion. The time for an activity can be reduced, for example, by adding more manpower (or overtime) or technology. Of course, the added manpower will increase the cost of the project, and the added cost must be compared to the potential gains. It is relatively easy to quantify the cost of added resources or technologies, but it is not so easy to quantify the strategic gains or potential benefits of early completion. Moreover, in certain situations organizations may face penalties for not completing projects expeditiously. For instance, a government regulation may have raised standards or established new patient safety processes (such as adopting bedside bar-coding technology), and if a provider organization has lagged in complying, then the due date can be accomplished only through condensing project times by investing more resources into the project. In such a case, clearly, paying stiff penalties versus paying the extra cost to meet the deadline and also being in compliance is the health care manager's choice in purely economic terms. The cost of the penalties (reversed rewards) would be well known. There are also situations in which the health care project managers cannot infuse resources to finishing projects earlier because certain activities simply cannot be completed before a set time. For example, to build a structure on a concrete footing, one must be sure to wait until the concrete hardens and settles. In practice, estimating how much an activity can be compressed yields only a rough approximation.

Close examination of a project's costs can clarify the dilemma a health care project manager faces. The main costs are of course the activity costs, and particularly their direct labor costs. Then there are indirect (overhead) costs. Finally, there can be project compression or crashing costs. Figure 13.8 illustrates the relationship among those costs.

The health care project manager's aim is to schedule the project so that the total expected costs are as low as possible or simply minimized. The cumulative project compression costs decrease as the project is scheduled for its normal completion time, but tracing the graph backwards from that point, one can observe that as the project duration is shortened, the cost of compression rises steeply. On the other hand, in that direction the overhead or indirect cost decreases as the project's duration is reduced. Thus, health care project managers must look at the overall cost picture, to settle on the best target date in terms of minimum total cost. Project managers would not opt for maximum crash time, since that has a steep cost, unless long-term potential benefits can be assessed and their net present value can be incorporated into the analysis. In a favorable long-term analysis, the shape of the total cost curve would shift toward the left, making such a decision appropriate.

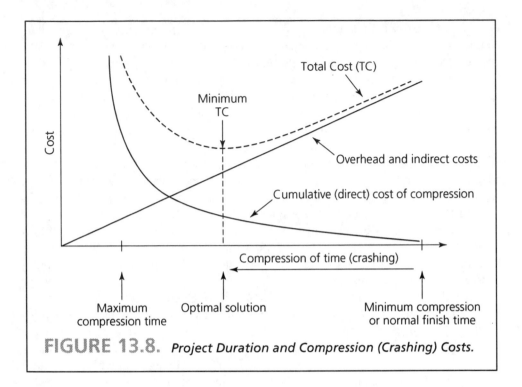

FIGURE 13.8. *Project Duration and Compression (Crashing) Costs.*

In order to carry out compression of the project, a project manager gathers estimates of the regular and the compression times and costs for each activity, and computes the lengths of all paths, including the critical path. Of course it makes sense to compress the activities on the critical path to reduce project completion time. However, if the lengths of the other paths are very close to that of the critical path, once the critical path length is seen to reach the length of one of those paths, then it will take working on multiple paths to reduce the project's completion time. In other words, in that case, there are multiple critical paths and the activity times have to be compressed on all of them. A general algorithm for project compression can be summarized as follows:

1. Compute path lengths and identify the critical path.

2. Rank the activities on critical path according to their compression costs.

3. Shorten the activity with the least compression cost and the critical path.

4. Calculate total costs.

5. Compare the total cost of the current compressed time to that of the previous compression time; if total cost has decreased, perform steps 1 through 4 again. Otherwise stop because optimum compression time has been achieved.

EXAMPLE 13.2

The indirect costs for design and implementation of a new health information system project are $8,000 per day. The project activities (A through I), their normal durations and compressed durations, and also the direct compression, or crashing, costs are shown in Figure 13.9. Find the optimal earlier project completion time.

Solution

We apply the algorithm shown earlier to this example in successive iterations to find the solution for the optimal earlier project completion time.

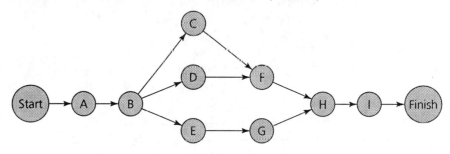

Activity	Normal time	Compressed time	Direct compression costs per day (in thousands)
A	20	19	11
B	75	74	8
C	42	40	6
D	45	44	10
E	28	26	7
F	21	18	20
G	40	40	0
H	20	19	18
I	20	19	20

FIGURE 13.9. *Project Compression.*

Iteration 1

Step 1: There are three paths. Adding the times of the activities, we obtain the path times. Since ABEGHI is the longest time path, with 203 days, it is the critical path.

Paths	Path Time
ABCFHI	198
ABDFHI	201
ABEGHI	203*

Step 2: Rank critical activities according to their costs.

Critical Activities	Compression Cost	Rank
A	11	3
B	8	2
E	7	1
G	n/a	n/a
H	18	4
I	20	5

Since activity G is not available for compression, it is not shown in the rankings. Among the remaining activities on the critical path, activity E has the lowest compression cost, and thus it is selected for time reduction.

Step 3: Since we can reduce this activity by two days, the new completion time considered for the project becomes (203 − 2 = 201) 201 days.

Step 4: The cost of compression for two days for activity E is 2 × $7,000 = $14,000. The indirect project cost for 201 days @ $8,000 per day amounts to $1,608,000 (201 × 8,000 = $1,608,000).

The total cost for 201 days then is equivalent to $1,622,000 (14,000 + 1,608,000).

Step 5: Without compressing the project, we would incur only the indirect costs, which would be for 203 days without the time reduction. The total cost for 203 days then would be $1,624,000 (203 × $8,000). Comparing that to the total cost for 201 days (see Step 4), $1,624,000 to $1,622,000, we observe a decrease. Thus we can continue compressing the project.

Iteration 2

Step 1: After compression of two days in Iteration 1, among the three paths we now have two paths with equivalent path times. Both ABDFHI and ABEGHI are the longest paths, with 201 days; thus both are critical paths.

Paths	Path Time
ABCFHI	198
ABDFHI	201*
ABEGHI	201*

Step 2: Rank critical activities according to their costs.

Critical Activities	Compression Cost	Critical Rank	Compression Activities	Cost	Rank
A	11	2	A	11	3
B	8	1	.B	8	1
E	7	n/a	D	10	2
G	n/a	n/a	F	20	5
H	18	3	H	18	4
I	20	4	I	20	5

Now we are considering critical activities from both paths simultaneously. In the ABEGHI path, we have exhausted compression time for activity E; hence it is no longer available for compression and is not shown in the rankings. Among the remaining activities on both critical paths, the activity B has the lowest compression cost, so it is selected for time reduction.

Step 3: Since we can reduce activity B by only one day, the new completion time to consider for the project becomes 200 (201 − 1) days.

Step 4: The cost of compression for activity B for one day is $1 \times \$8,000 = \$8,000$. The indirect cost for the project for 200 days @ \$8,000 per day amounts to \$1,600,000 ($200 \times \$8,000 = \$1,600,000$).

The total cost for 200 days, then, is equivalent to \$1,622,000 (\$14,000 + \$8,000 + \$1,600,000). Please note that the direct compression costs should be added in cumulatively; that is, for all three days of compression the project incurred \$22,000 (\$14,000 + \$8,000).

Step 5: From Iteration 1, the total cost for 201 days was \$1,622,000. Comparing that to the total cost for 200 days (see step 4), \$1,622,000 to \$1,622,000, we observe no change. Thus we can still continue compressing the project.

Iteration 3

Step 1: After compression by one day in Iteration 2, of the three paths we still have two paths, ABDFHI and ABEGHI, with 200 days each; both are critical paths.

Paths	Path Time
ABCFHI	197
ABDFHI	200*
ABEGHI	200*

Step 2: Rank critical activities according to their costs.

Critical Activities	Compression Cost	Critical Rank	Compression Activities	Cost	Rank
A	11	1	A	11	2
B	8	n/a	B	8	n/a
E	7	n/a	D	10	1
G	n/a	n/a	F	20	4
H	18	2	H	18	3
I	20	3	I	20	4

Again, we are considering the critical activities on both paths simultaneously. In both paths, we have exhausted compression time for activity B; hence it is no longer available for compression and is not shown in the rankings. Among the remaining activities on both critical paths, activity A ranks first in the ABEGHI path and activity D ranks first in the ABDFHI path. We must reduce both critical paths by one day to reduce completion time by the same amount. However, compressing Activity D from path ABDFHI and also activity A from path ABEGHI would cost $10,000 and $11,000, respectively, bringing the total compression cost for a one-day reduction to $21,000. Since activity A is common in both paths, choosing activity A to reduce time would cost only $11,000. Hence, activity A offers the lowest compression cost and is selected for time reduction.

Step 3: Since we can reduce activity A by only one day, the new completion time considered for the project becomes 199 (200 − 1) days.

Step 4: The cost of compression for a day for activity A is $1 \times \$11,000 = \$11,000$. The indirect costs of the project for 199 days @ $8,000 per day amount to $1,592,000 (199 × $8,000).

The total cost for 199 days, then, is equivalent to $1,625,000 ($14,000 + $8,000 + $11,000 + $1,592,000). Again, note that the direct compression cost should be added in cumulatively; that is, for all four days of compression, the project incurred $33,000 ($14,000 + $8,000 + $11,000).

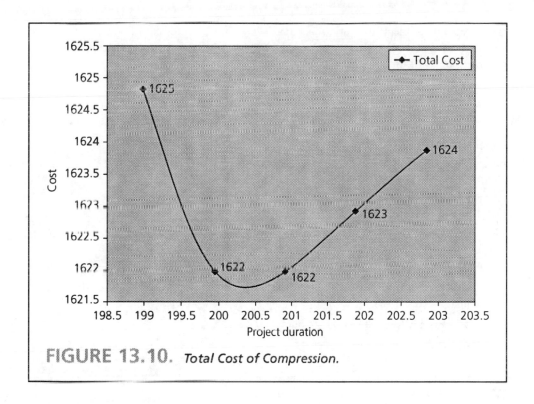

FIGURE 13.10. *Total Cost of Compression.*

Step 5: From Iteration 2, the total cost for 200 days was $1,622,000. Comparing the total cost for 199 days (see step 4): $1,625,000 to $1,622,000, we observe an increase. Thus we should stop compressing the project at Iteration 2. We should not spend $11,000 more to achieve completion at 199 days. Hence the optimum solution is 200 days. Figure 13.10 displays the total cost curve for project compression for this example.

SUMMARY

Project management is an approach for handling unique, one-time endeavors that may have long or short time horizons, significant costs, and significant effects on the organization's operation. Since these projects include many separate activities, planning and coordination are essential to complete them on time, within cost constraints, and with a high-quality result.

Projects are analyzed on the basis of the information that is available. If activity times and resource consumption are fairly certain, a deterministic analysis called the critical path method would be appropriate. On the other hand, if the activity times and resources are subject to variation, that leads also to variation in the project's completion, so in that case a probabilistic approach must be used.

This chapter examined each of those approaches and provided tools for early completion of projects.

KEY TERMS

Project Life Cycle
Project Manager
Gantt Chart
Critical Path
Probabilistic Approach

Beta Distribution
Joint Probability
PERT
CPM
Project Compression.

EXERCISES

13.1 Given the diagram shown in Figure EX 13.1, with activities A through G and duration times,

    a. Identify the paths and path duration times.

    b. Determine the critical path.

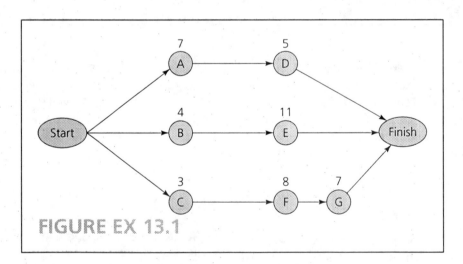

FIGURE EX 13.1

13.2 Given the diagram shown in Figure EX 13.2, with duration times for activities A through L:

    a. Identify the paths and path duration times.

    b. Determine the critical path.

13.3 Calculate ES, LS, EF, LF, and slack time for the activities in Exercise 13.1.

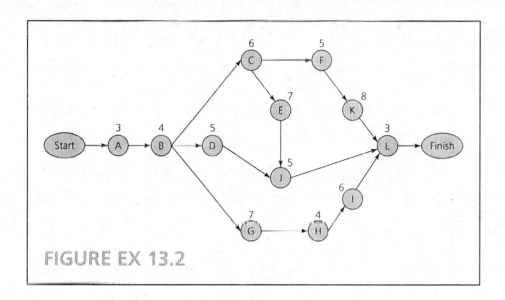

FIGURE EX 13.2

13.4 Calculate ES, LS, EF, LF, and slack time for the activities in Exercise 13.2.

13.5 Table EX 13.5 shows the precedence relationships among the activities to complete a project.

TABLE EX 13.5

Activity	Predecessor	Duration (days)
A	–	18
B	A	19
C	A	17
D	B	15
E	C	18
F	D	13
G	E	17
H	F, G	12

a. Construct an activity on node network for the project.

b. Identify the paths and path project durations.

c. Determine the critical path and the project completion time.

d. Calculate ES, LS, EF, LF, and slack time for each activity.

13.6 Table EX 13.6 shows the precedence relationships among the activities to complete a project.

TABLE EX 13.6

Activity	Predecessor	Duration (days)
A	–	23
B	–	20
C	–	29
D	A	8
E	B	18
F	D	15
G	C	19
H	D, E	16
I	F, G	12
J	H, I	14

a. Construct an activity on node network for the project.

b. Identify the paths and path project durations.

c. Determine the critical path and the expected project completion time.

d. Find the ES, LS, EF, LF, and slack time for each activity.

13.7 Table EX 13.7 shows the precedence relationships among the activities to complete a project.

Activity	Predecessor	Duration (weeks)
A	–	6
B	–	2
C	A	4
D	B	5
E	B	2
F	C, D	4
G	C, D	7
H	E, G	5
I	F	4

a. Construct an activity on node network for the project.

b. Identify the paths and path project durations.

   c. Determine the critical path and the expected project completion time.

   d. Find the ES, LS, EF, LF, and slack time for each activity.

13.8 Given the diagram of activities A through L shown in Figure EX 13.8, with their pessimistic, most likely, and optimistic duration times in weeks:

   a. Calculate the mean duration for each activity.

   h Calculate the variance for each activity time.

   c. Identify the mean and standard deviation for each path.

   d. Calculate the project completion probability for thirty, thirty-one, and thirty-two weeks.

13.9 There are four activities on the critical path of a network. The standard deviations of the four activities are one, two, four, and two days, respectively. Calculate the standard deviation of the critical path.

13.10 A health information systems company plans to design, market, and implement an information system that caters specifically to nephrology practices and interfaces with dialysis clinics, so that the physician's role in patient care can be proactive across the care continuum. Activities and their optimistic, pessimistic, and most likely activity durations in hours are shown in Table EX 13.10.

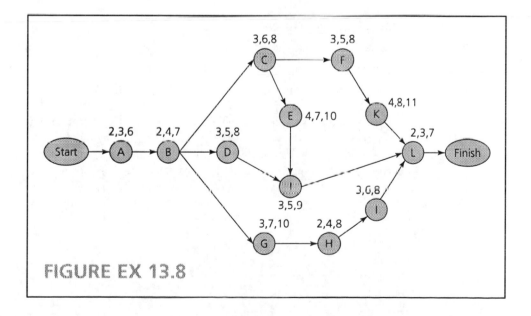

FIGURE EX 13.8

TABLE EX 13.10

Activity	Activity Description	Predecessor Activity	Optimistic	Most Likely	Pessimistic
A	Exploratory phase	–	65	157.5	250
B	Maestro modifications	A	590	940	1,290
C	Dialysis clinic interface	A	690	990	1,290
D	HL7 lab order interface	A	390	590	790
E	Scanned in documents	A	190	390	590
F	Standard phrase code set	A	8	29	50
G	Family history module	A	590	740	890
H	Outlook integration	A	1,090	1,690	2,290
I	Formulary import & check	A	390	590	790
J	Scheduler module	A	190	390	590
K	Physician encounter sheet	B	2,090	3,690	5,290
L	PDA module	K	1,090	3,190	5,290
M	Drug-drug & drug-allergy mod	I	390	590	790
N	Coordination of benefits	J	190	340	490
O	Referral tracking module	N	390	590	790
P	User training plan	C,D,E,F,G,H,L,M,O	40	50	60
Q	Marketing plan	L,P	60	150	240

   a. Calculate the mean duration for each activity.

   b. Calculate the variance for each activity time.

   c. Identify the mean and the standard deviation for each path.

   d. Calculate project completion probability for 8,200, 9,200, and 9,500 hours.

13.11 A hospital is planning to add a $60 million patient tower. In order to support both the existing hospital facility and the new patient tower, an existing energy plant will be expanded and upgraded. Equipment upgrades include a new generator, liquid oxygen tanks, cooling towers, boilers, and a chiller system to ensure adequate electricity, heating, air conditioning, hot water, and oxygen delivery systems. Existing fuel tanks will be relocated. The activities, their immediate predecessors, and the optimistic, most likely, and pessimistic times in weeks for this project are listed in Table EX 13.11.

TABLE EX 13.11

Activity	Activity Name	Predecessor	Optimistic	Most Likely	Pessimistic
A	Design	-	14	15	17
B	Budget estimate	A	2	3	4
C	Permits	B	14	16	19
D	Bid process	C	7	8	9
E	Subcontractor buyout	D	4	5	7
F	Startup	E	3	4	5
G	New additional construction	F	18	22	24
H	Cooling tower procurement	-	20	22	24
I	Cooling tower installation	G,H	9	11	12
J	LOX/fuel tank	I	1	1	3
K	Boiler procurement	-	29	30	31
L	Boiler installation	I,K	19	31	34
M	Abate old boiler	L	1	1	3
N	Chiller procurement	-	28	30	32
O	Chiller installation	M,N	25	29	34
P	Generator procurement	-	28	30	31
Q	Generator installation	P	12	16	20
R	Final inspection/testing	O,Q	1	1	2

    a. Calculate the mean duration time for each activity.

    b. Calculate the variance for each activity time.

    c. Identify the mean and the standard deviation for each path.

    d. Calculate project completion probability for 147, 150, and 152 weeks.

13.12 After some fifty years in the present location, Survival-Is-Our-Business Clinic (SIBC) is building satellite outpatient centers to increase its market share. After consultation with the general contractor and internal and external agencies, the activities have been identified for the outpatient clinic plan. For each activity, the most likely, optimistic, and pessimistic time estimates in weeks, as well as each activity's relationship to other activities are identified. In addition, the compressed time, normal costs, and compression costs for the activities are identified in Table EX 13.12.

TABLE EX 13.12

Activity	Description	Predecessor	Optimistic	Most Likely	Pessimistic	Compressed Time	Normal Cost	Compression Cost
A	Lease space	–	8	14	20	12	1000	2000
B	Hire director	–	12	16	18	14	2000	3000
C	Procure equipment	B	6	12	15	10	2500	4000
D	Renovate	A,B	5	6	8	5	3000	4000
E	Install equipment	C,D	1	2	5	1	1000	2000
F	Hire clinical staff	-	3	5	7	4	2000	6000
G	Staff training	F	2	4	5	3	2000	4500
H	Marketing	-	10	11	15	11	3000	3500
I	Final inspection	E,G,H	2	3	5	1	2000	5000

a. Calculate the mean duration for each activity.

b. Calculate the variance for each activity time.

c. Identify the mean and standard deviation for each path.

d. Calculate project completion probability for twenty-nine, thirty-two, and thirty-five weeks.

e. Calculate the total project cost.

13.13 If there is an incentive of $500 per week of early opening for the SIBC's satellite outpatient center in Exercise 13.2, determine the compression activities and compressed completion time.

13.14 The compression times and the compression costs for in-house development or outsource contracting for each activity in the health information project, Exercise 13.2, are given in Table EX 13.14.

TABLE EX 13.14

Activity	Activity Description	Mean Time (hours)	Compressed Time (hours)	Compression Cost (In-House: $80/hr)	Compression Cost (Outsource: 150/hr)
A	Exploratory phase	157.5	157.5	$ 12,600	$ 23,625
B	Maestro modifications	940	500	$ 75,200	$ 75,000
C	Dialysis clinic interface	990	800	$ 79,200	$ 120,000
D	HI7 lab order interface	590	590	$ 47,200	$ 88,500
E	Scanned in documents	390	350	$ 31,200	$ 52,500
F	Standard phrase code set	29	29	$ 2,320	$ 4,350
G	Family history module	740	600	$ 59,200	$ 90,000
H	Outlook integration	1690	1100	$ 135,200	$ 165,000
I	Formulary import & check	590	500	$ 47,200	$ 75,000
J	Scheduler module	390	390	$ 31,200	$ 58,500
K	Physician encounter sheet	3690	3000	$ 295,200	$ 450,000
L	PDA module	3190	2000	$ 255,200	$ 300,000
M	Drug-drug & drug-allergy module	590	590	$ 47,200	$ 88,500
N	Coordination of benefits	340	400	$ 27,200	$ 60,000
O	Referral tracking module	590	500	$ 47,200	$ 75,000
P	User training plan	50	50	$ 4,000	$ 7,500
Q	Marketing plan	150	150	$ 12,000	$ 22,500

   a. The software development department employs ten programmers. If all ten work exclusively on this project during an eight-hour work day, in how many days can the project be completed?

   b. What is the project completion cost if the work is completed in-house?

   c. Develop a project compression schedule using outsourcing to overseas employees; what is the reasonable completion time in days (assume that you can use up to fifteen overseas employees working eight-hour days), if company could receive $200,000 for early completion bonus?

13.15 The Memorial Hospital is creating a new patient-focused care system by redesigning a floor of the existing facility. The change involves changes in information systems, nurse responsibilities, various policies, and equipment. In sum, six major tasks must be undertaken. A PERT network diagram of the project, as well as optimistic, most likely, and pessimistic times (in weeks) for each activity are estimated and given in FIGURE EX 13.15.

TABLE EX 13.15

Activity	Optimistic	Most Likely	Pessimistic	Cost of Activity	Weekly Compression Costs
A	1	3	5	50	25
B	1	1	1	40	—
C	1	2	3	40	40
D	4.5	5	8	100	30
E	1.5	2	5	70	90
F	3	5	7	90	70

—activity cannot be compressed

   a. What is the total project completion time (in weeks), and which path is critical?

   b. What does it cost to complete this project?

   c. What is the probability that the transformation will take more than ten weeks? [Hint: No consideration is given to cost; illustrate with three normal curves as in the text examples, and compute the joint probability to justify your answer.]

   d. If the profit opportunity for each week that the project is completed early is $60, how many weeks earlier should the project be completed (how many weeks should we crash) to minimize the total costs of the project?

[Hint: Use Table EX 13.15 to show your work; total costs of completing the project include both profit opportunity and direct cost and cumulative crashing costs.]

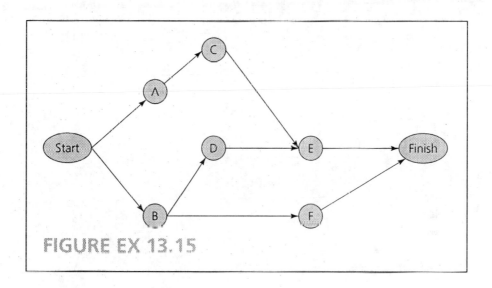

FIGURE EX 13.15

TABLE EX 13.15

(1)	(2)	(3)	(4)	(5)	(6)	(7)=(6)−(5)
Compressed Weeks	Total Weeks for Completion	Compressed Activities	Cost of Compression	Cumulative Compression Cost	Cumulative Profit Opportunity	Net Benefit
0	8	–	–	–		
1	7					
2	6					
3	5					

CHAPTER

14

QUEUING MODELS AND CAPACITY PLANNING

LEARNING OBJECTIVES

- Describe the queuing systems and their use in health care services.
- Recognize queuing concepts and their relationship to capacity planning.
- Describe various queuing model formulations that lend themselves to health care problems.
- Analyze the measures of performance in evaluation of queuing systems.
- Develop a model and solve a queuing problem in health services.

Queuing theory is a mathematical approach to the analysis of waiting lines. Waiting lines in health care organizations can be found wherever either patients or customers arrive randomly for services, such as walk-in patients and emergency room arrivals, or phone calls from physician offices to health maintenance organizations (HMO) for approvals. Patients arriving for health care services with appointments are not considered as waiting lines, even if they wait to see their health care provider. Most sorts of health care service systems have the capacity to serve more patients than they are called to over the long term. Therefore, customer waiting lines are a short-term phenomenon, and the employees who serve customers, or caregivers who serve patients, are frequently inactive while they wait for customers to arrive.

If service capacity is increased, waiting lines should become smaller, but then employees (called **servers**) will be idle more often as they wait for customers—or, in health care, patients (see Figure 14.1). A health care manager can examine the trade-off between capacity and service delays using **queuing analysis.** Specifically, when considering improvements in services, the health care manager weighs the cost of providing a given level of service against the potential costs from having patients wait.

Why must we wait in lines? The following example illustrates another waiting phenomenon. A hospital ER may have the capacity to handle an average of fifty patients an hour, and yet may have waiting lines even though the average number of patients is only thirty-five an hour. The key word is average. In reality, patients arrive at random intervals rather than at evenly spaced intervals, and some patients require more intensive treatment (longer service time) than others. In other words, both arrivals and length of service times exhibit great variability. As a result, the ER becomes temporarily overloaded at times, and patients have to wait. At other times, the ER is idle because there are no patients. Although a system may be underloaded from a macro viewpoint (long-term), variability in patient arrivals and medical service times sometimes causes the system to be overloaded from a micro standpoint (short-term). In systems where variability can be minimized—because of scheduled arrivals or constant service times—waiting lines should not ordinarily form. With the diversity of

FIGURE 14.1. *Queue Phenomenon.*

services and the arrival patterns in the health care sector, however, that condition is unattainable in many areas of delivery.

The goal of queuing is to minimize total costs. The two basic costs mentioned previously are those associated with patients or customers having to wait for service and those associated with capacity. **Capacity costs** are the costs of maintaining the ability to provide service. For example, physicians' and nurses' salaries, as well as other fixed costs, must be paid whether the ER is idle or not. **Waiting costs** include the salaries paid to employees while they wait for service from other employees (for example, a physician in a group practice, waiting for an exam room to be cleaned and readied for the next patient, or waiting for an X-ray or test result); the cost of waiting space (such as the size of a doctor's waiting room); and also the loss of business a health care organization can suffer when patients refuse to wait and go elsewhere in the future. Of course, society, too, incurs costs for more critical care when a patient has not been received soon enough because of congested waiting times or limited capacity.

It is difficult to accurately pin down the cost to the health care organization of patients' waiting time, so health care managers often treat waiting times or line lengths as a policy variable. An acceptable extent of waiting is specified, and the health care manager directs that capacity be established to meet that level. The goal of queuing analysis is to balance the cost of providing a level of health care service capacity with the cost to the health care organization of keeping patients waiting. The concept is illustrated in Figure 14.2.

Note that as service capacity increases, so does its cost; service capacity costs are shown as incremental (rising in steps for given service levels). As capacity increases, however, the number of patients waiting and the time they wait tend to decrease, so waiting costs decrease. A total cost curve is then added to the graph to reflect the trade-off

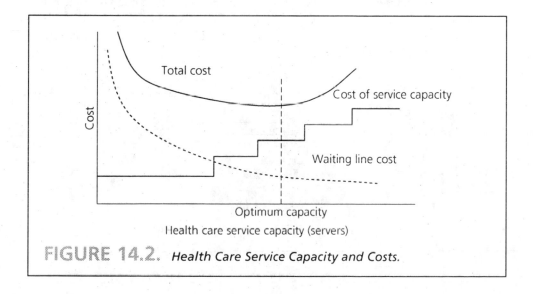

FIGURE 14.2. *Health Care Service Capacity and Costs.*

between those two costs. The goal of the analysis is to identify the level of service capacity that will minimize total cost.

Queuing System Characteristics

A health care manager can choose among many queuing models. Obviously, choosing the appropriate one is the key to solving the problem successfully. Model choice depends on the characteristics of the system under investigation. The main queuing model characteristics are: (1) the population source; (2) number of servers; (3) arrival patterns and service patterns; and (4) queue discipline.

Figure 14.3 illustrates a flu inoculation process as a simple queuing model: patients come from a population, enter on a queue (waiting line) for service, receive flu injections from a health care provider (server), and leave the system.

Population Source. The first characteristic to look at when analyzing a queuing problem is whether or not the potential number of patients is limited, that is, whether the population source is infinite or finite. In an **infinite source** situation, patient arrivals are unrestricted and can greatly exceed system capacity at any time. An infinite source exists when service (access) is unrestricted, such as at a public hospital ER. When potential patients are limited to small numbers, a **finite source** situation exists, for example when a mental health caseworker is assigned forty clients. When one or many clients leave or are added to the caseworker's assignment load, the probability changes of help being needed—a client needing therapeutic service. As seen in that example, then, finite source models require a formulation different than that of infinite source models. Other types of finite population situations are a health care facility (such as a PPO) contracted to serve the members of a given health insurance plan, or a physician practice with two thousand patients. For most of these queuing situations, however, infinite source models could be used, since the patient base is large enough not to cause any major shift in probabilities, and also would cause no significant errors. Hence, we will consider only infinite source models, as being usually more applicable to queuing and capacity problems in health care.

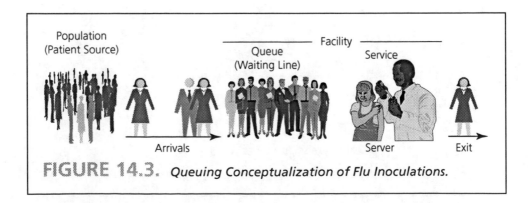

Population
(Patient Source)

──────────────── Facility ────────────────

Queue
(Waiting Line)

Service

Arrivals

Server

Exit

FIGURE 14.3. *Queuing Conceptualization of Flu Inoculations.*

Number of Servers. The capacity of queuing systems is determined by the capacity of each server (also known as a line or **channel**) and the number of servers being used. It is generally assumed that each channel can handle one customer at a time. Health care systems can be conceptualized as **single-line** or **multiple-line**, and may consist of **phases** (steps in a queuing system). Examples of single-line systems in health care facilities are rare. The flu inoculation example best illustrates one, in which a single health care provider carries out both administration (paperwork for consent, fee collection) and clinical care (inoculation) as a single server. In contrast, many solo health care providers (physicians, dentists, therapists) have offices with receptionists and nurses or other assistants; those are examples of single-line, multiphase systems. Figure 14.4 shows the conceptualization of a single-line, multiphase system. Patients arrive to see a receptionist, and if others are before them they wait until a receptionist is available [first queue]; eventually they reach a receptionist, process initial paperwork, and wait to see a nurse or physician assistant for initial examination of vital signs (blood pressure, temperature, complaint, and history taking) [second queue]; and they wait again until a physician is available [third queue].

Multiple-line systems are found in many health care facilities: hospitals, outpatient clinics, emergency services, and so on. Multiple-line queue systems can be either single-phase or multiphase. A single-phase, multiple-line system would be illustrated by an extension of flu inoculation to more than one server (three nurses giving inoculations and patients forming a single queue to wait) (see Figure 14.5). In actuality, most health care services are multiple-line, multiphase systems. For example, a nonurgent arrival to an emergency room can be conceptualized in several phases: (1) initial evaluation, (2) diagnostic tests, and (3) clinical interventions. Although the phases will vary from patient to patient, because each one receives care from several staff members in succession, the configuration in this case is a multiple-line queuing system. The lower half of Figure 14.5 illustrates the multiple-line, multiphase queuing example.

Arrival Patterns. Waiting lines occur because random, highly variable arrival and service patterns cause systems to be temporarily overloaded. Hospital emergency rooms

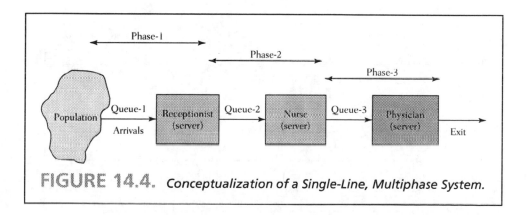

FIGURE 14.4. *Conceptualization of a Single-Line, Multiphase System.*

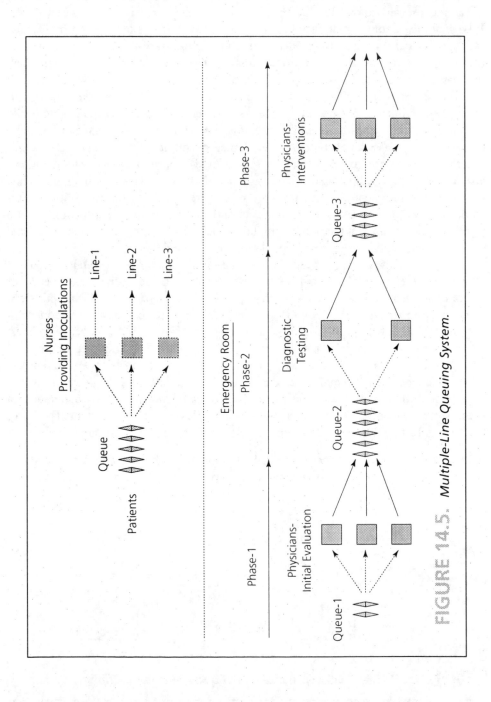

FIGURE 14.5. *Multiple-Line Queuing System.*

are very typical examples of erratic arrival patterns causing such variability. The arrival patterns might be different on mornings and afternoons, and even more so after physician offices close, in the evenings. In general, queues are more prevalent in evening hours and on weekends. Figure 14.6 illustrates the random behavior of arrivals at various times of the day and days of the week. The patterns on weekends are distributed more densely than those on weekdays, as are those during evening hours.

Besides that, in any block of time there are no discernible patterns, so the random nature of the arrivals—their numbers and the times between the arrivals—has to be measured. The variability can often be described by theoretical distributions.

The most commonly used models assume that the patient arrival rate can be described by a Poisson distribution and that the time between arrivals, inter-arrival time, can be described by a negative exponential distribution. Figure 14.7 conceptualizes the arrival rate and inter-arrival times.

Arrival rate is determined as the average arrivals for a given time period, as illustrated in Figure 14.7. During the hour of 9:00–10:00 P.M., there are six arrivals, and if that held true over the same time period for a number of days, then we could say that the average arrival rate is six patients per hour. The spacing between the arrivals, inter-arrival time, does not occur uniformly. The first patient arrives at ten minutes after the hour, the second fifteen minutes later, and so on. Such patterns are often characterized by negative exponential distribution. The mean of the negative exponential distribution,

FIGURE 14.6. *Emergency Room Arrival Patterns.*

average inter-arrival time, can be obtained by dividing the average number of patients arrived into the time period—in this case sixty minutes. Hence the average inter-arrival time for this example is 60 ÷ 6 = 10 minutes, which is interpreted as: patients are arriving on average ten minutes apart. One can convert arrival rate to inter-arrival time or vice versa, since arrival rates can be described with a Poisson distribution, which is more practical to use than negative exponential distribution. Poisson distribution, Figure 14.8, is a discrete distribution that shows the probability of arrivals in a given time period, where the mean and variance of the Poisson distribution are the same.

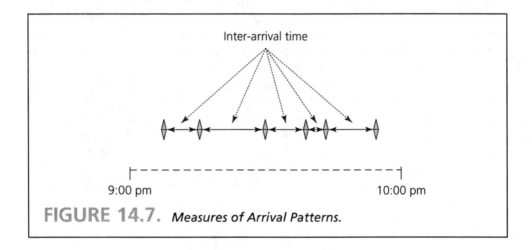

FIGURE 14.7. *Measures of Arrival Patterns.*

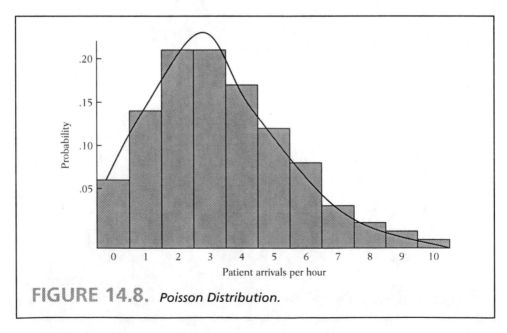

FIGURE 14.8. *Poisson Distribution.*

Service Patterns. Service to the arriving patients is another element that exhibits variability. Because of the varying nature of illnesses and patient conditions, the time required for clinical attention (service times) varies from patient to patient. Figure 14.9 illustrates a service pattern for ER patients when patient A requires over 100 minutes of direct clinical attention, but patient C requires about 25 minutes. As in the inter-arrival time, service time also can be described by negative exponential distribution. However, service rate and service times are also interchangeably used, so that the Poisson distribution can characterize the service rate.

In summary, the Poisson and the negative exponential distribution are alternate ways of presenting the same information. If service time is exponential, then the service rate is Poisson. Further, if the customer arrival rate is Poisson, then the inter-arrival rate (the time between arrivals) is exponential. In another example, if a lab processes ten customers per hour (rate), the average service time is six minutes. If the arrival rate is twelve per hour, then the average time between arrivals is five minutes. Thus, service and arrival rates are described by the Poisson distribution, and inter-arrival times and service times are described by a negative exponential distribution.

Queue Characteristics. Queues can be infinitely long or with limited capacity. A flu shot clinic with patients forming a queue around the block can be described as an infinite queue, whereas a physician office with fifteen chairs in a waiting room is an example of a limited-capacity queue.

A queue can be formed as a single line to one or more server(s), or it can be formed as separate lines for each server. In the second type, patients may jump from queue to queue to gain advantage in reaching a service point, but often lose more time because of service variability. Patients who arrive and see big lines (the flu shot example) may change their minds and not join the queue, but go elsewhere to obtain service; this is

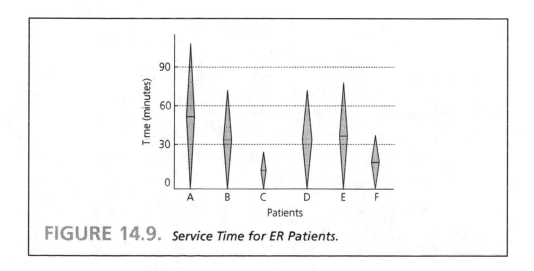

FIGURE 14.9. *Service Time for ER Patients.*

called **balking**. If they do join the queue and are dissatisfied with the waiting time, they may leave the queue; this is called **reneging.**

Queue discipline refers to the order in which customers are processed. The assumption that service is provided on a **first-come, first-served** basis is probably the most commonly encountered rule. First-come first-served, which is seen in many businesses, has special adaptations in health care queue discipline: shortest processing time first (for example, in the operating room simple or small surgeries may be scheduled first); reservation first (in the physician office); critical first (in the emergency room). Let us examine the example of the emergency room, which does not serve on a first-come basis. Patients do not all represent the same risk (or waiting costs); those with the highest risk (the most seriously ill) are processed first under a triage system, even though other patients may have arrived earlier.

Queuing models are identified by their characteristics. From a methods perspective, a nomenclature of A/B/C/D/E is used to describe them. Exhibit 14.1 provides details for each component of the nomenclature. The last two components, D and E, of the nomenclature are not used unless there is a specific waiting room capacity or a limited population of patients. Two examples of nomenclature in use are: (1) a queuing model with Poisson arrival and service rates with three servers is described by M/M/3; and (2) a physician office with waiting room capacity of fifteen, five physicians, and Poisson arrival and service rates is described by M/M/5/15.

Since infinite-patient-source models are our main focus, the last section of the nomenclature, "E," will be omitted in the ensuing discussions.

EXHIBIT 14.1. Queuing Model Classification.

A: specification of arrival process, measured by inter-arrival time or arrival rate.
    M: negative exponential or Poisson distribution
    D : constant value
    K : Erlang distribution
    G : a general distribution with known mean and variance

B: specification of service process, measured by inter-service time or service rate
    M: negative exponential or Poisson distribution
    D : constant value
    K : Erlang distribution
    G : a general distribution with known mean and variance

C: specification of number of servers — "s"

D: specification of queue or the maximum numbers allowed in a queuing system

E: specification of customer population

Measures of Queuing System Performance

The health care manager must consider five typical measures when evaluating existing or proposed service systems. Those measures are:

1. Average number of patients waiting (in queue or in the system)

2. Average time the patients wait (in queue or in the system)

3. Capacity utilization

4. Costs of a given level of capacity

5. Probability that an arriving patient will have to wait for service

The system utilization measure reflects the extent to which the servers are busy rather than idle. On the surface, it might seem that health care managers would seek 100 percent system utilization. However, increases in system utilization are achieved only at the expense of increases in both the length of the waiting line and the average waiting time, with values becoming exceedingly large as utilization approaches 100 percent. Under normal circumstances, 100 percent utilization may not be realistic; a health care manager should try to achieve a system that minimizes the sum of waiting costs and capacity costs. In queue modeling, the health care manager also must ensure that average arrival and service rates are stable, indicating that the system is in a **steady state,** a fundamental assumption.

Typical Infinite-Source Models

This section provides examples of the two commonly used models:

1. Single channel, M/M/s

2. Multiple channel, M/M/s > 1

where "s" designates the number of channels (servers).

These models assume steady state conditions and a Poisson arrival rate. The most commonly used symbols in queuing models are shown in Exhibit 14.2.

Model Formulations

Five key relationships provide the basis for queuing formulations and are common for all infinite-source models:

1. The average number of patients being served is the ratio of arrival to service rate.

$$r = \frac{\lambda}{\mu} \tag{14.1}$$

2. The average number of patients in the system is the average number in line plus the average number being served.

$$L = L_q + r \tag{14.2}$$

3. The average time in line is the average number in line divided by the arrival rate.

$$W_q = \frac{L_q}{\lambda} \tag{14.3}$$

4. The average time in the system is the sum of the time in line plus the service time.

$$W = W_q + \frac{1}{\mu} \tag{14.4}$$

5. System utilization is the ratio of arrival rate to service capacity.

$$\rho = \frac{\lambda}{s\mu} \tag{14.5}$$

Single Channel, Poisson Arrival, and Exponential Service Time (M/M/1). The simplest model represents a system that has one server (or possibly a single surgical team). The queue discipline is first-come, first-served, and it is assumed that the customer arrival rate can be approximated by a Poisson distribution, and service time by a negative exponential distribution, or Poisson service rate. The length of queue can be endless, just as the demand for medical services is. The formulas (performance measures) for the single-channel model are as follows:

$$L_q = \frac{\lambda^2}{\mu(\mu - \lambda)} \tag{14.6}$$

$$P_0 = 1 - \frac{\lambda}{\mu} \qquad\qquad (14.7)$$

$$P_n = P_0 \left(\frac{\lambda}{\mu}\right)^n \qquad\qquad (14.8)$$

or

$$P_n = \left(1 - \frac{\lambda}{\mu}\right)\left(\frac{\lambda}{\mu}\right)^n.$$

Once arrival (λ) and service (μ) rates are determined, length of the queue (L_q), probability of no arrival (P_0), and n arrivals (P_n) can be determined easily from the formulas.

EXAMPLE 14.1

A hospital is exploring the level of staffing needed for a booth in the local mall, where they would test and provide information on diabetes. Previous experience has shown that, on average, every fifteen minutes a new person approaches the booth. A nurse can complete testing and answering questions, on average, in twelve minutes. If there is a single nurse at the booth, calculate system performance measures including the probability of idle time and of one or two persons waiting in the queue. What happens to the utilization rate if another workstation and nurse are added to the unit?

Solution

Arrival rate: λ = 1(hour) ÷ 15 = 60(minutes) ÷ 15 = 4 persons per hour.
Service rate: μ = 1(hour) ÷ 12 = 60(minutes) ÷ 12 = 5 persons per hour.
Using formula (14.1), we get:

$$r = \frac{\lambda}{\mu} = \frac{4}{5} = .8 \text{ average persons served at any given time.}$$

Then using formula (14.6), we obtain

$$L_q = \frac{4^2}{5(5 - 4)} = 3.2 \text{ persons waiting in the queue.}$$

Formula (14.2) helps us to calculate number of persons in the system as:

$$L = L_q + \frac{\lambda}{\mu} = 3.2 + .8 = 4 \text{ persons.}$$

Using formulas (14.3) and (14.4) we obtain wait times:

$$W_q = \frac{L_q}{\lambda} = \frac{3.2}{4} = 0.8 = 48 \text{ minutes of waiting time in the queue}$$

$$W = W_q + \frac{1}{\mu} = 48 + \frac{60}{5} = 48 + 12 = 60 \text{ minutes in the system}$$
(waiting and service).

Using formulas (14.7) and (14.8), we calculate queue lengths of zero, one, and two persons:

$$P_0 = 1 - \frac{\lambda}{\mu} = 1 - \frac{4}{5} = 1 - .8 = .2, \text{ 20 percent probability of idle time}$$

$$P_1 = P_0 \left(\frac{\lambda}{\mu}\right)^1 = (.2)\left(\frac{4}{5}\right)^1 = (.2)(.8)^1 = (.2)(.8) = .16 \text{ or } 16\%$$

$$P_2 = P_0 \left(\frac{\lambda}{\mu}\right)^2 = (.2)\left(\frac{4}{5}\right)^2 = (.2)(.8)^2 = (.2)(.64) = .128 \text{ or } 12.8\%.$$

Finally, using formula (14.5) for utilization of servers:
Current system utilization (s 5 1);

$$\rho = \frac{\lambda}{s\mu} = \frac{4}{1 \times 5} = 80\%.$$

System utitilization with an additional nurse (s 5 2);

$$\rho = \frac{\lambda}{s\mu} = \frac{4}{2 \times 5} = 40\%.$$

System utilization decreases as we add more resources to it.

In M/M/1 queue models, arrival time cannot be greater than service time. Since there is only one server, the system can tolerate up to 100% utilization. If arrival rates are more than service rates, then a multi-channel queue system is appropriate.

Excel Solution. Using Excel queuing template, a simple M/M/1 queue problem setup and solution are shown in Figure 14.10. Readers can observe the same system performance measures as obtained via the formulas above, from the Excel. The probabilities for numbers of persons in the system at any given time can be observed at cell "C14" by changing the "n" value in cell "C13." Figure 14.11 depicts the probabilities of "n" persons in the system, where "n" is changed from 0 to 10.

Queuing analysis formulations for more than one server and other extensions require intensive formulations for queue length (L_q) and idle system (P_0) as shown in (14.9) and (14.10), respectively.

$$L_q = \frac{\lambda\mu\left(\dfrac{\lambda}{\mu}\right)^s}{(s-1)!(s\mu-\lambda)^2}P_0 \qquad (14.9)$$

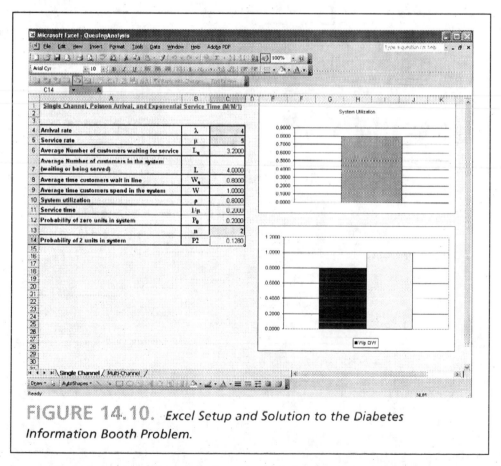

FIGURE 14.10. *Excel Setup and Solution to the Diabetes Information Booth Problem.*

Source: Screen shots reprinted by permission from Microsoft Corporation.

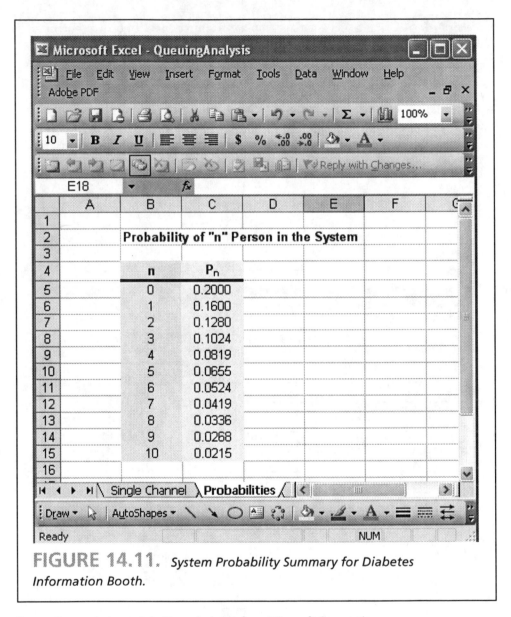

FIGURE 14.11. *System Probability Summary for Diabetes Information Booth.*

Source: Screen shots reprinted by permission from Microsoft Corporation.

$$P_0 = \cfrac{1}{\left[\displaystyle\sum_{n=0}^{s-1} \cfrac{\left(\cfrac{\lambda}{\mu}\right)^n}{n!} + \cfrac{\left(\cfrac{\lambda}{\mu}\right)^s}{s!\left(1 - \cfrac{\lambda}{s\mu}\right)} \right]}$$ (14.10)

In multi-server models, two additional performance measures can be calculated as shown in (14.11) and (14.2)

$$W_a = \frac{1}{s\mu - \lambda}$$ (14.11)

$$P_w = \frac{W_q}{W_a}$$ (14.12)

where

W_a = the average time for an arrival not immediately served, and

P_w = probability that an arrival will have to wait for service.

Hand-solving such problem is beyond both the intent of this text and the time available to health care managers. However, using Excel queuing template, that incorporates these formulas, one can employ such higher-order models for their capacity formulations and for measuring existing and redesigned systems' performance.

Multi-Channel, Poisson Arrival, and Exponential Service Time (M/M/s > 1). Expanding on Example 14.1: The hospital found that among the elderly, this free service had gained popularity, and now, during weekday afternoons, arrivals occur on average every 6 minutes 40 seconds (or 6.67 minutes), making the effective arrival rate 9 per hour. To accommodate the demand, the booth is staffed with two nurses working during weekday afternoons at the same average service rate. What are the system performance measures for this situation?

Solution. This is an M/M/2 queuing problem. The Excel solution provided in Figure 14.12 shows the 90 percent utilization. It is noteworthy that now each person has to wait on average one hour before they can be served by any of the nurses. On the basis of these results, the health care manager may consider expanding the booth further during those hours.

The M/M/3 solution of adding another workstation staffed with a nurse is shown in Figure 14.13. Increasing the capacity of the system from two to three servers improves the system performance measures significantly. Now, with three nurses, the average wait is reduced from .8526 hour (51 minutes) to .0591 hour (3.5 minutes), and the total time spent in the system is now 15.5 minutes, compared to 63 minutes (1.0526 hours) with two nurses. Of course, the expansion also reduces congestion in system utilization, which used to be 90 percent and is now at 60 percent. While these are improvements in the system, the probability of idle time for the nurses increases from 5.2 percent to 14.5 percent.

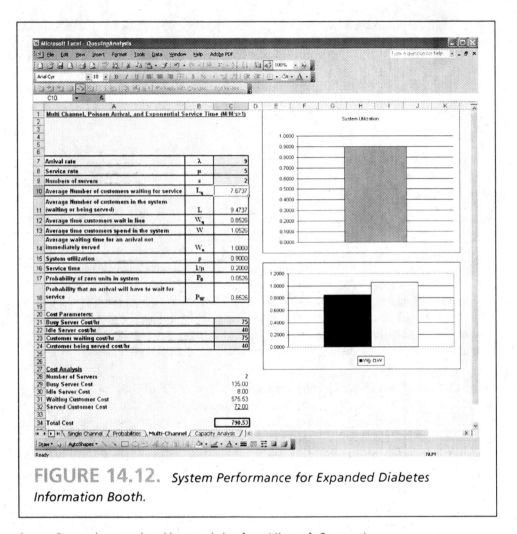

FIGURE 14.12. *System Performance for Expanded Diabetes Information Booth.*

Source: Screen shots reprinted by permission from Microsoft Corporation.

CAPACITY ANALYSIS AND COSTS

Up to this point we have explored system performance measures, but not considered costs. Health care information booths are marketing tools for health care organizations and as such should be assessed for cost-effectiveness. Total cost of a queuing system is calculated adding various costs involved. Here, we will consider busy server, idle server, waiting customer, and served customer costs as part of total cost. Calculation of the costs is shown in formulas (14.13) through (14.16) as follows:

$$C_B = c_b(L - L_q) \qquad (14.13)$$

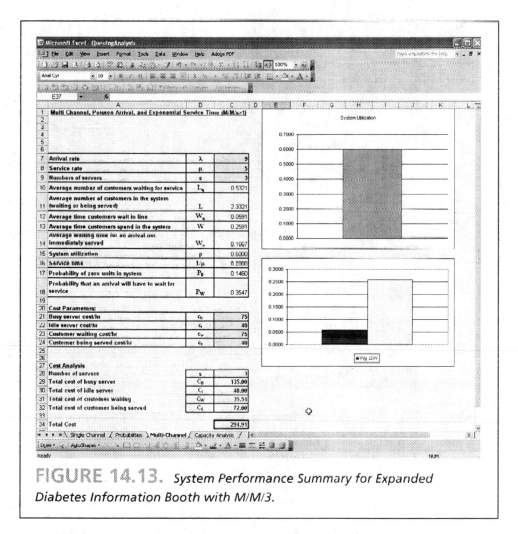

FIGURE 14.13. *System Performance Summary for Expanded Diabetes Information Booth with M/M/3.*

Source: Screen shots reprinted by permission from Microsoft Corporation and Yih-Long Chang (author of WinQSB).

where

C_B = Total cost of busy server

c_b = Busy server cost/hr

$$C_I = c_i(s - L + L_q)$$

(14.14)

where

C_I = Total cost of idle server

c_i = Idle server cost/hr

$$C_W = c_w W_q \lambda \qquad (14.15)$$

where

C_w = Total cost of customer waiting

c_w = Customer waiting cost/hr

$$C_S = c_s (W - W_q) \lambda \qquad (14.16)$$

C_w = Total cost of customer waiting

where

C_s = Total cost of customer being served

c_s = Customer being served cost/hr.

Total cost (TC) for the system is given by:

$$TC = C_B + C_I + C_W + C_S \qquad (14.17)$$

The health care manager should assess the impact of not serving potential patients appropriately (long waiting times in booths creating dissatisfied customers) against the capacity costs of the information booth (setting up terminals and staffing the booth with nurses).

Assuming an operational cost per hour of $40 (for the idle or busy server), and customer waiting costs (or busy-server cost) of $75/hour, one can evaluate the best capacity alternative for this problem. Figure 14.14 shows the data entry and solution to the optimum capacity calculation. The total costs column for each server number is the sum of costs associated with servers and customers. Here, the total cost of two servers (s = 2) is $790.53; with three servers the total cost goes down to $294.91 per hour; and when capacity increased to four servers, the total cost per hour increases to $302.89. Table 14.1 provides a summary of the M/M/s queue performance results under three capacities (s = 2, 3, 4) so the health care manager can evaluate them and conclude on a capacity. Three servers not only provide the minimum total cost per hour for this system, but also suggest a reasonable waiting time, queue length, and utilization rate. Thus, the optimal solution for the "diabetes information booth" capacity decision is three servers.

SUMMARY

The realities of health care organizations can be abstracted and analyzed using various queuing models, of which M/M/s is the most common. The key to this abstraction is to identify the bottleneck in operations and evaluate that portion of the

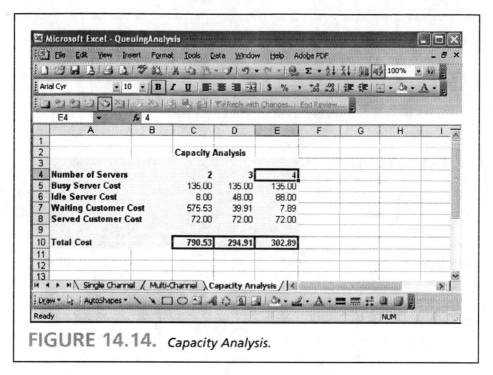

FIGURE 14.14. Capacity Analysis.

Source: Screen shots reprinted by permission from Microsoft.

TABLE 14.1. Summary Analysis for M/M/s Queue for Diabetes Information Booth.

Performance Measure	2 Stations	3 Stations	4 Stations
Patient arrival rate	9	9	9
Service rate	5	5	5
System utilization	90%	60%	45%
l (system)	9.5	2.3	1.9
L_q	7.7	0.5	0.1
W (system) — in hours	1.05	.26	0.21
W_q—in hours	0.85	.06	0.01
P_o (idle)	5.3%	14.6%	16.2%
P_w (busy)	85.3%	35.5%	12.8%
Total system cost in $ per hour	790.53	294.91	302.89

operation. For example, an emergency room may be responding to the needs of patients adequately during weekdays, but difficulties may be arising over the weekends and in certain hours of the evening. Then two separate models can be identified to solve the capacity requirements for those particular time periods by measuring the arrival rates at those times and the other particulars (costs).

Queue discipline is another factor especially important in health care. Health care managers must look at multiple priorities and process patient service according to the most urgent and least urgent. This problem, too, can be evaluated as separate problems in queuing situations—with varying arrival and service rates. That is, even in the same system, queue problems can be identified for different categories of patients. The case study provided at the end of the chapter is an example for this situation.

KEY TERMS

Capacity

Waiting Costs

Population Source

Server

Phases

Arrival Pattern

Service Pattern

Queue Discipline

Balking

Reneging

Steady State

Poisson Arrival

Exponential Service Time

Infinite Source

EXERCISES

14.1 People call a suburban hospital's health hotline at the rate of eighteen per hour on Monday mornings; this can be described by Poisson distribution. Providing general information or chaneling to other resources takes an average of three minutes per call and varies exponentially. There is one nurse agent on duty on Mondays. Determine each of the following:

   a. System utilization

   b. Average number in line

   c. Average time in line

   d. Average time in the system

14.2 One physician on duty full time works in a hospital emergency room. Previous experience has shown that emergency patients arrive according to a Poisson distribution with an average rate of four per hour. The physician can provide emergency treatment for approximately six patients per hour. The distribution of the physician's service time is approximately a negative exponential. Assume that the queue length can be infinite with FCFS discipline. Answer the following questions.

a. Determine the arrival and service rates.

b. Calculate the average probability of the system utilization and idle time.

c. Calculate the probability of no patients in the system and the probability of three patients in the system.

d. What are the average numbers of patients in the waiting line (L_q) and in the system (L)?

e. What are the average times that patients will spend in the waiting line (W_q) and in the system (W)?

14.3 On average, six nurses work per shift at a community hospital emergency service. Patients arrive at the emergency service according to Poisson distribution with a mean of six per hour. Service time is exponential, with a mean of thirty minutes per patient. Assume that there is one patient per nurse. Find each of the performance measures listed below, using Excel queuing template.

a. Compute the average number of patients in a queue.

b. Compute the probability of zero units in the system.

c. Compute the average waiting time for patients in a queue and in the system.

d. Compute the system utilization rate.

e. On the weekend, emergency service averages four patients per hour, and the service rate is expected to be forty minutes. How many nurses will be needed to achieve an average time in line of thirty minutes or less?

14.4 Ocean View General Hospital operates five cardiac catheterization labs. The hours of operation are ideally 7:00 A.M. to 4:30 P.M., but because of the nature of the work, the day doesn't end until all scheduled cases are completed. Patients are scheduled in the labs in ninety-minute time slots. Although each cardiologist performs at his or her own rate, the average time requirement for a diagnostic study is sixty minutes, and an interventional case including a stent requires about ninety minutes.

Patients are rarely scheduled more than three to four days in advance, and most are scheduled about forty-eight hours before the procedure. The patient mix is 60 percent outpatient and 40 percent inpatient. Outpatients are asked to arrive two hours in advance of their scheduled time, in order to prepare them for the catheterization lab, but also to provide flexibility in the schedule if a physician finishes early and cases can be moved up. The hardest part of managing this area is the unpredictable nature of the schedule. Emergency patients with an acute myocardial infarction have priority and are immediately taken into the lab, bumping scheduled patients.

Each lab is staffed with a team of three or four members, who are responsible for the care of the patient during the procedure and also for room turnover. They are not responsible for recovery of the patient or for the line-extraction process. This system enables them to turn the room over for the next patient in fifteen to twenty minutes postprocedure, increasing lab throughput.

The recovery room has fourteen staff assigned to cardiac catheterization patients. The lab performs 8,052 procedures per year and is open for 234 days a year. Catheterization labs are open for six hours of operations. Patients stop arriving two hours before the last scheduled case. The average procedure time is 87 minutes.

The following costs are associated with catheterization lab:

1.   Cost of the catheterization team idle: the four-member team of Registered Cardiovascular Invasive Specialists with an hourly rate of $22.00/hour. Total: $88.00/hour.

2.   Cost of waiting: the cost of care provided in the preprocedure area. A two-person team of an RN and an EMT are able to care for six preprocedure patients waiting to go to the catheterization lab. Hourly salaries: RN: $28.00 and EMT: $12.00. Total: $6.66/hour.

3.   Cost of customers being served: the average cost of performing a cardiac catheterization procedure is $800.00.

Using Excel queuing template, determine the optimum capacity for the Ocean View General Hospital's catheterization labs.

14.5   A major operation in an outpatient medical office is answering the telephones. This is especially true in primary care, such as pediatrics. Patients mostly use the telephone to communicate with the physician's office. In pediatrics, such interactions include calling for appointments, refills, medical advice, referrals, and forms (for example: school forms, camp forms.) Because of the frequent use of the telephone in outpatient pediatrics, it is an important focus for assessing productivity and efficiency.

A pediatric practice consists of nine physicians and two nurse practitioners. The practice has two offices. The patient population is approximately ten thousand children, with nearly fifty thousand visits per year. The phone system consists of sixteen telephone lines, most of them at the main office.

As the practice has grown, there have been increasing complaints from patients about wait time on the phone lines. All incoming calls are routed to the main office. When a patient dials the practice's office telephone number, a voicemail system directs the caller to press a number according to the purpose of the call (for example, "Press 'one' for appointments"). The system also distributes the phone calls according to whether the person calling is a patient, physician, laboratory, or hospital.

During the winter months, when the volume of sick patients is highest, a patient's wait can sometimes be as long as ten to fifteen minutes on the appointment line before speaking to a person. Since most customer service guidelines recommend telephone hold times no longer than one minute, this is an area that greatly needs improvement.

Telephone calls form a single waiting line and are served on a first-come, first-served basis. Arrival rates can be described by Poisson distribution, and service times can be described by negative exponential distribution. With these characteristics, a multiple-channel model for queuing analysis is most appropriate.

The queuing analysis of the practice's phone system can be divided into three parts of the work-day, which lasts from 8:00 A.M. to 5:00 P.M. For the first hour of the day (8:00 A.M. to 9:00 A.M.) there are usually three receptionists working to answer telephone calls only. For the last hour of the day (4:00 P.M. to 5:00 P.M.), there are usually five receptionists answering phones as well as checking patients in and out. For the bulk of the day, there are usually six receptionists working. The use of fewer servers during the first and last hours is primarily because fewer patients are being seen during those hours, so fewer servers are needed for checking patients in and out.

To determine the customer arrival rate (or phone calls/hour), incoming monthly phone call data for the previous year were obtained from the telephone company (Table EX 14.5.1).

From examining previous studies of the office's phone call volume distribution, it is estimated that 30 percent of the phone calls occur between 8 A.M. and 9 A.M., 40 percent between 9 A.M. and 4 P.M., and the remaining 30 percent arriving from 4 P.M. to 5 P.M. (Table 14.5.2).

TABLE EX 14.5.1

Month	Phone Calls
January	6,640
February	6,756
March	6,860
April	6,226
May	6,671
June	7,168
July	6,802
August	6,971
September	7,205
October	6,944
November	6,623
December	6,875
Total	81,741

To estimate the service rate (or phone calls/hour/receptionist), several sample studies were performed by an office administrator. It is important to note that the receptionists perform functions other than answering phones, such as checking patients in and out. Therefore, the number of phone calls that a server can answer per hour depends on the other responsibilities that the person has that day. In order to arrive at a service rate, the assumption was made that

TABLE EX 14.5.2

Customer Arrival Rates (λ)

8:00 A.M. to 9:00 A.M.	31 phone calls/hr
9:00 A.M. to 4:00 P.M.	42 phone calls/hr
4:00 P.M. to 5:00 P.M.	31 phone calls/hr
8:00 A.M. to 9:00 A.M.	31 phone calls/hr

the average maximum of phone calls per hour for the sample days would represent the servers operating at the maximum phone-call-answering capacity when having other responsibilities. While this assumption may underestimate actual server rate, for purposes of this study, the conservative estimate is acceptable in the absence of further data.

There is one exception to this assumption. During the first hour of the day, from 8:00 A.M. to 9:00 A.M., patients are not yet being seen in the office. Therefore, during that hour the servers have a faster telephone service rate, since they have no other primary duties (Table EX 14.5.3). From samples studied, we have determined that the maximum service capability when only answering phones is approximately four minutes per phone call, or fifteen calls per hour per server. This number was used for the service rate for the first hour (8:00 A.M. to 9:00 P.M.).

Cost studies were then performed based on the financial data from the previous year. Capacity costs were calculated based on salary and benefits per server and a percentage of the equipment maintenance, phone line costs, rent, and other capital expenditures (Table EX 14.5.4).

TABLE EX 14.5.3

Service Rate (μ)

8:00 A.M. to 9:00 A.M.	15 phone calls/hr*
9:00 A.M. to 4:00 P.M.	8 phone calls/hr
4:00 P.M. to 5:00 P.M.	8 phone calls/hr

With a total of fifty employees and a total of thirty full-time equivalents (FTEs), the portion of capital expenditures was determined as 1/30 of costs. Phone line charges were determined by a per-line charge, since one server would utilize one line each day.

Capacity cost or busy server cost would be equivalent to idle server cost. Regardless of whether or not the receptionist is answering the phone, she is paid the same salary and benefits and is using the same space and utilities. In addition, the practice must pay the phone line and equipment maintenance charges, regardless of usage.

For calculation purposes, a value was assigned to the cost of the customer of waiting. A value of $50/hour was assigned to customer waiting costs. In reality, though, customer waiting costs

TABLE EX 14.5.4

Total Hourly Cost for Busy Server Summary	
Salary	$13.00
Benefit	$3.75
Telephone Charges	$4.73
Capital Expenses	$4.83
Total Hourly Cost for Busy Server	$26.31

are likely to vary with the length of time waited, with a steep exponential increase in cost to the patient for longer times waited.

Using Excel queuing template, perform a queuing analysis for the pediatric practice's telephone system to determine the optimal server capacity for the volume of phone calls that they receive. Are there enough servers/receptionists and enough phone lines?

TABLE EX 14.5.5

Cost Summary	
Busy server cost/hr	$26.31
Idle server cost/hr	$26.31
Customer waiting cost/hr	$50

14.6 An outpatient clinic that is open two hundred days/year receives twelve thousand visits per year, or approximately sixty patients per day. These visits are divided over two wings, for thirty patients per wing. Appointments are made for two three-hour sessions per day. Thus, the patient arrival rate averages five patients per hour, $(\lambda) = 5$ patients/hour.

By observing the check-in and checkout processes, the service rate can be determined. Each check-in requires that the patient be retrieved from the waiting area, contact and insurance information be reviewed, and possibly a copay collected. This process takes approximately ten minutes, so the service rate for check-ins is six patients per hour. Thus, the service rate for check-ins is $(\mu) = 6$ patients/hour.

Checkout takes approximately twenty minutes per patient and involves scheduling follow-up appointments, ordering tests, and answering questions. Hence the service rate for checkouts is $(\lambda) = 3$ patients/hour.

Currently, three employees perform the administrative duties. One is assigned check-in duties, and the other two mostly check out patients. All are cross-trained on both roles, and in reality the staff varies from day to day in who performs which role.

To address the long wait times, the clinic administrator wants to evaluate hiring additional staff members. Assuming that both service rates approximate Poisson distribution, and using Excel queuing template, calculate the optimal staffing pattern for the clinic and the system performance measures.

14.7 Emergency room use at "SAVE-ME!!" Hospital peaks on Saturday nights during the period from 7:00 P.M. to 2:00 A.M. Historically, the hospital has provided space for five stations (examining rooms) for nonemergency cases and two stations for emergency cases during that period. Nonemergency patients are examined on a first-come, first-served basis, and emergency cases are treated on a most-serious, first-served basis, after a triage nurse has screened all cases. An area competitor hospital recently announced discontinuation of emergency services within six months. "SAVE-ME!!" estimates that current arrival patterns during the 7:00 P.M.–2:00 A.M. period would increase by one-third for nonemergency cases and would double for emergency cases. The hospital wants to know how additional resources in the ER might reduce congestion and waiting time, as well as the overall cost of operations for nonemergency and for emergency patients.

The past year's operating data were gathered from the information systems; they included records of arrival and service times. Preliminary examination of the data revealed little seasonal variation in ER use for that year, and ER personnel stated that their protocols and procedures had remained relatively constant since the reorganization of the ER two years ago.

The arrival pattern of patients, tabulated for twenty Saturday nights (total of one hundred hours), showed that 900 nonemergency and 150 emergency patients came to the ER during that time. The arrival pattern approximates a Poisson distribution. After a lengthy time-motion study, the average service time was found to be thirty minutes per nonemergency and seventy-five minutes per emergency patient. A separate study conducted by the finance/accounting department provided estimates for relevant costs as shown in Table EX 14.7.

TABLE EX 14.7

Cost type\Patient Type	NonEmergency	Emergency
Busy server cost/hr	100	200
Idle server cost/hr	450	800
Customer waiting cost/hr	200	400
Customer being served cost/hr	100	300

a. Using Excel queuing template, analyze both the emergency and the nonemergency capacity requirements for current conditions and for six months later, and fill in the Performance Evaluation Table.

Performance Measure	NonEmergency			Emergency		
	Current Capacity 3-Stations	Optimal Capacity ?-Stations	6-Months Optimal ? Stations	Current Capacity 2-Stations	Optimal Capacity ? Stations	6-Months Optimal ? Stations
Patient Arrival Rate						
Service Rate						
Overall System Utilization						
L (system)						
L_q						
W (system)						
W_q						
P_o (idle)						
P_w (busy)						
Total System Cost						

Note: Replace "?" marks on the table with optimal capacity.

b. Recommend the number of examining rooms for current and the future conditions on the basis of the above performance-evaluation statistics.

CHAPTER

SIMULATION

LEARNING OBJECTIVES

- Describe the concept of simulation and its use in health care services.
- Review the components of simulation modeling.
- Design a simple simulation problem in a health services organizational setting.

Simulation can be applied to a wide range of problems in health care management and operations. In its simplest form, health care managers can use simulation to explore solutions with a model that duplicates a real process, using a *what if* approach. In this way they can enhance decision making by capturing situations that are too complicated to model mathematically (like queuing problems). Consider construction of a spreadsheet with a financial planning model of a health care institution with many parameters. Suppose that the model is built in such a way that by changing forecast demand levels one can calculate the revenue and cost information associated with each. This, in its simplest form, is "what if" analysis: each time a parameter value is changed, a new solution is obtained. That is the essence of simulation.

SIMULATION PROCESS

Simulation models, like any other decision-making tool, must be constructed in a systematic way. The first step is to define the problem on hand and the objectives being sought. Once a health care manager has a good handle on that, she or he can start developing the technical aspects of the model (see the Monte Carlo described on page 391). Testing the model is the next step in simulation modeling, a very important one: the developed model should mimic reality, or the situation being modeled, very closely.

If the simulation outcomes are out of the expected range, then the conceptual model and its parameters have to be refined until they do produce satisfactory results.

To illustrate development of a simple simulation model, we will emulate patient arrivals at a public health clinic. As in queuing applications, performance measures for this situation will be tracked. We assume the patient arrival patterns and service process are random. Hence, we need an instrument to randomly simulate this situation. Let's call this the "simulator."

Imagine a coin as a simple "simulator" with two outcomes. For example, if the coin toss is heads "H," we will assume that one patient arrives during a determined time period (assumed to be one hour). If the outcome of the toss is tails "T," we assume no arrivals. Similarly, we must simulate service patterns. Let us assume that if the outcome of the coin toss is heads, it will take two hours to care for the patient (service time), and if it is tails it will take one hour. Table 15.1 displays this simple experiment for eight hours in which we toss the coin only once each hour. In the example, outcome of the coin toss for the first hour (8:00–8:59) is "H," for patient #1, and let us assume that patient arrives at the beginning of the hour. Now we have to follow that patient until he or she exits the system (clinic). Since there is no one before that patient, patient #1 proceeds to the physician for care, and the coin toss for service is "H," indicating two hours of service. Therefore the patient will be with physician from 8:00 to 9:59 and exits the system at 9:59, as reflected in the last column.

The coin toss for the second hour of business (9:00–9:59) is also "H," indicating the arrival of patient #2. However, this patient cannot see the physician right away because

TABLE 15.1. **Simple Simulation Experiment for Public Clinic.**

Time	Coin Toss for Arrival	Arriving Patient	Queue	Coin Toss for Service	Physician	Departing Patient
1) 8:00–8:59	H	#1		H	#1	–
2) 9:00–9:59	H	#2	#2	T	#1	#1
3) 10:00–10:59	H	#3	#3	T	#2	#2
4) 11:00–11:59	T	–	–	–	#3	#3
5) 12:00–12:59	H	#4		H	#4	–
6) 1:00–1:59	H	#5	#5	H	#4	#4
7) 2:00–2:59	T	–	–	–	#5	
8) 3:00–3:59	H	#6	#6	T	#5	#5

the physician is providing care for patient #1, so patient #2 must wait in the queue. We must know how long patient #2 needs service, and the coin toss is "T," indicating only one hour of service.

In the following hour (10:00–10:59), while patient #2 is seeing the physician, patient #3 arrives and joins the queue. Patient #3 also requires one hour of service. During the fourth period, there are no arrivals (coin toss is "T"); patient #3 moves out of the queue to the physician's care and exits the system at the end of the fourth period.

During the next two periods, patients #4 and #5 arrive, each needing two hours of service. Patient #5 waits in the queue until patient #4 clears the system. During the last period (3:00–3:59), another patient arrives (patient #6). That patient waits for patient #5 to clear the system, so when the clinic closes at the end of the hour, one patient is still in the system.

From the above simulation experiment we can collect the familiar performance measures: number of arrivals, average number waiting, average time in queue, service utilization, and average service time. The statistics of this experiment from the patients' perspective are summarized in Table 15.2.

Using the information from Tables 15.1 and 15.2, we can delineate the performance measures for this simulation experiment as:

▪ *Number of arrivals:* A total of six arrivals.

▪ *Average number waiting:* Four of the patients waited, over a total of eight periods; hence the average number waiting is 4/8 = 0.5 patient.

TABLE 15.2. **Summary Statistics for Public Clinic Experiment.**

Patient	Queue Wait Time	Service Time	Total Time in System
#1	0	2	2
#2	1	1	2
#3	1	1	2
#4	0	2	2
#5	1	2	3
#6	1	1	2
Total	4	9	13

- *Average time in queue:* Four of the patients waited one hour each; hence the average wait time for all patients is 2/3 hour or 4 minutes: 4 hours ÷ 6 patients = 2/3 hours or 40 minutes.

- *Service utilization:* For this case, utilization of physician services, the physician was busy for all 8 periods and had to stay one additional hour to take care of patient #6; hence the service utilization is 112.5 percent, 9 hours out of the available 8: 9 ÷ 8 = 112.5 percent.

- *Average service time:* Three of the patients required 2 hours of service each, and the other three patients only 1 hour of service each totaling 9 hours of service time; hence the average service time is 90 minutes, calculated by dividing total service time by the number of patients: 9 ÷ 6 = 1.5 hours or 90 minutes.

- *Average time in system:* To calculate patients' time spent in the clinic, we must add patient wait time in the queue to the duration of the physician's care time. From Table 13.2, the total time for all patients in the system is 13 hours. The average time in the system is 2.166 hours or 130 minutes, calculated by dividing 13 hours by the number of patients: 13 ÷ 6 = 2.166.

The experiment demonstrates that with simulation we can derive the solution to a problem without actually living through it. Here we can assess whether the system was over- or underutilized and the patient wait was tolerable. Keep in mind that this was only one experiment and that many more experiments must be conducted, and performance measures averaged over all of them, to obtain a reasonable approximation of real life situations. Furthermore, we must ask how realistic it is to use as the simulation a coin toss, which provides only two possible outcomes, as simulator. In real life we certainly can experience more than one—indeed, many arrivals in a given hour and also a wider range of service times.

Of course we could use a pair of dice, which could provide random arrival and service times for up to twelve different outcomes, but still the outcomes will be restricted by the shape of the object we were using. To overcome such limitations, we could use Monte Carlo simulation and a random number table.

Monte Carlo Simulation Method

Monte Carlo is a probabilistic simulation technique that is used when a process has a random component. The method requires developing a probability distribution that reflects the random component of the system being studied.

Process of Monte Carlo Method. Monte Carlo simulation follows these general steps:

Step 1: Selection of an appropriate probability distribution.

Step 2: Determining the correspondence between distribution and random numbers.

Step 3: Obtaining (generating) random numbers and running simulation.

Step 4: Summarizing the results and drawing conclusions.

To illustrate, we can simulate service at the public health clinic using Monte Carlo technique. The first step is to choose an appropriate probability distribution. Two popular techniques to generate arrival patterns from probability distributions are empirical and theoretical distribution.

Empirical Distribution. If managers have no clue pointing to the type of probability distribution to use, they may use an empirical distribution, which can be built using the arrivals log at the clinic. For example, out of 1,000 observations, the following frequencies, shown in Table 15.3, were obtained for arrivals in a busy public health clinic.

Here, each frequency has to be converted to a probability by dividing the frequency by the sum of frequencies (1,000). Then we can develop a cumulative probability table by summing the successive probabilities, as shown in Table 15.4.

The next step is to assign random number intervals to each cumulative probability breakdown. For no patient arrival (zero arrival), we must find from 0 to 18 percent probability, hence we must designate 18 percent of the random numbers to this event, or the numbers 1 to 180. Similarly, for the 1-patient-arrival category, we must assign 40 percent of all numbers, so we use 181 to 580, and so on.

Theoretical Distribution. The second popular method for constructing arrivals is to use known theoretical statistical distributions that would describe patient arrival patterns. From queuing theory, we learned that Poisson distribution characterizes such arrival patterns. However, in order to use theoretical distributions, one must have an idea about the distributional properties for the Poisson distribution, namely its mean. In the absence of such information, the expected mean of the Poisson distribution can

TABLE 15.3. Patient Arrival Frequencies.

Number of Arrivals	Frequency
0	180
1	400
2	150
3	130
4	90
5 & more	50
Sum	1,000

TABLE 15.4. **Probability Distribution for Patient Arrivals.**

Number of Arrivals	Frequency	Probability	Cumulative Probability	Corresponding Random Numbers
0	180	.180	.180	1 to 180
1	400	.400	.580	151 to 580
2	150	.150	.730	581 to 730
3	130	.130	.860	731 to 860
4	90	.090	.950	861 to 950
5 & more	50	.050	1.00	951 to 000

also be estimated from the empirical distribution by summing the products of each number of arrivals times its corresponding probability (multiplication of number of arrivals by probabilities). In the public health clinic example, we get:

$$\lambda = (0 \times .18) + (1 \times .25) + (2 \times .30) + (3 \times .15) + (4 \times .10) + (5 \times .05) = 1.7$$

The cumulative Poisson probability distribution for $\lambda = 1.7$ is shown in Table 15.5 along with the range of random numbers that have to be assigned for this purpose.

Random numbers must both be uniformly distributed and not follow any pattern. They must be picked in packs of three digits. Furthermore, we must avoid starting at the same spot on a random number table. Two of the best approaches are to use either a dollar bill or a die to determine the starting point on a random number table, approaches which can be found in any standard statistics text or can be generated using spreadsheet software (such as Excel).

Random Number Look-Up. For instance, using a random number table (such as that shown in Figure 15.1) if the serial number on a dollar bill starts with the digits 2,419, use the first digit to locate the row, and the second digit to locate the column. In this case the number would be 616. To select the next number, move through either rows or columns. Suppose we decide to move along columns, using the third number in the dollar bill serial number. If this number is odd, move downward; if the number is even, move upward. In this case, moving through the column, since the third number is odd (1), we move downward, picking the next series of numbers as 862, 56, 583, and so on until we reach 875, the end of the column. When the column is finished, we should move to the next column, based on the fourth digit of the serial number. If this number is odd, move

TABLE 15.5. Cumulative Poisson Probabilities for λ = 1.7.

Arrivals x	Cumulative Probability	Corresponding Random Numbers
0	.183	1 to183
1	.493	184 to 493
2	.757	494 to 757
3	.907	758 to 907
4	.970	908 to 970
5 & more	1.00	970 to 000

	1	2	3	4	5	6	7	8	9	10
1	519	135	800	898	971	317	236	511	530	165
2	737	545	641	616	969	573	423	250	878	977
3	338	586	352	862	91	388	316	231	689	964
4	558	722	683	56	764	52	412	597	33	101
5	618	228	307	583	180	830	415	993	46	665
6	941	672	488	908	903	880	85	164	958	669
7	511	664	510	848	780	761	623	683	677	102
8	857	665	998	38	164	444	696	387	894	675
9	303	427	696	536	546	994	619	61	945	727
10	821	302	483	668	351	254	170	435	260	85
11	171	692	569	255	900	562	938	774	240	860
12	300	595	220	142	915	541	381	874	602	145
13	648	139	382	776	955	606	520	750	178	411
14	669	270	298	324	683	948	230	930	115	865
15	113	871	190	646	989	29	403	186	182	835
16	124	611	494	59	230	77	79	587	251	47
17	687	467	707	354	283	850	899	985	866	832
18	20	718	520	455	487	808	430	736	937	425
19	595	355	282	245	158	154	544	77	92	830
20	535	538	165	674	38	351	610	711	787	680
21	934	27	356	201	73	660	561	905	000	188
22	262	699	596	91	87	11	838	775	465	827
23	284	6	24	454	203	790	453	968	402	66
24	326	873	349	177	141	784	840	619	808	96
25	629	254	121	875	965	905	251	220	675	807

Random number generator formula: =RAND()*1000

FIGURE 15.1. *Random Numbers*.
*Random numbers are generated using Excel.

Source: Screen shots reprinted by permission of Microsoft Corporation.

right; if even, move to the left column to find the next number. Since the number is odd (9), we move to the right column (column number 5), start with 965 and go upward.

If movement through rows is desired, then if the number is odd, move right; if even, move to the left column to find the next number. In this case, moving row-wise, since the third number is odd, we move right, picking the next series numbers as 969, 573, 423, and so on until we end the row with 977. Once the row is finished, we should move either up or down depending upon the value of the fourth digit in the bill serial number. If the number is odd, move down; if even, move up to find the next number. Since the number is odd (9), we move down one row (row number 3). We start with 964 and go left, picking other numbers as 689, 231, and 316 and so on until that row ends.

Going back to the public health clinic example, we can use the numbers, 616, 862, 56, 583, 908, 848, 38, and 536 obtained from Figure 15.1 to determine the arrival numbers, as we cross-reference our list of numbers with the corresponding numbers on Table 15.6 (Poisson distribution $\lambda = 1.7$) to generate a number for arrivals in each time period. Table 15.7 depicts the random numbers and their corresponding arrival

TABLE 15.6. Cumulative Poisson Probabilities for Arrivals: $\lambda = 1.7$.

Patients Arrived	Cumulative Probability	Corresponding Random Numbers
0	.183	1–183
1	.493	184–493
2	.757	494–757
3	.907	758–907
4 & more	1.000	908–000

SERVICE: $\mu = 2.0$

Patients Served	Cumulative Probability	Corresponding Random Numbers
0	.135	1–135
1	.406	136–406
2	.677	407–677
3	.857	678–857
4 & more	1.000	858–000

TABLE 15.7. Monte Carlo Simulation Experiment for Public Health Clinic

Time	Random Numbers (& Arrivals)	Arriving Patients	Queue	Random Numbers (& Service)	Physician	Departing Patients
1) 8:00-8:59	616 (2)	#1,#2	–	764 (3)	#1,#2	#1,#2
2) 9:00-9:59	862 (3)	#3,#4,#5	#4,#5	180 (1)	#3	#3
3) 10:00-10:59	55 (0)	–	–	903 (4+)	#4,#5	#4,#5
4) 11:00-11:59	583 (2)	#6,#7	–	780 (3)	#6,#7	#6,#7
5) 12:00-12:59	908 (4)	#8,#9,#10,#11	#9,#10,#11	164 (1)	#8	#8
6) 1:00-1:59	848 (3)	#12,#13,#14	#11,#12,#13,#14	546 (2)	#9,#10	#9,#10
7) 2:00-2:59	38 (0)	–	#12,#13,#14	351 (1)	#11	#11
8) 3:00-3:59	536 (2)	#15,#16		900 (4+)	#12,#13,#14,#15,#16	#12,#13,#14,#15,#16

λ column 2   serial # 248

μ column 3   serial #. 4572

numbers, as well as the patient numbers from the simulation experiment. Now, for each patient, we need to generate varying service times based on random numbers. Let us assume that the visit time with the physician has the characteristics of negative exponential distribution, with a mean service time of thirty minutes. Recall that a Poisson distribution can describe the service rate (reciprocal of the negative exponential distribution mean). Hence, the mean service rate $\mu = 2.0$ patients per hour (60 min ÷ 30 min = 2). The corresponding cumulative Poisson probabilities shown in Table 15.6 describe how many patients can be served in an hour.

Let us use another dollar bill to determine the starting point for picking random numbers for service times for the eight time slots. Assuming that the serial number is 4,572, we pick 764 as the starting point going downward. We record the numbers and their corresponding numbers for patients that can be served in the "Random Numbers (& Service)" column of Table 15.7.

Using information from Tables 15.7 and 15.8, we can delineate the performance measures for this simulation experiment as:

▪ *Number of arrivals:* There are a total of sixteen arrivals.

▪ *Average number waiting:* Of those sixteen arriving patients, in twelve instances patients were counted as waiting during the eight periods, so the average number waiting is 12/16 = .75 patient.

▪ *Average time in queue:* The average wait time for all patients is the total open hours, 12 hours ÷ 16 patients = .75 hour or 45 minutes.

▪ *Service utilization:* For, in this case, utilization of physician services, the physician was busy for all eight periods, so the service utilization is 100 percent, 8 hours out of the available 8: 8 ÷ 8 = 100 percent.

▪ *Average service time:* The average service time is 30 minutes, calculated by dividing the total service time by number of patients: 8 ÷ 16 = 0.5 hour or 30 minutes.

▪ *Average time in system:* From Table 15.8, the total time for all patients in the system is 20 hours. The average time in the system is 1.25 hours or 1 hour 15 minutes, calculated by dividing 20 hours by the number of patients: 20 ÷ 16 = 1.25.

This Monte Carlo simulation experiment demonstrates more realistic outcomes for the clinical example. However, simulations have to be repeated over and over again to obtain stable results in the long run. Of course it is impractically time-consuming to perform the analysis as described above. There are many computer-based simulation packages that can perform such analysis on very sophisticated problems by simulating the situations thousands or even millions of times to obtain solutions. These programs are also capable of reporting all performance statistics.

In practice, building simulation programs became very easy using icon-based process, distribution, and other parameter generators. Variations of GPSS, SIMSCRIPT,

TABLE 15.8. **Summary Statistics for Public Clinic Monte Carlo Simulation Experiment.**

Patient	Queue Wait Time +	Service Time =	Total Time in System
#1	0	0.5	0.5
#2	0	0.5	0.5
#3	0	1.0	1.0
#4	1	0.5	1.5
#5	1	0.5	1.5
#6	0	0.5	0.5
#7	0	0.5	0.5
#8	0	1.0	1.0
#9	1	0.5	1.5
#10	1	0.5	1.5
#11	2	1.0	3
#12	2	0.2	2.2
#13	2	0.2	2.2
#14	2	0.2	2.2
#15	0	0.2	0.2
#16	0	0.2	0.2
Total	12	8	20

and RESQ simulation programs are widely used. However, there is a significant learning curve for using such programs. Some health care managers may prefer to use spreadsheets to program their simulation models. Using Poisson distribution with $\lambda = 1.7$, patient arrivals for 100 simulated time periods (cases) were generated. In Figure 15.2, each random number and its corresponding simulated arrivals are displayed.

FIGURE 15.2. *Excel-Based Simulated Arrivals.*

Figure 15.3 demonstrates the programming for each cell for the first twenty-five cases, for random numbers and simulated arrivals.

PERFORMANCE MEASURES AND MANAGERIAL DECISIONS

One of the objectives in simulation modeling is to generate a solution to support health care managerial decision making. By examining performance measures, health care managers can choose among various operational, tactical, and strategic decisions. To closely examine such possible choices, especially in capacity decisions, let us define some parameters:

r_1 = Busy time during regular business hours ÷ Total regular hours open.

r_2 = Total busy time, including during overtime ÷ Total regular hours open.

r_t = Target utilization rate (for example, 90 percent).

The health care provider's current output (busy hours) rates, r_1 and r_2, compared to the target utilization rate, r_t, could provide basis for the managerial decisions. Figure 15.4 illustrates the possible decisions under such circumstances.

Template downloaded on Sakai

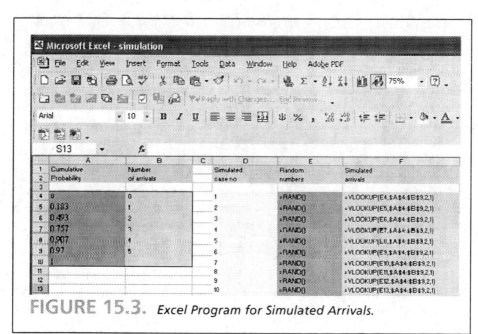

FIGURE 15.3. *Excel Program for Simulated Arrivals.*

Source: All screen shots reprinted by permission from Microsoft Corporation.

	$r_1 < r_t$	$r_1 >= r_t$
$r_2 < r_t$	Marketing and Referral Systems to Increase Business Volume	Status Quo
$r_2 >= r_t$	Appointment Scheduling	Increase Capacity

$$r_1 = \frac{\text{Busy time during regular hours}}{\text{Total regular hours open}}$$

$$r_2 = \frac{\text{Total busy time, including during over time}}{\text{Total regular hours open}}$$

r_t = Target utilization rate (e.g., 90%)

FIGURE 15.4. *Performance-Measure-Based Managerial Decision Making.*

The left side of the decision alternatives box shows two rows: values for busy rate with overtime, r_2, and for busy rate without overtime, r_1, in relation to the target utilization rate. If the utilization rate without overtime is greater than the target utilization rate $(r_1 > r_t)$; and the utilization rate with overtime is still less than target utilization rate $(r_2 < r_t)$, then the health care provider is functioning well within designed capacity. In that case, keeping the status quo would be the most appropriate decision. On the other hand, if the health care manager finds lower utilization rates both with regular time and with overtime and thus is not achieving the target utilization, $r_2 < r_t$ and $r_1 < r_t$, then effort and resources should be expanded on marketing and referral systems as tactical decisions to increase patient volume.

If a health care facility is using too much overtime but has lower volume, the situation could occur as $r_1 < r_t$ and $r_2 > r_t$—here the problem is operational: scheduling patients appropriately. The health care manager must adopt sound appointment scheduling and minimize the no-shows by using follow-up calls to scheduled patients for their appointments.

The last situation portrays a strategic decision where both r_1 and r_2 are greater than the utilization target—that is even with overtime the health care facility cannot catch up with demand. Under that circumstance, increasing capacity is appropriate.

SUMMARY

Like any method, simulation has both advantages and limitations. Simulation is advantageous for problems that are difficult to solve mathematically. Moreover, with simulation, health care managers can expeditiously experiment with system behavior without having to experiment with the actual system. A variety of simulation techniques can be useful in clinical decision making or in training medical decision makers: no harm can occur to patients from simulated scenarios.

Despite these advantages, simulation does require considerable effort to develop a suitable model, and even then does not guarantee an optimum solution. However, any respectable solution obtained through simulation, as long as it captures the reality as closely as possible, is better than spending vast amounts of time to build sophisticated mathematical models.

KEY TERMS

Simulator
Monte Carlo Method
Empirical Distribution

Performance Measures
Managerial Decisions.

Sakai - Figure 15.1

EXERCISES

15.1 Arrivals to a flu shot clinic held by a local grocery store follow Poisson distribution with a mean of 10. Including paperwork, it takes eight minutes to complete the flu shot process once a person's turn comes up. Using Monte Carlo simulation:

   a.   Simulate the process for the first twenty persons arriving for flu shots. *#15 1*
   b.   Determine the average time in queue. *⁎*
   c.   Determine the service utilization. *⁻*
   d.   Determine the average time in the system. *= Poisson distribution mean × 8 : 50*

15.2 Arrivals to a solo pediatric practice follow Poisson distribution with a mean of four patients per hour. Visit times for children depend on their condition and follow a negative exponential distribution with a mean of twenty minutes. Using Monte Carlo simulation:

   a.   Simulate the pediatric practice for twenty-five patients.
   b.   Determine the average time in queue.
   c.   Determine the service utilization.
   d.   Determine the average time in system. *4 Y*

15.3 Using Excel, simulate the flu clinic process in Exercise 15.1 for one thousand hours, and *– extra credit* answer the following:

   a.   How many persons arrived for flu shots?
   b.   How many balked due to queues?
   c.   What is the average number of persons in the system (L)?
   d.   What is the average waiting time (Wq)?
   e.   What is the average total time in the system (W)?

15.4 Using Excel, simulate the pediatric clinic process in Exercise 15.2 for one thousand hours, and answer the following:

   a.   How many children arrived for a visit?
   b.   How many balked due to queues?
   c.   What is the average number of children in the system (L)?
   d.   What is the average waiting time (Wq)?
   e.   What is the average total time in the system (W)?

15.5 Using Excel, simulate Exercise 14.1 for one thousand hours.

   a.   How many calls were received by the nurse?
   b.   How many callers hung up (were balked) due to the queue?
   c.   What is the average number of calls in the system (L)?
   d.   What is the average waiting time for a call (Wq)?
   e.   What is the average total time for a call (W)?

15.6 Using Excel, simulate Exercise 14.2 for one thousand hours.

   a.   How many patients arrived at the emergency room?
   b.   How many were balked due to the queue?
   c.   What is the average number of patients in the system (L)?
   d.   What is the average waiting time for an emergency room visit (Wq)?
   e.   What is the average total time for an emergency room visit (W)?

15.7 Using Excel, develop a simulation model for Exercise 14.6 and simulate for one thousand hours. Report the performance measures at the current capacity and make recommendations.

APPENDIX

Standard Normal Distribution P(o < z < x)

z	0.00	0.01	0.02	0.03	0.04	0.05	0.06	0.07	0.08	0.09
0.0	0.0000	0.0040	0.0080	0.0120	0.0160	0.0199	0.0239	0.0279	0.0319	0.0359
0.1	0.0398	0.0438	0.0478	0.0517	0.0557	0.0596	0.0636	0.0675	0.0714	0.0753
0.2	0.0793	0.0832	0.0871	0.0910	0.0948	0.0987	0.1026	0.1064	0.1103	0.1141
0.3	0.1179	0.1217	0.1255	0.1293	0.1331	0.1368	0.1406	0.1443	0.1480	0.1517
0.4	0.1554	0.1591	0.1628	0.1664	0.1700	0.1736	0.1772	0.1808	0.1844	0.1879
0.5	0.1915	0.1950	0.1985	0.2019	0.2054	0.2088	0.2123	0.2157	0.2190	0.2224
0.6	0.2257	0.2291	0.2324	0.2357	0.2389	0.2422	0.2454	0.2486	0.2517	0.2549
0.7	0.2580	0.2611	0.2642	0.2673	0.2704	0.2734	0.2764	0.2794	0.2823	0.2852
0.8	0.2881	0.2910	0.2939	0.2967	0.2995	0.3023	0.3051	0.3078	0.3106	0.3133
0.9	0.3159	0.3186	0.3212	0.3238	0.3264	0.3289	0.3315	0.3340	0.3365	0.3389
1.0	0.3413	0.3438	0.3461	0.3485	0.3508	0.3531	0.3554	0.3577	0.3599	0.3621
1.1	0.3643	0.3665	0.3686	0.3708	0.3729	0.3749	0.3770	0.3790	0.3810	0.3830
1.2	0.3849	0.3869	0.3888	0.3907	0.3925	0.3944	0.3962	0.3980	0.3997	0.4015
1.3	0.4032	0.4049	0.4066	0.4082	0.4099	0.4115	0.4131	0.4147	0.4162	0.4177
1.4	0.4192	0.4207	0.4222	0.4236	0.4251	0.4265	0.4279	0.4292	0.4306	0.4319
1.5	0.4332	0.4345	0.4357	0.4370	0.4382	0.4394	0.4406	0.4418	0.4429	0.4441
1.6	0.4452	0.4463	0.4474	0.4484	0.4495	0.4505	0.4515	0.4525	0.4535	0.4545

(Continued)

411

Standard Normal Distribution P(o < z < x)

z	0.00	0.01	0.02	0.03	0.04	0.05	0.06	0.07	0.08	0.09
1.8	0.4641	0.4649	0.4656	0.4664	0.4671	0.4678	0.4686	0.4693	0.4699	0.4706
1.9	0.4713	0.4719	0.4726	0.4732	0.4738	0.4744	0.4750	0.4756	0.4761	0.4767
2.0	0.4772	0.4778	0.4783	0.4788	0.4793	0.4798	0.4803	0.4808	0.4812	0.4817
2.1	0.4821	0.4826	0.4830	0.4834	0.4838	0.4842	0.4846	0.4850	0.4854	0.4857
2.2	0.4861	0.4864	0.4868	0.4871	0.4875	0.4878	0.4881	0.4884	0.4887	0.4890
2.3	0.4893	0.4896	0.4898	0.4901	0.4904	0.4906	0.4909	0.4911	0.4913	0.4916
2.4	0.4918	0.4920	0.4922	0.4925	0.4927	0.4929	0.4931	0.4932	0.4934	0.4936
2.5	0.4938	0.4940	0.4941	0.4943	0.4945	0.4946	0.4948	0.4949	0.4951	0.4952
2.6	0.4953	0.4955	0.4956	0.4957	0.4959	0.4960	0.4961	0.4962	0.4963	0.4964
2.7	0.4965	0.4966	0.4967	0.4968	0.4969	0.4970	0.4971	0.4972	0.4973	0.4974
2.8	0.4974	0.4975	0.4976	0.4977	0.4977	0.4978	0.4979	0.4979	0.4980	0.4981
2.9	0.4981	0.4982	0.4982	0.4983	0.4984	0.4984	0.4985	0.4985	0.4986	0.4986
3.0	0.4987	0.4987	0.4987	0.4988	0.4988	0.4989	0.4989	0.4989	0.4990	0.4990
3.1	0.4990	0.4991	0.4991	0.4991	0.4992	0.4992	0.4992	0.4992	0.4993	0.4993
3.2	0.4993	0.4993	0.4994	0.4994	0.4994	0.4994	0.4994	0.4995	0.4995	0.4995
3.3	0.4995	0.4995	0.4995	0.4996	0.4996	0.4996	0.4996	0.4996	0.4996	0.4997
3.4	0.4997	0.4997	0.4997	0.4997	0.4997	0.4997	0.4997	0.4997	0.4997	0.4998
3.5	0.4998	0.4998	0.4998	0.4998	0.4998	0.4998	0.4998	0.4998	0.4998	0.4998

Generated using Excel. Column A provides z-values and Row 1 provides the second decimal for the z-values.

Formula for cell B2 is = NORMSDIST ($A1+B$1)−0.5. Copying this formula to rest of the cells generates the table.

APPENDIX

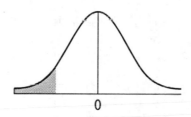

Standard Normal Distribution P(−3.5 < z < 3.5)

z	0.00	0.01	0.02	0.03	0.04	0.05	0.06	0.07	0.08	0.09
−3.5	0.0002	0.0002	0.0003	0.0003	0.0003	0.0003	0.0003	0.0003	0.0003	0.0003
−3.4	0.0003	0.0003	0.0004	0.0004	0.0004	0.0004	0.0004	0.0004	0.0005	0.0005
−3.3	0.0005	0.0005	0.0005	0.0005	0.0006	0.0006	0.0006	0.0006	0.0006	0.0007
−3.2	0.0007	0.0007	0.0007	0.0008	0.0008	0.0008	0.0008	0.0009	0.0009	0.0009
−3.1	0.0010	0.0010	0.0010	0.0011	0.0011	0.0011	0.0012	0.0012	0.0013	0.0013
−3.0	0.0013	0.0014	0.0014	0.0015	0.0015	0.0016	0.0016	0.0017	0.0018	0.0018
−2.9	0.0019	0.0019	0.0020	0.0021	0.0021	0.0022	0.0023	0.0023	0.0024	0.0025
−2.8	0.0026	0.0026	0.0027	0.0028	0.0029	0.0030	0.0031	0.0032	0.0033	0.0034
−2.7	0.0035	0.0036	0.0037	0.0038	0.0039	0.0040	0.0041	0.0043	0.0044	0.0045
−2.6	0.0047	0.0048	0.0049	0.0051	0.0052	0.0054	0.0055	0.0057	0.0059	0.0060
−2.5	0.0062	0.0064	0.0066	0.0068	0.0069	0.0071	0.0073	0.0075	0.0078	0.0080
−2.4	0.0082	0.0084	0.0087	0.0089	0.0091	0.0094	0.0096	0.0099	0.0102	0.0104
−2.3	0.0107	0.0110	0.0113	0.0116	0.0119	0.0122	0.0125	0.0129	0.0132	0.0136
−2.2	0.0139	0.0143	0.0146	0.0150	0.0154	0.0158	0.0162	0.0166	0.0170	0.0174
−2.1	0.0179	0.0183	0.0188	0.0192	0.0197	0.0202	0.0207	0.0212	0.0217	0.0222
−2.0	0.0228	0.0233	0.0239	0.0244	0.0250	0.0256	0.0262	0.0268	0.0274	0.0281
−1.9	0.0287	0.0294	0.0301	0.0307	0.0314	0.0322	0.0329	0.0336	0.0344	0.0351

(Continued)

Standard Normal Distribution P(−3.5 < z < 3.5)

z	0.00	0.01	0.02	0.03	0.04	0.05	0.06	0.07	0.08	0.09
−1.8	0.0359	0.0367	0.0375	0.0384	0.0392	0.0401	0.0409	0.0418	0.0427	0.0436
−1.7	0.0446	0.0455	0.0465	0.0475	0.0485	0.0495	0.0505	0.0516	0.0526	0.0537
−1.6	0.0548	0.0559	0.0571	0.0582	0.0594	0.0606	0.0618	0.0630	0.0643	0.0655
−1.5	0.0668	0.0681	0.0694	0.0708	0.0721	0.0735	0.0749	0.0764	0.0778	0.0793
−1.4	0.0808	0.0823	0.0838	0.0853	0.0869	0.0885	0.0901	0.0918	0.0934	0.0951
−1.3	0.0968	0.0985	0.1003	0.1020	0.1038	0.1056	0.1075	0.1093	0.1112	0.1131
−1.2	0.1151	0.1170	0.1190	0.1210	0.1230	0.1251	0.1271	0.1292	0.1314	0.1335
−1.0	0.1587	0.1611	0.1635	0.1660	0.1685	0.1711	0.1736	0.1762	0.1788	0.1814
−0.9	0.1841	0.1867	0.1894	0.1922	0.1949	0.1977	0.2005	0.2033	0.2061	0.2090
−0.8	0.2119	0.2148	0.2177	0.2206	0.2236	0.2266	0.2296	0.2327	0.2358	0.2389
−0.7	0.2420	0.2451	0.2483	0.2514	0.2546	0.2578	0.2611	0.2643	0.2676	0.2709
−0.6	0.2743	0.2776	0.2810	0.2843	0.2877	0.2912	0.2946	0.2981	0.3015	0.3050
−0.5	0.3085	0.3121	0.3156	0.3192	0.3228	0.3264	0.3300	0.3336	0.3372	0.3409
−0.4	0.3446	0.3483	0.3520	0.3557	0.3594	0.3632	0.3669	0.3707	0.3745	0.3783
−0.3	0.3821	0.3859	0.3897	0.3936	0.3974	0.4013	0.4052	0.4090	0.4129	0.4168
−0.2	0.4207	0.4247	0.4286	0.4325	0.4364	0.4404	0.4443	0.4483	0.4522	0.4562
−0.1	0.4602	0.4641	0.4681	0.4721	0.4761	0.4801	0.4840	0.4880	0.4920	0.4960
0.0	0.5000	0.5040	0.5080	0.5120	0.5160	0.5199	0.5239	0.5279	0.5319	0.5359
0.1	0.5398	0.5438	0.5478	0.5517	0.5557	0.5596	0.5636	0.5675	0.5714	0.5753
0.2	0.5793	0.5832	0.5871	0.5910	0.5948	0.5987	0.6026	0.6064	0.6103	0.6141
0.3	0.6179	0.6217	0.6255	0.6293	0.6331	0.6368	0.6406	0.6443	0.6480	0.6517
0.4	0.6554	0.6591	0.6628	0.6664	0.6700	0.6736	0.6772	0.6808	0.6844	0.6879
0.5	0.6915	0.6950	0.6985	0.7019	0.7054	0.7088	0.7123	0.7157	0.7190	0.7224
0.6	0.7257	0.7291	0.7324	0.7357	0.7389	0.7422	0.7454	0.7486	0.7517	0.7549
0.7	0.7580	0.7611	0.7642	0.7673	0.7704	0.7734	0.7764	0.7794	0.7823	0.7852
0.8	0.7881	0.7910	0.7939	0.7967	0.7995	0.8023	0.8051	0.8078	0.8106	0.8133
0.9	0.8159	0.8186	0.8212	0.8238	0.8264	0.8289	0.8315	0.8340	0.8365	0.8389
1.0	0.8413	0.8438	0.8461	0.8485	0.8508	0.8531	0.8554	0.8577	0.8599	0.8621
1.1	0.8643	0.8665	0.8686	0.8708	0.8729	0.8749	0.8770	0.8790	0.8810	0.8830
1.2	0.8849	0.8869	0.8888	0.8907	0.8925	0.8944	0.8962	0.8980	0.8997	0.9015
1.3	0.9032	0.9049	0.9066	0.9082	0.9099	0.9115	0.9131	0.9147	0.9162	0.9177
1.4	0.9192	0.9207	0.9222	0.9236	0.9251	0.9265	0.9279	0.9292	0.9306	0.9319
1.5	0.9332	0.9345	0.9357	0.9370	0.9382	0.9394	0.9406	0.9418	0.9429	0.9441
1.6	0.9452	0.9463	0.9474	0.9484	0.9495	0.9505	0.9515	0.9525	0.9535	0.9545
1.7	0.9554	0.9564	0.9573	0.9582	0.9591	0.9599	0.9608	0.9616	0.9625	0.9633
1.8	0.9641	0.9649	0.9656	0.9664	0.9671	0.9678	0.9686	0.9693	0.9699	0.9706
1.9	0.9713	0.9719	0.9726	0.9732	0.9738	0.9744	0.9750	0.9756	0.9761	0.9767
2.0	0.9772	0.9778	0.9783	0.9788	0.9793	0.9798	0.9803	0.9808	0.9812	0.9817
2.1	0.9821	0.9826	0.9830	0.9834	0.9838	0.9842	0.9846	0.9850	0.9854	0.9857
2.2	0.9861	0.9864	0.9868	0.9871	0.9875	0.9878	0.9881	0.9884	0.9887	0.9890
2.3	0.9893	0.9896	0.9898	0.9901	0.9904	0.9906	0.9909	0.9911	0.9913	0.9916

2.4	0.9918	0.9920	0.9922	0.9925	0.9927	0.9929	0.9931	0.9932	0.9934	0.9936
2.5	0.9938	0.9940	0.9941	0.9943	0.9945	0.9946	0.9948	0.9949	0.9951	0.9952
2.6	0.9953	0.9955	0.9956	0.9957	0.9959	0.9960	0.9961	0.9962	0.9963	0.9964
2.7	0.9965	0.9966	0.9967	0.9968	0.9969	0.9970	0.9971	0.9972	0.9973	0.9974
2.8	0.9974	0.9975	0.9976	0.9977	0.9977	0.9978	0.9979	0.9979	0.9980	0.9981
2.9	0.9981	0.9982	0.9982	0.9983	0.9984	0.9984	0.9985	0.9985	0.9986	0.9986
3.0	0.9987	0.9987	0.9987	0.9988	0.9988	0.9989	0.9989	0.9989	0.9990	0.9990
3.1	0.9990	0.9991	0.9991	0.9991	0.9992	0.9992	0.9992	0.9992	0.9993	0.9993
3.2	0.9993	0.9993	0.9994	0.9994	0.9994	0.9994	0.9994	0.9995	0.9995	0.9995
3.3	0.9995	0.9995	0.9995	0.9996	0.9996	0.9996	0.9996	0.9996	0.9996	0.9997
3.4	0.9997	0.9997	0.9997	0.9997	0.9997	0.9997	0.9997	0.9997	0.9997	0.9998
3.5	0.9998	0.9998	0.9998	0.9998	0.9998	0.9998	0.9998	0.9998	0.9998	0.9998

Generated using Excel. Column A provides z−values and Row 1 provides the second decimal for the z−values.

Formula for cell B2 is = NORMSDIST($A1+B$1). Copying this formula to rest of the cells generates the table.

APPENDIX

Cumulative Poisson Probabilities

μ/x	0	1	2	3	4	5	6	7	8	9	10
0.05	0.951	0.999	1.000	1.000	1.000	1.000	1.000	1.000	1.000	1.000	1.000
0.1	0.905	0.995	1.000	1.000	1.000	1.000	1.000	1.000	1.000	1.000	1.000
0.15	0.861	0.990	0.999	1.000	1.000	1.000	1.000	1.000	1.000	1.000	1.000
0.2	0.819	0.982	0.999	1.000	1.000	1.000	1.000	1.000	1.000	1.000	1.000
0.25	0.779	0.974	0.998	1.000	1.000	1.000	1.000	1.000	1.000	1.000	1.000
0.3	0.741	0.963	0.996	1.000	1.000	1.000	1.000	1.000	1.000	1.000	1.000
0.35	0.705	0.951	0.994	1.000	1.000	1.000	1.000	1.000	1.000	1.000	1.000
0.4	0.670	0.938	0.992	0.999	1.000	1.000	1.000	1.000	1.000	1.000	1.000
0.45	0.638	0.925	0.989	0.999	1.000	1.000	1.000	1.000	1.000	1.000	1.000
0.5	0.607	0.910	0.986	0.998	1.000	1.000	1.000	1.000	1.000	1.000	1.000
0.55	0.577	0.894	0.982	0.998	1.000	1.000	1.000	1.000	1.000	1.000	1.000
0.6	0.549	0.878	0.977	0.997	1.000	1.000	1.000	1.000	1.000	1.000	1.000
0.65	0.522	0.861	0.972	0.996	0.999	1.000	1.000	1.000	1.000	1.000	1.000
0.7	0.497	0.844	0.966	0.994	0.999	1.000	1.000	1.000	1.000	1.000	1.000
0.75	0.472	0.827	0.959	0.993	0.999	1.000	1.000	1.000	1.000	1.000	1.000
0.8	0.449	0.809	0.953	0.991	0.999	1.000	1.000	1.000	1.000	1.000	1.000

μ/x	11	12	13	14	15	16	17	18	19	20
0.05	1.000	1.000	1.000	1.000	1.000	1.000	1.000	1.000	1.000	1.000
0.1	1.000	1.000	1.000	1.000	1.000	1.000	1.000	1.000	1.000	1.000
0.15	1.000	1.000	1.000	1.000	1.000	1.000	1.000	1.000	1.000	1.000
0.2	1.000	1.000	1.000	1.000	1.000	1.000	1.000	1.000	1.000	1.000
0.25	1.000	1.000	1.000	1.000	1.000	1.000	1.000	1.000	1.000	1.000
0.3	1.000	1.000	1.000	1.000	1.000	1.000	1.000	1.000	1.000	1.000
0.35	1.000	1.000	1.000	1.000	1.000	1.000	1.000	1.000	1.000	1.000
0.4	1.000	1.000	1.000	1.000	1.000	1.000	1.000	1.000	1.000	1.000
0.45	1.000	1.000	1.000	1.000	1.000	1.000	1.000	1.000	1.000	1.000
0.5	1.000	1.000	1.000	1.000	1.000	1.000	1.000	1.000	1.000	1.000
0.55	1.000	1.000	1.000	1.000	1.000	1.000	1.000	1.000	1.000	1.000
0.6	1.000	1.000	1.000	1.000	1.000	1.000	1.000	1.000	1.000	1.000
0.65	1.000	1.000	1.000	1.000	1.000	1.000	1.000	1.000	1.000	1.000
0.7	1.000	1.000	1.000	1.000	1.000	1.000	1.000	1.000	1.000	1.000
0.75	1.000	1.000	1.000	1.000	1.000	1.000	1.000	1.000	1.000	1.000
0.8	1.000	1.000	1.000	1.000	1.000	1.000	1.000	1.000	1.000	1.000

(Continued)

μ/x	0	1	2	3	4	5	6	7	8	9	10
0.85	0.427	0.791	0.945	0.989	0.998	1.000	1.000	1.000	1.000	1.000	1.000
0.9	0.407	0.772	0.937	0.987	0.998	1.000	1.000	1.000	1.000	1.000	1.000
0.95	0.387	0.754	0.929	0.984	0.997	1.000	1.000	1.000	1.000	1.000	1.000
1	0.368	0.736	0.920	0.981	0.996	0.999	1.000	1.000	1.000	1.000	1.000
1.1	0.333	0.699	0.900	0.974	0.995	0.999	1.000	1.000	1.000	1.000	1.000
1.2	0.301	0.663	0.879	0.966	0.992	0.998	1.000	1.000	1.000	1.000	1.000
1.3	0.273	0.627	0.857	0.957	0.989	0.998	1.000	1.000	1.000	1.000	1.000
1.4	0.247	0.592	0.833	0.946	0.986	0.997	0.999	1.000	1.000	1.000	1.000
1.5	0.223	0.558	0.809	0.934	0.981	0.996	0.999	1.000	1.000	1.000	1.000
1.6	0.202	0.525	0.783	0.921	0.976	0.994	0.999	1.000	1.000	1.000	1.000
1.7	0.183	0.493	0.757	0.907	0.970	0.992	0.998	1.000	1.000	1.000	1.000
1.8	0.165	0.463	0.731	0.891	0.964	0.990	0.997	0.999	1.000	1.000	1.000
1.9	0.150	0.434	0.704	0.875	0.956	0.987	0.997	0.999	1.000	1.000	1.000
2	0.135	0.406	0.677	0.857	0.947	0.983	0.995	0.999	1.000	1.000	1.000
2.2	0.111	0.355	0.623	0.819	0.928	0.975	0.993	0.998	1.000	1.000	1.000
2.4	0.091	0.308	0.570	0.779	0.904	0.964	0.988	0.997	0.999	1.000	1.000
2.6	0.074	0.267	0.518	0.736	0.877	0.951	0.983	0.995	0.999	1.000	1.000
2.8	0.061	0.231	0.469	0.692	0.848	0.935	0.976	0.992	0.998	0.999	1.000
3	0.050	0.199	0.423	0.647	0.815	0.916	0.966	0.988	0.996	0.999	1.000
3.2	0.041	0.171	0.380	0.603	0.781	0.895	0.955	0.983	0.994	0.998	1.000
3.4	0.033	0.147	0.340	0.558	0.744	0.871	0.942	0.977	0.992	0.997	0.999
3.6	0.027	0.126	0.303	0.515	0.706	0.844	0.927	0.969	0.988	0.996	0.999
3.8	0.022	0.107	0.269	0.473	0.668	0.816	0.909	0.960	0.984	0.994	0.998
4	0.018	0.092	0.238	0.433	0.629	0.785	0.889	0.949	0.979	0.992	0.997
4.2	0.015	0.078	0.210	0.395	0.590	0.753	0.867	0.936	0.972	0.989	0.996
4.4	0.012	0.066	0.185	0.359	0.551	0.720	0.844	0.921	0.964	0.985	0.994
4.6	0.010	0.056	0.163	0.326	0.513	0.686	0.818	0.905	0.955	0.980	0.992
4.8	0.008	0.048	0.143	0.294	0.476	0.651	0.791	0.887	0.944	0.975	0.990
5	0.007	0.040	0.125	0.265	0.440	0.616	0.762	0.867	0.932	0.968	0.986
5.2	0.006	0.034	0.109	0.238	0.406	0.581	0.732	0.845	0.918	0.960	0.982
5.4	0.005	0.029	0.095	0.213	0.373	0.546	0.702	0.822	0.903	0.951	0.977
5.6	0.004	0.024	0.082	0.191	0.342	0.512	0.670	0.797	0.886	0.941	0.972
5.8	0.003	0.021	0.072	0.170	0.313	0.478	0.638	0.771	0.867	0.929	0.965
6	0.002	0.017	0.062	0.151	0.285	0.446	0.606	0.744	0.847	0.916	0.957

μ/x	11	12	13	14	15	16	17	18	19	20
0.85	1.000	1.000	1.000	1.000	1.000	1.000	1.000	1.000	1.000	1.000
0.9	1.000	1.000	1.000	1.000	1.000	1.000	1.000	1.000	1.000	1.000
0.95	1.000	1.000	1.000	1.000	1.000	1.000	1.000	1.000	1.000	1.000
1	1.000	1.000	1.000	1.000	1.000	1.000	1.000	1.000	1.000	1.000
1.1	1.000	1.000	1.000	1.000	1.000	1.000	1.000	1.000	1.000	1.000
1.2	1.000	1.000	1.000	1.000	1.000	1.000	1.000	1.000	1.000	1.000
1.3	1.000	1.000	1.000	1.000	1.000	1.000	1.000	1.000	1.000	1.000
1.4	1.000	1.000	1.000	1.000	1.000	1.000	1.000	1.000	1.000	1.000
1.5	1.000	1.000	1.000	1.000	1.000	1.000	1.000	1.000	1.000	1.000
1.6	1.000	1.000	1.000	1.000	1.000	1.000	1.000	1.000	1.000	1.000
1.7	1.000	1.000	1.000	1.000	1.000	1.000	1.000	1.000	1.000	1.000
1.8	1.000	1.000	1.000	1.000	1.000	1.000	1.000	1.000	1.000	1.000
1.9	1.000	1.000	1.000	1.000	1.000	1.000	1.000	1.000	1.000	1.000
2	1.000	1.000	1.000	1.000	1.000	1.000	1.000	1.000	1.000	1.000
2.2	1.000	1.000	1.000	1.000	1.000	1.000	1.000	1.000	1.000	1.000
2.4	1.000	1.000	1.000	1.000	1.000	1.000	1.000	1.000	1.000	1.000
2.6	1.000	1.000	1.000	1.000	1.000	1.000	1.000	1.000	1.000	1.000
2.8	1.000	1.000	1.000	1.000	1.000	1.000	1.000	1.000	1.000	1.000
3	1.000	1.000	1.000	1.000	1.000	1.000	1.000	1.000	1.000	1.000
3.2	1.000	1.000	1.000	1.000	1.000	1.000	1.000	1.000	1.000	1.000
3.4	1.000	1.000	1.000	1.000	1.000	1.000	1.000	1.000	1.000	1.000
3.6	1.000	1.000	1.000	1.000	1.000	1.000	1.000	1.000	1.000	1.000
3.8	0.999	1.000	1.000	1.000	1.000	1.000	1.000	1.000	1.000	1.000
4	0.999	1.000	1.000	1.000	1.000	1.000	1.000	1.000	1.000	1.000
4.2	0.999	1.000	1.000	1.000	1.000	1.000	1.000	1.000	1.000	1.000
4.4	0.998	0.999	1.000	1.000	1.000	1.000	1.000	1.000	1.000	1.000
4.6	0.997	0.999	1.000	1.000	1.000	1.000	1.000	1.000	1.000	1.000
4.8	0.996	0.999	1.000	1.000	1.000	1.000	1.000	1.000	1.000	1.000
5	0.995	0.998	0.999	1.000	1.000	1.000	1.000	1.000	1.000	1.000
5.2	0.993	0.997	0.999	1.000	1.000	1.000	1.000	1.000	1.000	1.000
5.4	0.990	0.996	0.999	1.000	1.000	1.000	1.000	1.000	1.000	1.000
5.6	0.988	0.995	0.998	0.999	1.000	1.000	1.000	1.000	1.000	1.000
5.8	0.984	0.993	0.997	0.999	1.000	1.000	1.000	1.000	1.000	1.000
6	0.980	0.991	0.996	0.999	0.999	1.000	1.000	1.000	1.000	1.000

(Continued)

μ/x	0	1	2	3	4	5	6	7	8	9	10
6.2	0.002	0.015	0.054	0.134	0.259	0.414	0.574	0.716	0.826	0.902	0.949
6.4	0.002	0.012	0.046	0.119	0.235	0.384	0.542	0.687	0.803	0.886	0.939
6.6	0.001	0.010	0.040	0.105	0.213	0.355	0.511	0.658	0.780	0.869	0.927
6.8	0.001	0.009	0.034	0.093	0.192	0.327	0.480	0.628	0.755	0.850	0.915
7	0.001	0.007	0.030	0.082	0.173	0.301	0.450	0.599	0.729	0.830	0.901
7.2	0.001	0.006	0.025	0.072	0.156	0.276	0.420	0.569	0.703	0.810	0.887
7.4	0.001	0.005	0.022	0.063	0.140	0.253	0.392	0.539	0.676	0.788	0.871
7.6	0.001	0.004	0.019	0.055	0.125	0.231	0.365	0.510	0.648	0.765	0.854
7.8	0.000	0.004	0.016	0.048	0.112	0.210	0.338	0.481	0.620	0.741	0.835
8	0.000	0.003	0.014	0.042	0.100	0.191	0.313	0.453	0.593	0.717	0.816
8.2	0.000	0.003	0.012	0.037	0.089	0.174	0.290	0.425	0.565	0.692	0.796
8.4	0.000	0.002	0.010	0.032	0.079	0.157	0.267	0.399	0.537	0.666	0.774
8.6	0.000	0.002	0.009	0.028	0.070	0.142	0.246	0.373	0.509	0.640	0.752
8.8	0.000	0.001	0.007	0.024	0.062	0.128	0.226	0.348	0.482	0.614	0.729
9	0.000	0.001	0.006	0.021	0.055	0.116	0.207	0.324	0.456	0.587	0.706
9.2	0.000	0.001	0.005	0.018	0.049	0.104	0.189	0.301	0.430	0.561	0.682
9.4	0.000	0.001	0.005	0.016	0.043	0.093	0.173	0.279	0.404	0.535	0.658
9.6	0.000	0.001	0.004	0.014	0.038	0.084	0.157	0.258	0.380	0.509	0.633
9.8	0.000	0.001	0.003	0.012	0.033	0.075	0.143	0.239	0.356	0.483	0.608
10	0.000	0.000	0.003	0.010	0.029	0.067	0.130	0.220	0.333	0.458	0.583

Generated using Excel. Column A provides μ-values and Row 1 provides the x-numbers of arrivals.
Formula for cell B2 is = POISSON(B$1+$A2, TRUE). Copying this formula to rest of the cells generates the table.

μ/x	11	12	13	14	15	16	17	18	19	20
6.2	0.975	0.989	0.995	0.998	0.999	1.000	1.000	1.000	1.000	1.000
6.4	0.969	0.986	0.994	0.997	0.999	1.000	1.000	1.000	1.000	1.000
6.6	0.963	0.982	0.992	0.997	0.999	0.999	1.000	1.000	1.000	1.000
6.8	0.955	0.978	0.990	0.996	0.998	0.999	1.000	1.000	1.000	1.000
7	0.947	0.973	0.987	0.994	0.998	0.999	1.000	1.000	1.000	1.000
7.2	0.937	0.967	0.984	0.993	0.997	0.999	1.000	1.000	1.000	1.000
7.4	0.926	0.961	0.980	0.991	0.996	0.998	0.999	1.000	1.000	1.000
7.6	0.915	0.954	0.976	0.989	0.995	0.998	0.999	1.000	1.000	1.000
7.8	0.902	0.945	0.971	0.986	0.993	0.997	0.999	1.000	1.000	1.000
8	0.888	0.936	0.966	0.983	0.992	0.996	0.998	0.999	1.000	1.000
8.2	0.873	0.926	0.960	0.979	0.990	0.995	0.998	0.999	1.000	1.000
8.4	0.857	0.915	0.952	0.975	0.987	0.994	0.997	0.999	1.000	1.000
8.6	0.840	0.903	0.945	0.970	0.985	0.993	0.997	0.999	0.999	1.000
8.8	0.822	0.890	0.936	0.965	0.982	0.991	0.996	0.998	0.999	1.000
9	0.803	0.876	0.926	0.959	0.978	0.989	0.995	0.998	0.999	1.000
9.2	0.783	0.861	0.916	0.952	0.974	0.987	0.993	0.997	0.999	0.999
9.4	0.763	0.845	0.904	0.944	0.969	0.984	0.992	0.996	0.998	0.999
9.6	0.741	0.828	0.892	0.936	0.964	0.981	0.990	0.995	0.998	0.999
9.8	0.719	0.810	0.879	0.927	0.958	0.977	0.988	0.994	0.997	0.999
10	0.697	0.792	0.864	0.917	0.951	0.973	0.986	0.993	0.997	0.998

APPENDIX

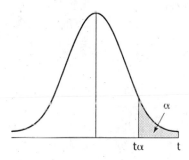

t Distribution

t Distribution					Values of α				
df	0.1	0.05	0.025	0.01	0.005	0.0025	0.001	0.0005	0.0001
1	3.08	6.31	12.71	31.82	63.66	127.32	318.31	636.62	3183.10
2	1.89	2.92	4.30	6.96	9.92	14.09	22.33	31.60	70.70
3	1.64	2.35	3.18	4.54	5.84	7.45	10.21	12.92	22.20
4	1.53	2.13	2.78	3.75	4.60	5.60	7.17	8.61	13.03
5	1.48	2.02	2.57	3.36	4.03	4.77	5.89	6.87	9.68
6	1.44	1.94	2.45	3.14	3.71	4.32	5.21	5.96	8.02
7	1.41	1.89	2.36	3.00	3.50	4.03	4.79	5.41	7.06
8	1.40	1.86	2.31	2.90	3.36	3.83	4.50	5.04	6.44
9	1.38	1.83	2.26	2.82	3.25	3.69	4.30	4.78	6.01
10	1.37	1.81	2.23	2.76	3.17	3.58	4.14	4.59	5.69
11	1.36	1.80	2.20	2.72	3.11	3.50	4.02	4.44	5.45
12	1.36	1.78	2.18	2.68	3.05	3.43	3.93	4.32	5.26
13	1.35	1.77	2.16	2.65	3.01	3.37	3.85	4.22	5.11

(Continued)

423

t Distribution   Values of α

df	0.1	0.05	0.025	0.01	0.005	0.0025	0.001	0.0005	0.0001
14	1.35	1.76	2.14	2.62	2.98	3.33	3.79	4.14	4.99
15	1.34	1.75	2.13	2.60	2.95	3.29	3.73	4.07	4.88
16	1.34	1.75	2.12	2.58	2.92	3.25	3.69	4.01	4.79
17	1.33	1.74	2.11	2.57	2.90	3.22	3.65	3.97	4.71
18	1.33	1.73	2.10	2.55	2.88	3.20	3.61	3.92	4.65
19	1.33	1.73	2.09	2.54	2.86	3.17	3.58	3.88	4.59
20	1.33	1.72	2.09	2.53	2.85	3.15	3.55	3.85	4.54
21	1.32	1.72	2.08	2.52	2.83	3.14	3.53	3.82	4.49
22	1.32	1.72	2.07	2.51	2.82	3.12	3.50	3.79	4.45
23	1.32	1.71	2.07	2.50	2.81	3.10	3.48	3.77	4.42
24	1.32	1.71	2.06	2.49	2.80	3.09	3.47	3.75	4.38
25	1.32	1.71	2.06	2.49	2.79	3.08	3.45	3.73	4.35
26	1.31	1.71	2.06	2.48	2.78	3.07	3.43	3.71	4.32
27	1.31	1.70	2.05	2.47	2.77	3.06	3.42	3.69	4.30
28	1.31	1.70	2.05	2.47	2.76	3.05	3.41	3.67	4.28
29	1.31	1.70	2.05	2.46	2.76	3.04	3.40	3.66	4.25
30	1.31	1.70	2.04	2.46	2.75	3.03	3.39	3.65	4.23
60	1.30	1.67	2.00	2.39	2.66	2.91	3.23	3.46	3.96
100	1.29	1.66	1.98	2.36	2.63	2.87	3.17	3.39	3.86
200	1.29	1.65	1.97	2.35	2.60	2.84	3.13	3.34	3.79
300	1.28	1.65	1.97	2.34	2.59	2.83	3.12	3.32	3.77
400	1.28	1.65	1.97	2.34	2.59	2.82	3.11	3.32	3.75
500	1.28	1.65	1.96	2.33	2.59	2.82	3.11	3.31	3.75

Generated using Excel. Column A provides μ-values and Row 1 provides the probability values.
Formula for cell B2 is = TINV(2*B$1+$A2). Copying this formula to rest of the cells generates the table.

REFERENCES

Addams, H. L., Bracci, L., and Overfelt, F. "Bar Coding: An Effective Productivity Concept." *Journal of Nursing Administration, 21*(10), October 1991.

Altman, S. H., Goldberger, S., and Crane, S. "The Need for a National Focus on Health Care Productivity." *Health Affairs,* Spring 1990.

Anderson, T. D. "Special Issues in Productivity Programs." *Topics in Health Care Financing, 15*(3), 1989.

Ashby, J. L., Jr. and Altman, S. H. "The Trend in Hospital Output and Labor Productivity, 1980–1989." *Inquiry, 29,* Spring 1992.

Becker, C. "Raising the Bar: FDA Issues Final Regulations on Bar-Code Adoption." *Modern Health Care,* March 1, 2004.

Bendix, R. "Operating scheduling for the OR." *Modern Healthcare, 5*:16m–16o, June 1976.

Bergman, R. "Reengineering Health Care." *Hospitals & Health Networks,* February 5, 1994.

Breslawski, S. and Hamilton D. "Operating Room Scheduling: Choosing the Best System." *Association of Perioperative Registered Nurses Journal, 53*(5), May 1991.

Brown, P. "Punching the Body Clock." *Nursing Times, 84*(44), 1988.

Budget Reconciliation Act of 1987 (Public Law 100–203). *Provisions Affecting the Federal-State Unemployment Compensation Program,* U.S. DEPARTMENT OF LABOR, Employment and Training Administration, Washington, D.C. 20210.

Burns, L. R. *The Health Care Value Chain.* San Francisco: Jossey-Bass, 2002.

Cadbury, A. *Industry and Employment.* London: Foundation for Business Responsibilities, 1987.

Cerne, F. "Study Finds Bedside Terminals Prove Their Worth." *Hospitals,* February 5, 1989.

Chase, R. B. and Aquilano, N. J. *Production and Operations Management: A Life Cycle Approach.* Boston: Richard D. Irwin, Inc., 1989.

Chassin, M. R. "Is Health Care Ready for Six Sigma Quality?" *Milbank Quarterly, 76*(4), 1998.

Childs, B. "Bedside Terminals: A New Player." *U.S. Healthcare,* May 1989, pp. 6–7.

Cooper, W. W., Seiford, L. M., and Tone, K. *Data Envelopment Analysis: A Comprehensive Text with Models, Applications, References and DEA-Solver Software.* Boston: Kluwer Academic Publishers, 2000.

Corsi, L. A. "Ten Hour Shifts." Letter to the editor of *Nursing Management, 22*(9), 1991.

Dartmouth Medical School. *The Dartmouth Atlas of Health Care.* Chicago, IL: American Hospital Publishing, 1998 [http://www.dartmouthatlas.org].

Daughtery, J. "Premium Shift: A Solution to an Expensive Option." *Nursing Management, 23*(1), 1992.

Davis, M. A. "On Nursing Home Quality: A Review and Analysis." *Medical Care Review, 48*(2), Summer 1991.

Denbor, R. W. and Kubic, F. T. *Report of Special Study of Scheduling of Surgical Operations and the Utilization of the ORs in the Washington Hospital Center.* Washington, D.C., June 1963.

Dexter, F. and Traub, R. D. "How to Schedule Elective Surgical Cases into Specific Operating Rooms to Maximize the Efficiency of Use of Operating Room Time." *Anesthesia & Analgesia, 94,* 2002, pp. 933–42.

Dexter, F., Abouleish, A. E., Epstein, R., Whitten, C. H., and Lubarsky, D. A. "Use of Operating Room Information System Data to Predict the Impact of Reducing Turnover Times on Staffing Costs." *Anesthesia & Analgesia, 97,* 2003, pp. 1119–26.

Dexter, F., Macario, A., Traub, R. D., Hopwood, M., and Lubarsky, D. A. "An Operating Room Scheduling Strategy to Maximize the Use of Operating Room Block Time: Computer Simulation of Patient Scheduling and Survey of Patients' Preferences for Surgical Procedure Times." *Anesthesia & Analgesia, 89,* 1999, pp. 7–20.

Findlay, J. "Shifting Time." *Nursing Times, 90*(2), 1994.

Fitzsimmons, J. A. and Fitzsimmons, M. J. *Service Management, Operations, Strategy and Information Technology.* 4th ed. Boston: McGraw-Hill/Irwin, 2004.

Francis, R. L. and White, J. A. *Facility Layout and Location: An Analytical Approach.* Englewood Cliffs, NJ: Prentice-Hall, 1974.

Goldman, H., Knappenberger, H. A., and Shearon, A. T. "A Study of the Variability of Surgical Estimates." *Hospital Management, 110,* September 1970.

Goodman, D. C., and others. "Primary Care Service Areas: A New Tool for the Evaluation of Primary Care Services." *Health Services Research,* 2003, *38*(1), pp. 287–309.

Gordon, T., and others. "Surgical Unit Time Utilization Review: Resource Utilization and Management Implications." *Journal of Medical Systems, 12,* 1988.

Gross, M. "The Potential of Professional Nursing Information Systems." *U.S. Healthcare,* 6(9), 1989a.

Gross, M. "The Potential of Information Systems in Nursing." *Nursing Health Care,* 9(9), 1989b.

Hackey, B. A., Casey, K. L. and Narasimhan, S. L. "Maximizing Resources: Efficient Scheduling in the OR." *Association of Perioperative Registered Nurses Journal, 39,* 1984.

Hammer, M. and Champy, J. *Re-engineering the Corporation: A Manifesto for Business Revolution.* New York: Harper Business, 1993.

Herzberg, F. *The Motivation to Work.* New York: John Wiley, 1959.

Institute of Medicine. *Medicare: A Strategy for Quality Assurance.* Washington, D.C.: National Academy Press, 1990.

Kahl, K., Ivancin, L. and Fuhrmann, M. "Automated Nursing Documentation System Provides a Favorable Return on Investment." *Journal of Nursing Administration, 21*(11), November 1991.

Kelley, M. G., Easham, A. and Bowling, G. S. "Efficient OR Scheduling: A Study to Reduce Cancellations." *Association of Perioperative Registered Nurses Journal, 41,* March 1985.

Kerzner, H. *Advanced Project Management, Best Practices on Implementation, 2nd ed.* Hoboken, N. J.: Wiley, 2004.

Kimber, A. "Trapped on a Nine to Five Treadmill." *Personnel Today,* 9(7), 1991.

Kinney, M. "Flexible Scheduling and Part-Time Work: What Price Do We Pay?" *Journal of Nursing Administration, 17*(6), 1990.

Kirk, R. *Nurse Staffing and Budgeting: Practical Management Tools.* Frederick, MD: Aspen Publications, 1986.

Kirk, R. "Using Workload Analysis and Acuity Systems to Facilitate Quality and Productivity." *Journal of Nursing Administration, 20*(3), March 1990.

Klastorin, T. *Project Management: Tools and Trade-Offs.* Hoboken, N.J.: Wiley, 2004.

Kowalski, J. C. "Inventory to Go: Can Stockless Deliver Efficiency?" *Health Care Financial Management,* November, 1991, pp. 21–34.

Krumrey, N. A. and Byerly, G. E. "A Step-By-Step Approach to Identifying a Partner and Making the Partnership Work." *Hospital Material Management Quarterly, 16*(3), 1995.

Lamkin, L. R. and Sleven, M. "Staffing Standards: Why Not? A Report from the ONS Administration Committee." *Oncology Nursing Forum, 18*(7), 1991, 1241.

Magerlein, J. M. and Martin, J. B. "Surgical Demand Scheduling: A Review." *Health Services Research, 13,* Winter 1978.

Marie, M. "Staffing and Productivity." *Nursing Management, 22*(12), 20–21.

McFadden, C. D. and Leahy, T. M. *US Healthcare Distribution: Positioning the Healthcare Supply Chain for the 21st Century.* New York: Goldman Sachs, 2000.

Medical Group Management Association. [www.mgma.com], 2004.

Medicus System Corporation. (1987). *Patient Classification Indicator Applications (Med/Surg/Peds/OB).* Evanston, IL: Medicus System Corporation.

Meyer, D. "Work Load Management System Ensures Stable Nurse-Patient Ratio." *Hospitals, 52,* 1978, 81–85.

Miller, M. L. "Implementing Self-Scheduling." *The Journal of Nursing Administration, 14*(3), 1984.

Morrisey, J. "Doubling their Measures." *Modern Health Care,* p. 12. March 22, 2004.

Muther, R. and Wheeler, J. "Simplified Systematic Layout Planning." *Factory 120,* nos. 8, 9, and 10 (August, September, and October, 1962) pp. 68–77, 111–119, 101–113.

National Cancer Institute. *Cancer Mortality Maps and Graphs* [http://cancercontrolplanet.cancer.gov/atlas/index.jsp].

Newstrom, J. W. and Pierce, J. L. "Alternative Work Schedules: The State of the Art." *The Personnel Administration,* October 1979.

Niebel, B. W. *Motion and Time Study, 8th ed.* Burr Ridge, Ill: Richard D. Irwin, 1988.

Organization for Economic Cooperation and Development. "Health Data 2004–Frequently Requested Data. Table 10: Total Expenditure on Health, %GDP." [http://www.oecd.org/document/16/0,2340,en_2825_ 495642_2085200_1_1_1,00.html].

Olmstead, B. and Smith, S. *Creating a Flexible Workforce: How to Select and Manage Alternative Work Options.* New York: Amacon, 1989.

Ozcan, Y. A. "Physician Benchmarking: Measuring Variation in Practice Behavior in Treatment of Otitis Media." *Health Care Management Science, 1*(1), 1998.

Ozcan, Y. A. and Lynch, J. R. "Rural Hospital Closures: An Inquiry into Efficiency." *Advances in Health Economics and Health Services Research, 13,* 1993.

Ozcan, Y. A. and Luke, R. D. "National Study of the Efficiency of Hospitals in Urban Markets." *Health Services Research, 27*(6), 1993.

Ozcan, Y. A. and McCue, M. J. "Financial Performance Index for Hospitals." *Journal of Operational Research Society, 47,* 1996.

Ozcan, Y. A., Merwin, E., Lee, K., and Morrisey, J. P. "Benchmarking Using DEA: The Case of Mental Health Organizations." Chapter 7. In M. L. Brandeau, F. Sainfort, and W. P. Pierskalla (eds.). *Operations Research and Health Care: A Handbook of Methods and Applications.* Boston: Kluwer Academic Publishers, 2004.

Ozcan, Y. A. Health Care Benchmarking and Performance Evaluation An Assessment using Data Envelopment Analysis (DEA). Springer, Newton, MA, 2008.

Ozgen, H. and Ozcan, Y. A. "A National Study of Efficiency for Dialysis Centers: An Examination of Market Competition and Facility Characteristics for Production of Multiple Dialysis Outputs." *Health Services Research, 37*(3), 2002.

Ozgen, H. and Ozcan, Y. A. "Longitudinal Analysis of Efficiency in Multiple Output Dialysis Markets." *Health Care Management Science, 7*(4), 2004.

Page, J. A. and McDougall, M. D. "Staffing for High Productivity." In M. D. McDougall, R. P. Covert, and V. B. Melton (eds.), *Productivity and Performance Management in Health Care Institutions.* Chicago, IL: American Hospital Publishing Co., 1989.

Palmer, J. "Eight and 12 Hour Shifts: Comparing Nurses' Behavior Patterns." *Nursing Management, 22*(9), 1991.

Phillips, K. T. "Operating Room Utilization." *Hospital Topics, 53,* March/April 1975.

Piper, L. R. "Patient Acuity Systems and Productivity." *Topics in Health Care Finance, 15*(3), 1989.

Rasmussen, S. R. "Staffing and Scheduling Options." *Critical Care Quarterly,* June 1982.

Redinius, D. L. "Six Sigma Trends in Health Care." [www.advanceforhie.com/Common/editorial/editorial. aspx?CC=30666] Mar. 17, 2004.

Ringl, K. and Dotson, L. "Self-Scheduling for Professional Nurses." *Nursing Management, 20*(2), 1989.

Rose, M. and Baker, N. "Flexibility Pays." *Employment Gazette, 9*(8), 1991.

Rose, M. B. and Davies, D. C. "Scheduling in the Operating Theater." *Annals of the Royal College of Surgeons of England, 66,* 1984.

Russell, R. S. and Taylor, B. W. *Operations Management, 2nd ed.* New Jersey: Prentice Hall, 1995.

Salvage, J. "Double Shift." *Nursing Standard, 6*(2), 1990.

Sanders, T. "Materiel Management in the 1990s: A New Paradigm." *Hospital Material Management Quarterly, 11*(3), 1990.

Schonberger, R. J. and Knod, E. M. Jr. *Operations Management: Continuous Improvement.* Boston: Richard D. Irwin, Inc., 1994.

Scottish Office Home and Health Department, National Nursing and Midwifery – Consultative Committee. *The Role and Function of the Professional Nurse.* Edinburgh: HSMO, 1992.

Seal, K. C. (2201) "A Generalized PERT/CPM Implementation in a Spreadsheet," *INFORMS Transactions on Education* 2:1 (16–26).

Sheehan, P. E. "Purchasing: A Necessary Partnership." *Hospital Material Management Quarterly, 16*(3), 1995.

Sinclair, V. G. "The Impact of Information Systems on Nursing Performance and Productivity." *Journal of Nursing Administration, 21*(2), February 1991.

Shukla, R. K. "Theory of Support Systems and Nursing Performance." In E. Lewis (ed.), *Human Resource Management.* Aspen Publications, 1987.

Shukla, R. K. Theories and Strategies of Healthcare: Technology-Strategy-Performance. Chapters 2 & 4. Unpublished manuscript, 1991.

Shukla, R. K. "Admissions Monitoring and Scheduling to Improve Work Flow in Hospitals." Inquiry, 22, 1992.

Shukla, R. K., Ketcham J. S., and Ozcan, Y. A. "Comparison of Subjective Versus Database Approaches for Improving Efficiency of Operating Room Scheduling." *Health Services Management Research, 3,* July 1990.

Skinner, W. C. "The Productivity Paradox," *Harvard Business Review,* July, 1986.

Stack, R. T. "Leadership Ought to be Easy." Remarks of R. Timothy Stack at the Medical College of Virginia [http://www.had.vcu.edu/alumni/stack_talk.html]. Mar. 2004.

Stahl, R., Schultz, B., and Pexton, C. "Healthcare's Horizon." *Six Sigma Forum Magazine,* ASQ Publications 2(2), 2003.

Stevenson, W. J. *Operations Management, 7th ed.* Boston: McGraw-Hill/Irwin, 2002.

Taylor, F. W. Principles of Scientific Management. [http://melbecon.unimelb.edu.au/het/taylor/sciman.htm] (Originally published in 1911.)

U.S. Department of Labor. "The 2004–05 Career Guide to Industries: Health." [http://www.bls.gov/oco/cg/cgs035.htm], Dec. 2004.

U.S. Department of Labor. [www.bls.gov/oco/cg/cgs035.htm#nature], 2006.

Velianoff, G. "Establishing a 10-Hour Schedule." *Nursing Management, 22*(9), 1991.

Virginia Atlas of Community Health. [http://vaatlas.vahealthycommunities.com/login.aspx].

Walker, E. K. "Staffing Accommodations to Hospital Unit Admissions." *Nursing Economics, 8*(5), 1990.

Warner, M. D. "Nurse Staffing, Scheduling, and Reallocation in the Hospital." *Hospital and Health Services Administration,* Summer 1976.

Williams, W. L. "Improved Utilization of the Surgical Suite." *Hospitals, 45,* March 1, 1971.

Young, S. T. *Multiple Productivity Approaches to Management. Health Care Management Review, 17*(2), 1992.

INDEX

Page references followed by *fig* indicate an illustrated figure; followed by *t* indicate a table; followed by *e* indicate an exhibit.

429

Printed in the United States of America
ED-09-25-12